2012
YEAR BOOK OF
HAND AND UPPER
LIMB SURGERY®

The 2012 Year Book Series

Year Book of Anesthesiology and Pain Management™: Drs Chestnut, Abram, Black, Gravlee, Lien, Mathru, and Roizen

Year Book of Cardiology®: Drs Gersh, Cheitlin, Elliott, Gold, Graham, and Thourani

Year Book of Critical Care Medicine®: Drs Dries, Zanotti-Cavazzoni, Latenser, Martinez, Rincon, and Zwank

Year Book of Dermatology and Dermatologic Surgery™: Dr Del Rosso

Year Book of Diagnostic Radiology®: Drs Elster, Abbara, Oestreich, Offiah, Rosado de Christenson, Stephens, and Strickland

Year Book of Emergency Medicine®: Drs Hamilton, Bruno, Handly, Minczak, Mullin, Quintana, and Ramoska

Year Book of Endocrinology®: Drs Schott, Apovian, Clarke, Eugster, Meikle, Oetgen, Ovalle, Schteingart, and Toth

Year Book of Hand and Upper Limb Surgery®: Drs Yao, Adams, Isaacs, Lee, and Rizzo

Year Book of Medicine®: Drs Barker, Garrick, Gersh, Khardori, LeRoith, Panush, Talley, and Thigpen

Year Book of Neonatal and Perinatal Medicine®: Drs Fanaroff, Benitz, Donn, Neu, Papile, Polin, and Van Marter

Year Book of Neurology and Neurosurgery®: Drs Klimo, Minagar, Gandhi, House, Kevill, Liu, Mazia, Panagariya, Ragel, Riesenburger, Robottom, Schwendimann, Shafazand, Uhm, and Yang

Year Book of Obstetrics, Gynecology, and Women's Health®: Drs Dungan and Shulman

Year Book of Oncology®: Drs Arceci, Bauer, Chiorean, Gordon, Lawton, Murphy, Thigpen, and Tsao

Year Book of Ophthalmology®: Drs Rapuano, Cohen, Flanders, Hammersmith, Milman, Myers, Nagra, Nelson, Penne, Pyfer, Sergott, Shields, Talekar, and Vander

Year Book of Orthopedics®: Drs Morrey, Huddleston, Rose, Swiontkowski, and Trigg

Year Book of Otolaryngology-Head and Neck Surgery®: Drs Sindwani, Balough, Franco, Gapany, and Mitchell

Year Book of Pathology and Laboratory Medicine®: Drs Raab and Bissell

Year Book of Pediatrics®: Dr Stockman

Year Book of Plastic and Aesthetic Surgery™: Drs Miller, Gosman, Gurtner, Gutowski, Ruberg, Salisbury, and Smith

2012

The Year Book of HAND AND UPPER LIMB SURGERY®

Editors
Jeffrey Yao, MD
Assistant Professor of Orthopaedic Surgery, Robert A. Chase Hand and Upper Limb Center, Stanford, California

Associate Editors
Julie Adams, MD
Assistant Professor of Orthopedic Surgery, University of Minnesota, Minneapolis, Minnesota
Jonathan Isaacs, MD
Chair, Division of Hand Surgery, Associate Professor, Department of Orthopedic Surgery, VCU Medical Center, Richmond, Virginia
Steve K. Lee, MD
Associate Professor of Orthopedic Surgery, Hospital for Special Surgery, Weill Cornell Medical College, New York, New York
Marco Rizzo, MD
Associate Professor, Department of Orthopedic Surgery, Mayo Clinic College of Medicine, Rochester, Minnesota

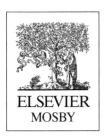

ELSEVIER
MOSBY

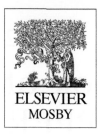

ELSEVIER
MOSBY

Vice President, Continuity: Kimberly Murphy
Developmental Editor: David Parsons
Production Supervisor, Electronic Year Books: Donna M. Skelton
Electronic Article Manager: Mike Sheets
Illustrations and Permissions Coordinator: Dawn Vohsen

2012 EDITION

Printed and bound by CPI Group (UK) Ltd, Croydon, CR0 4YY

Composition by TNQ Books and Journals Pvt Ltd, India

Editorial Office:
Elsevier
Suite 1800
1600 John F. Kennedy Blvd.
Philadelphia, PA 19103-2899

International Standard Serial Number: 1551-7977
International Standard Book Number: 978-0-323-08881-7

Transferred to Digital Printing, 2012

Editors Emeritus

Peter C. Amadio, MD

Lloyd A. and Barbara A. Amundson Professor of Orthopedics; Consultant, Department of Orthopedic Surgery, Mayo Clinic, Rochester, Minnesota

Richard A. Berger, MD, PhD

Professor of Orthopedic Surgery and Anatomy; Dean, Mayo School of Continuous Professional Development; Chair, Division of Hand Surgery, Mayo Clinic, Rochester, Minnesota

James Chang, MD

Professor of Surgery and Orthopedic Surgery, Chief of Plastic Surgery, Stanford University Medical Center, Stanford, California

Robert A. Chase, MD

Emile Holman Professor of Surgery (Emeritus), Stanford University School of Medicine, Stanford, California

James H. Dobyns, MD

Emeritus Professor (Academic) of Orthopedic Surgery, United States Air Force, Emeritus Professor (Academic) of Orthopedic Surgery, Mayo Foundation, Rochester, Minnesota; Emeritus Professor (Clinical) of Orthopedic Surgery, University of Texas Health Science Center, San Antonio, Texas

Vincent R. Hentz, MD

Emeritus Professor of Surgery, Stanford University School of Medicine, Robert A. Chase Hand and Upper Limb Center, Division of Plastic Surgery, Stanford University Medical Center, Stanford, California

Amy L. Ladd, MD

Professor of Orthopaedic Surgery and Plastic Surgery, Robert A. Chase Hand and Upper Limb Center; Chief, Pediatric Hand Clinic, Lucile Packard Children's Hospital, Stanford, California

Contributing Editors

Keith A. Bengtson, MD
Assistant Professor, Department of Physical Medicine and Rehabilitation, Mayo Clinic, Rochester, Minnesota

Philip Blazar, MD
Assistant Professor, Department of Orthopaedic Surgery, Brigham and Women's Hospital, Boston, Massachusetts

Lance M. Brunton, MD
Professor, Department of Orthopaedic Surgery, University of Medicine and Dentistry of New Jersey, Newark, New Jersey

John T. Capo, MD
Assistant Professor of Orthopaedic Surgery, University of Pittsburgh Medical Center, Pittsburgh, Pennsylvania

Louis Catalano, MD
Assistant Professor of Clinical Orthopaedic Surgery, Columbia University College of Physicians and Surgeons, C.V. Starr Hand Surgery Center, New York, New York

R. Chris Chadderdon, MD
OrthoCarolina, Charlotte, North Carolina

Neal C. Chen, MD
Assistant Professor in Orthopaedic Surgery, Thomas Jefferson University Hospital, The Philadelphia Hand Center, P.C., Philadelphia, Pennsylvania

Emilie Cheung, MD
Assistant Professor, Robert A. Chase Hand & Upper Limb Center, Department of Orthopaedic Surgery, Redwood City, California

Matthew Seung Suk Choi, MD
Associate Professor, Chief, Department of Plastic and Reconstructive Surgery, Hanyang University Guri Hospital, Guri, Gyunggi-do, Korea

Alphonsus Chong, MD
Associate Consultant, Department of Hand & Reconstructive Microsurgery, National University Hospital, Singapore

Susan J. Clark, OTR/L, CHT
Certified Hand Therapist, Stanford University Medical Center, Redwood City, California

J. Henk Coert, MD, PhD
Associate Professor, Department of Plastic and Reconstructive Surgery, Rotterdam, The Netherlands

Catherine Curtin, MD
Assistant Professor, Robert A. Chase Hand and Upper Limb Center, Division of Plastic Surgery, Stanford University Medical Center, Stanford, California

Aaron Daluiski, MD
Assistant Professor of Orthopaedic Surgery, Hospital for Special Surgery, Weill Cornell Medical College, New York, New York

Charles S. Day, MD, MBA

Associate Professor of Orthopedic Surgery, Harvard Medical School, Chief of the Division of Hand and Upper Extremity Surgery, Department of Orthopaedic Surgery, Beth Israel Deaconess Medical Center, Boston, Massachusetts

Antonio M. Foruria, MD, PhD

Shoulder Elbow Reconstructive Surgery Unit, Orthopedic Surgery and Trauma Service, Fundacion Jimenez Diaz, Madrid, Spain

Michael Fox, MBBS

Consultant Orthopaedic Surgeon, Peripheral Nerve Injury Unit, Royal National Orthopaedic Hospital, Brockley Hill, Stanmore, Middlesex, United Kingdom

Jessica Frankenhoff, MD

Assistant Professor, Department of Orthopaedic Surgery, VCU Medical Center, Richmond, Virginia

Jeffrey B. Friedrich, MD, FACS

Associate Professor of Surgery and Orthopedics, Division of Plastic Surgery, University of Washington, Seattle, Washington

R. Glenn Gaston, MD

Chief of Hand Surgery, Carolinas Medical Center, Department of Orthopedic Surgery, OrthoCarolina, Charlotte, North Carolina

Ruby Grewal, MD, MSc, FRCSC

Assistant Professor, The Hand and Upper Limb Centre, St. Joseph's Health Centre, London, Ontario, Canada

Warren Hammert, MD

Associate Professor of Orthopaedic and Plastic Surgery, University of Rochester Medical Center, Rochester, New York

Alicia K. Harrison, MD

Assistant Professor, Orthopaedic Surgery, University of Minnesota, Minneapolis, Minnesota

Thomas Hughes, MD

Assistant Professor, AGH Department of Orthopedics, Allegheny Orthopedics Associates, Pittsburgh, Pennsylvania

Sidney M. Jacoby, MD

Assistant Professor in Orthopaedic Surgery, Thomas Jefferson University Hospital, The Philadelphia Hand Center, P.C., Philadelphia, Pennsylvania

Sanjeev Kakar, MD

Assistant Professor, Department of Orthopedic Surgery, Mayo Clinic, Rochester, Minnesota

Ryosuke Kakinoki, MD, PhD

Associate Professor, Chief, Hand Surgery and Microsurgery, Department of Orthopedic Surgery and Rehabilitation Medicine, Graduate School of Medicine, Kyoto University, Kyoto, Japan

F. Thomas D. Kaplan, MD

Indiana Hand to Shoulder Center, Indianapolis, Indiana

Jeffrey Macalena, MD
Assistant Professor, Orthopaedic Surgery, University of Minnesota, Minneapolis, Minnesota

Timothy R. McAdams, MD
Assistant Professor, Robert A. Chase Hand and Upper Limb Center, Department of Orthopaedic Surgery, Stanford, California

Kai Megerle, MD
Postdoctoral Fellow, Division of Plastic Surgery, Stanford University Medical Center, Palo Alto, California

Peter M. Murray, MD
Professor, Department of Orthopedic Surgery, Mayo Clinic, Jacksonville, Florida

Virginia H. O'Brien, OTD, OTR/L, CHT
Supervisor, Hand and Physical Therapy, Fairview Hand Center, University Orthopaedics Therapy Center, University of Minnesota Medical Center, Fairview, Minneapolis, Minnesota

Rick F. Papendrea, MD
Assistant Clinical Professor, Department of Orthopaedic Surgery, Medical College of Wisconsin, Orthopedic Associates of Wisconsin, Waukesha, Wisconsin

Martin A. Posner, MD
Clinical Professor of Orthopaedic Surgery, Chief, Division of Hand Surgery, NYU Hospital for Joint Diseases, New York University School of Medicine, New York, New York

Tamara D. Rozental, MD
Assistant Professor of Orthopaedic Surgery, Harvard Medical School, Beth Israel Deaconess Medical Center, Carl J. Shapiro Department of Orthopaedics, Boston, Massachusetts

Eon K. Shin, MD
Assistant Professor in Orthopaedic Surgery, Thomas Jefferson University Hospital, The Philadelphia Hand Center, PC, Philadelphia, Pennsylvania

Steven S. Shin, MD, MMS
Director, Hand Surgery, Chief Financial Officer, Kerlan-Jobe Orthopaedic Clinic, Los Angeles, California

John Sperling, MD, MBA
Professor, Department of Orthopedic Surgery, Mayo Clinic, Rochester, Minnesota

Jin Bo Tang, MD
Professor and Chair, Department of Hand Surgery, Affiliated Hospital of Nantong University; Chair, Hand Surgery Research Center, Nantong University, Jiangsu, China

Peter Tang, MD, MPH
Assistant Professor of Clinical Orthopaedic Surgery, Columbia University College of Physicians and Surgeons, Columbia University Medical Center, New York, New York

Christopher J. Tuohy, MD
Assistant Professor, Department of Orthopaedic Surgery, Wake Forest University, Winston-Salem, North Carolina

Christina M. Ward, MD
Assistant Professor, Orthopaedic Surgery, University of Minnesota, Regions Hospital, St. Paul, Minnesota

J. Michael Wiater, MD
Chief of Shoulder Surgery, Associate Professor, Department of Orthopaedic Surgery, William Beaumont Hospital, Royal Oak, Michigan

Aviva Wolff, OT, CHT
Chief, Section of Hand Therapy, Hospital for Special Surgery, Weill Cornell Medical College, New York, New York

Thomas W. Wright, MD
Professor of Orthopedic Surgery, University of Florida Orthopaedic and Sports Medicine Institute, Gainesville, Florida

Dan Zlotolow, MD
Department of Orthopaedic Surgery, University of Maryland, Baltimore, Maryland

Table of Contents

Journals Represented

Journals represented in this YEAR BOOK are listed below.

Acta Orthopaedica
AJR American Journal of Roentgenology
American Journal of Sports Medicine
Annals of Plastic Surgery
Archives of Physical Medicine and Rehabilitation
Arthroscopy
Clinical Biomechanics
Clinical Neurology and Neurosurgery
Clinical Orthopaedics and Related Research
Hand
Injury
Journal of Applied Physiology
Journal of Bone and Joint Surgery (American)
Journal of Bone and Joint Surgery (British)
Journal of Hand Surgery
Journal of Hand Surgery, European Volume
Journal of Hand Therapy
Journal of Neurosurgery
Journal of Orthopaedic Research
Journal of Orthopaedic Trauma
Journal of Pediatric Orthopedics
Journal of Plastic, Reconstructive & Aesthetic Surgery
Journal of Reconstructive Microsurgery
Journal of Shoulder and Elbow Surgery
Journal of Trauma
Microsurgery
Neurosurgery
Orthopedics
Plastic and Reconstructive Surgery
Radiology
Skeletal Radiology

STANDARD ABBREVIATIONS

The following terms are abbreviated in this edition: acquired immunodeficiency syndrome (AIDS), cardiopulmonary resuscitation (CPR), central nervous system (CNS), cerebrospinal fluid (CSF), computed tomography (CT), deoxyribonucleic acid (DNA), electrocardiography (ECG), health maintenance organization (HMO), human immunodeficiency virus (HIV), intensive care unit (ICU), intramuscular (IM), intravenous (IV), magnetic resonance (MR) imaging (MRI), ribonucleic acid (RNA), and ultrasound (US).

NOTE

The YEAR BOOK OF HAND AND UPPER LIMB SURGERY® is a literature survey service providing abstracts of articles published in the professional literature. Every effort is made to assure the accuracy of the information presented in these pages. Neither the editors nor the publisher of the YEAR BOOK OF HAND AND UPPER LIMB SURGERY®

can be responsible for errors in the original materials. The editors' comments are their own opinions. Mention of specific products within this publication does not constitute endorsement.

To facilitate the use of the YEAR BOOK OF HAND AND UPPER LIMB SURGERY® as a reference tool, all illustrations and tables included in this publication are now identified as they appear in the original article. This change is meant to help the reader recognize that any illustration or table appearing in the YEAR BOOK OF HAND AND UPPER LIMB SURGERY® may be only one of many in the original article. For this reason, figure and table numbers will often appear to be out of sequence within the YEAR BOOK OF HAND AND UPPER LIMB SURGERY®.

Introduction

We are proud to bring you the 28th edition of the YEAR BOOK OF HAND AND UPPER LIMB SURGERY. It is our honor to continue a Mayo Clinic and Stanford University collaborative editorial tradition begun by Drs James Dobyns and Robert Chase and continued by Drs Peter Amadio and Vincent Hentz, and most recently by Drs Richard Berger, Amy Ladd, James Chang and Scott Steinmann.

This is the first year the YEAR BOOK has enlisted an editorial board, with associate editors chosen for their expertise in the field of upper limb surgery, as well as for their geographic diversity around the United States. Dr Jeffrey Yao remains the editor-in-chief and is indebted to the editorial board (Drs Julie Adams, Jonathan Isaacs, Steve K Lee and Marco Rizzo) for their contributions.

As the number of available sources of information regarding upper limb surgery or the busy surgeon increases, the goal of the YEAR BOOK is to distill the previous year's most salient journal articles into a shorter, more digestible form. Recently, upper limb surgeons have expressed a growing interest in pathology of the entire limb, including the shoulder, elbow, wrist and hand. The content of this year's YEAR BOOK OF HAND AND UPPER LIMB SURGERY continues to reflect this trend. The literature surveyed by this year's YEAR BOOK covers a diverse subject matter, stretching from the brachial plexus to the fingertip. Many articles have addressed current concepts regarding topics ranging from arthroplasty, reconstruction, trauma, arthroscopy, and congenital concerns of the entire upper limb.

We are deep within the Internet generation, with information readily at a surgeon's fingertips. As a result, the YEAR BOOK OF HAND AND UPPER LIMB SURGERY strives to evolve as well. This year we continue to embrace a "real-time" electronic eClips Consult format (www.eclips.consult.com), which keeps us even more up to date and makes the information from the YEAR BOOK more accessible and current. Moving forward, the goal of the editorial board will be to have a year-long continuous updating of the YEAR BOOK with the most current and salient articles uploaded online shortly after they are published. This format will allow the subscribing physician to access the YEAR BOOK electronically all year long to obtain the most up-to-date reviews and commentaries available.

As with every year, we would like to acknowledge the immense effort of the contributing editors to the YEAR BOOK, without whom this edition would not be possible. All of the contributing editors have been selected for their known national and international expertise in particular areas of the upper extremity. We are indebted to them for their commentary printed on these pages.

Finally, we would like to thank Mr David Parsons from Elsevier for his stewardship in helping guide us through this edition, and into the future.

Jeffrey Yao, MD

Introduction

We are proud to bring you the 28th edition of the YEAR BOOK OF HAND and Upper Limb Surgery. It is our honor to continue a major effort and...

Finally, we would like to thank MaryBeth Vsquone from Elsevier for her steadfast help in helping guide us through this edition, and into the future.

Jeffrey Yao, MD

1 Hand Trauma

Anticoagulation Following Digital Replantation
Buckley T, Hammert WC (Univ of Rochester Med Ctr, NY)
J Hand Surg 36A:1374-1376, 2011

Background.—Replanting amputated digits is associated with success rates as high as 90%. The most common complications are venous insufficiency and arterial thrombosis. Artery-only replantation has reasonable success, but can be complicated by arterial thrombi, 90% of which occur in the first 24 hours, or venous thrombosis, 42% of which occurs after the first 24 hours. Surgeons vary widely concerning methods of systemic anticoagulation and duration of therapy. Aspirin, intravenous (IV) heparin, low-molecular-weight heparin (LMWH), IV dextran, and local heparin through direct injection or continuous drip on an open incision are all methods currently used to achieve anticoagulation.

> *Case Report.*—Man, 28, sustained a guillotine-type amputation of his left index and middle fingers through the middle phalanx while preparing food. The digits were wrapped in gauze immediately, stored on ice in a plastic bag, and taken to the emergency room with the patient within an hour of the injury. Replantation was attempted.

Assessment of Anticoagulation Methods.—Available evidence covers the use of systemic thromboprophylaxis, local heparinization, artery-only replantation, and no thromboprophylaxis. Among the systemic approaches, success rates are comparably high for LMWH and 325 mg of aspirin. Microvascular thrombosis and flap failure are less likely with the use of postoperative subcutaneous heparin. Intraoperative heparin boluses of 3000 units 10 minutes before pedicle ligation achieves rates of microvascular thrombosis, total or partial flap loss, hematoma, seroma, pulmonary embolism, and death comparable to those with no anticoagulant intervention. IV heparin boluses of 2500 to 5000 U has achieved complete survival of 7 of 13 digits and partial survival of 11 of 13 digits. Studies of postoperative dextran for patients having free tissue transfer and replantation show no significant difference in success rates.

Local heparin offers a way to resolve venous congestion and is a safe alternative to systemic heparinization or leeches. Continuous heparinized saline drip onto a paraungual stab incision to stimulate bleeding yields a replantation survival rate of 64%, which is lower than the overall 76% rate for patients with and without the continuous drip.

Artery-only replantation has achieved 100% survival rates. Replantation was not aided by any other alternative means to reduce venous congestion in these patients. Survival rates obtained when patients had no intraoperative or postoperative anticoagulation interventions are comparable to those when anticoagulation is used, suggesting these interventions offer no survival benefit.

Conclusions.—The recommended method for the patient in question is 325 mg of aspirin daily for 5 days while the patient is monitored in the hospital. Subcutaneous LMWH is added for prophylaxis against lower extremity deep vein thrombosis for nonambulatory patients. IV LMWH can be used with intraoperative complications, then warfarin or LMWH is instituted for about 30 days after discharge. Dextran carries a potential for allergic reactions and intravascular volume expansion, so it is avoided.

▶ This concise evidence-based review addresses the role of various forms of anticoagulation following digital replantation to reduce the risk of microvascular thrombosis.

In their survey of the published literature, the authors find much variation in anticoagulation practice following replantation and reconstructive microsurgery. They attribute this to a lack of definitive evidence supporting any particular treatment. The various forms of anticoagulation for digital replantation and reconstructive microsurgery practiced and published in the literature are also described. These range from no anticoagulation, local measures, and systemic anticoagulation.

The authors finally present their own approach toward anticoagulation for both replantation and free tissue transfer. In the standard case, they use aspirin. Low-molecular-weight heparin (LMWH) for 5 days is added for nonambulatory patients. If there are intraoperative difficulties, intravenous heparin is used in place of LMWH, with conversion to warfarin or LMWH for about 30 days.

Their work succinctly presents the current state of knowledge and opinion about anticoagulation. As the authors discuss in their article, there is a paucity of good comparison studies and the need for better-designed research to address this question. These studies are critical if we are to have a better basis to make decisions about anticoagulation in finger replantation. In the absence of good data supporting their use, microsurgeons should consider a "primum non nocere" approach, where omitting anticoagulation might not actually adversely affect the outcome of replantation but avoid its complications.

A. Chong, MD

Posttraumatic Reconstruction of the Hand—A Retrospective Review of 87 Toe-to-Hand Transfers Compared With an Earlier Report

Kvernmo HD, Tsai T-M (Univ of Louisville School of Medicine, KY; Kleinert Kutz and Associates Hand Surgery Group, Louisville, KY)
J Hand Surg 36A:1176-1181, 2011

Purpose.—The purpose of this study was to retrospectively review the results of 87 toe-to-hand transfers performed in 73 procedures, compare them to the report published by the senior author in 1983, and confirm the hypothesis that results of toe-to-hand transfers at our center have improved over time.

Methods.—The results of 87 toe-to-hand transfers performed between 1981 and 2001 were reviewed and compared with the results of 54 toe-to-hand transfers performed between 1974 and 1980. The measured parameters were type of reconstruction performed, anticoagulation therapy, vascular patency, frequency of secondary surgery, and strength of thumb reconstructions.

Results.—In the recent time period, 11% of the procedures had complications with revascularization of the transferred digit, and long-term survival was seen in 98% of the toe-to-hand transfers. This is a significant improvement over earlier results, in which 33% of the cases had some microvascular compromise and the survival of grafts was lower (91%). Pinch strength for thumb reconstructions improved, and the number of secondary surgeries performed dropped, but neither of these parameters reached a significant level. Toes used for reconstruction changed, with an 18% decrease in use of big toe for thumb reconstruction and a similar increase in use of the second toe. For non-thumb digital reconstructions there was a 60% decrease in use of second and third toe combined, whereas use of the second toe alone increased similarly.

Conclusions.—This study showed reduction of the incidence of vascular compromise compared to the previous report. Improved strength of thumb reconstructions and reduced need for secondary surgery was also displayed. These findings are likely attributed to refinements in reconstructive procedures and operative techniques.

Type of Study/Level of Evidence.—Therapeutic IV (Table 2).

▶ This review of a series of toe-to-hand transfers is interesting because the same author had earlier published a similar series of cases. This allows for some comparison between the 2 series. It provides a useful record of one surgeon's practice and outcomes in complex microsurgical toe transfer over a long period.

There were some changes in the types of reconstruction done over time. In the later series, there was an increase in the use of the second toe over the big toe and also less use of combined second and third toes. This reflected a recognition of the increased morbidity of the big toe or combined toe block transfers. There was also a change in the flaps used before toe transfer, with other flaps chosen in preference to the groin flap in the newer series.

TABLE 2.—Comparison of Secondary Surgery Between the Previous and Current Study

Type of Secondary Procedures	Previous (1976–1980)[7]	Current (1981–2001)
Total number of procedures	40	73
Number of secondary procedures	26 (68%)	37 (51%)*
Number of secondary surgeries	26	58
Tenolysis	19	19
Osteotomies with bone graft	4	5
Deepening of first web space	3	9
Tendon reconstructions	—	9
De-bulking of flaps	—	9
Interphalangeal joint arthrodesis	—	6
Free vascular joint transfer		1

Editor's Note: Please refer to original journal article for full references.
*$P=.143$.

The main difference in outcome was a decreased need for re-exploration. Other outcome measures, such as survival, strength, and need for secondary surgery (Table 2), were assessed, but the results did not reach significance.

The main weakness of this study is that it used a historical cohort for comparison. Randomization and blinding were not done. Therefore, the conditions of the two groups might not have been the same.

The author was already a very experienced microsurgeon when he wrote his results for the first case series. This second study shows that there is a continual learning curve with complex microsurgery cases. Even beyond the first 54 transfers published in the earlier series, there was still room for refinement of judgment, surgical technique, and postoperative treatment. It suggests that such cases should be performed by the most experienced microsurgeon available.

A. Chong, MD

Remodeling Potential of Phalangeal Distal Condylar Malunions in Children
Puckett BN, Gaston RG, Peljovich AE, et al (Childrens Healthcare of Atlanta, GA; Atlanta Med Ctr Orthopaedic Residency Program, GA; Hand and Upper Extremity Ctr of Georgia, Atlanta; et al)
J Hand Surg 37A:34-41, 2012

Purpose.—Distal condylar phalangeal (DCP) fractures in children are uncommon, but their periarticular location makes them problematic. Malunions are particularly difficult to treat. These fractures are generally thought to have a poor remodeling potential because their location is far from the phalangeal physis. We present 8 cases of DCP malunion in children with a mean 5-year follow-up demonstrating consistent remodeling.

Methods.—In this study, DCP fractures were defined as those occurring at or distal to the collateral ligament recess of the proximal or middle phalanx in skeletally immature patients. Radiographic parameters examined at the time of established malunion and at final follow-up included coronal and sagittal plane deformity and translational malalignment of the distal fragment in relation to the proximal shaft. Range of motion was measured, and a brief questionnaire was implemented to establish patient satisfaction.

Results.—We examined 8 patients with a minimum 1-year follow-up (mean, 5.3 y). Average age at injury was 8.8 years (range, 2−14 y). In the sagittal plane, fractures remodeled from an initial mean deformity of 30.9° to 0.0°; in the coronal plane, from 10.5° to 3.9°. Fracture translation in the sagittal plane corrected, as well, from a mean 57.5% at injury to 0.0% at final follow-up. There was no functionally limiting loss of motion of the digit in any patient. Subjectively, only 2 patients complained of cosmetic deformity, both of which were coronal plane deformities of the small finger.

Conclusions.—In this case series, DCP malunions in children remodeled significantly and completely in the sagittal plane, and all patients had good final range of motion. Furthermore, patients were satisfied with nonsurgical

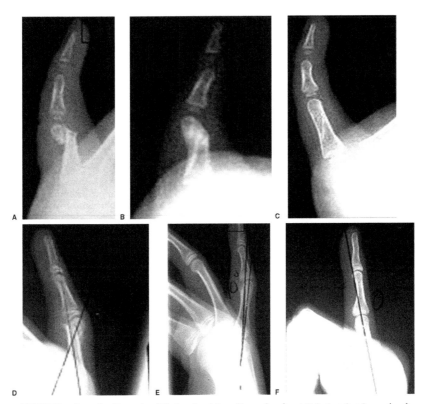

FIGURE 2.—Lateral radiographs. **A** Patient 8 at injury (6 months of age). **B** Patient 8 at 2 months after injury. **C** Patient 8 at 11 months after injury, demonstrating full remodeling. **D** Patient 3 at 14 years of age. **E** Patient 3 at 2 months after injury. **F** Patient 3 at 82 months after injury, demonstrating full remodeling. (Reprinted from Puckett BN, Gaston RG, Peljovich AE, et al. Remodeling potential of phalangeal distal condylar malunions in children. *J Hand Surg.* 2012;37A:34-41, Copyright 2012, with permission from the American Society for Surgery of the Hand.)

treatment at long-term follow-up. This series describes the remodeling potential of DCP fractures in children, lending support to the previously reported cases. These findings support treating late-presenting pediatric DCP malunions nonsurgically.

Type of Study/Level of Evidence.—Therapeutic IV (Fig 2).

▶ Although the numbers are small and the study is retrospective, this article should change your practice. There has been a long-held and promoted belief by many that phalangeal neck fractures in children do not remodel because they are too far from the growth plate.[1] Proximity to a physis has been thought to be a major determinant of remodeling potential for all fractures. It appears that the thickened and bioactive skeletally immature periosteum, in conjunction with Wolff's law acting on the bone in the plane of motion of the nearest joint, can affect remodeling even at the opposite end of the bone from the physis in these fractures. Previous demonstrations of phalangeal neck fracture remodeling were scattered case reports in young children.[2] This study demonstrates complete or nearly complete remodeling in the plane of motion of the nearest joint for all mal-unions seen in their practice, even in children nearing skeletal maturity. Fractures did not remodel in the coronal plane, however. Based on their findings, they no longer treat malunions with subcondylar fossa recession. Instead, they allow established malunions to remodel with time if the physes are open. I agree with the authors that acute fractures should still be reduced and pinned if displaced, and that impending malunions should still be treated with osteoclasis and pinning. Although remodeling may be certain over time, earlier motion can be recovered by percutaneous fixation methods.

D. A. Zlotolow, MD

References

1. Waters PM, Taylor BA, Kuo AY. Percutaneous reduction of incipient malunion of phalangeal neck fractures in children. *J Hand Surg Am.* 2004;29:707-711.
2. Cornwall R, Waters P. Remodeling of phalangeal neck fracture malunions in children: case report. *J Hand Surg Am.* 2004;29:458-461.

Interobserver Reliability of Computed Tomography to Diagnose Scaphoid Waist Fracture Union
Buijze GA, The Science of Variation Group (Massachusetts General Hosp, Boston)
J Hand Surg 37A:250-254, 2012

Purpose.—To determine the interobserver agreement and diagnostic performance characteristics of computed tomography (CT) for determining union of scaphoid waist fractures.

Methods.—A total of 59 orthopedic and trauma surgeons rated for union a set of 30 sagittal CT scans of 30 scaphoid waist fractures. Of these fractures, 20 were treated nonoperatively, were imaged between 6 and 10 weeks after injury, and were known to have eventually achieved union.

Ten were operatively confirmed to be ununited. We rated each scan as united or ununited using a Web-based rating application. We assessed interobserver reliability using Siegel's multirater Kappa. We calculated diagnostic performance characteristics using Bayesian formulas.

Results.—The interobserver agreement among 59 raters was substantial. The average sensitivity, specificity, and accuracy of diagnosing union of scaphoid waist fractures on sagittal CT scans were 78%, 96%, and 84%, respectively. Assuming a 90% prevalence of fracture union of the scaphoid, the positive predictive value of a diagnosis of union on sagittal CT scan was 0.99 and the negative predictive value was 0.41.

Conclusions.—Our results suggest that CT scans are accurate and reliable for diagnosis of union but inadequate for ruling out nonunion of scaphoid waist fractures between 6 and 10 weeks after injury.

Type of Study/Level of Evidence.—Diagnostic III.

▶ Diagnosing scaphoid union after fracture remains challenging for hand surgeons. The authors are to be commended to address this problem. Because of the position of the scaphoid in 3-dimensional space, plain films have shown limited reliability. CT scan may be able to visualize nonunions of the scaphoid. This article lacks the statement that the nonunited scaphoid fractures were symptomatic and the united fractures were asymptomatic. In clinical practice on CT scan, nonunited fracture of the scaphoid that is asymptomatic may not require treatment, or the patient may not seek treatment.

The study design is a level 3B: this would be an individual case-control study with nonconsecutive patients. It is not known with which criteria the observers scored the scans. Also, the dropout rate of the observers is not known because they received 3 reminders during a period of 6 weeks. It would also be interesting to see whether the lost observers were evenly distributed in experience.

The CT scans were performed on different machines. The position of the wrist was different for united and nonunited fractures. The expertise and experience of the observer varied: 50% saw fewer than 10 fractures per year, and 25% saw 0 to 5 fractures per year. It would be interesting to learn how many observers saw only one fracture per year in the 0 to 5 fractures group. How was this distributed? The participation of a musculoskeletal radiologist in the observer team was also lacking.

The advantage of CT over plain films is multiplanar reconstruction. By providing only sagittal views, the superior benefit of this technique has not been fully used. In my experience, it would be favorable to take advantage of the multiplanar information provided by CT scans.

H. Coert, MD, PhD

Intrafocal Pin Plate Fixation of Distal Ulna Fractures Associated With Distal Radius Fractures

Foster BJ, Bindra RR (Loyola Univ Med Ctr, Maywood, IL)
J Hand Surg 37A:356-359, 2012

Subcapital ulnar fractures in association with distal radius fractures in elderly patients increase instability and pose a treatment challenge. Fixation of the ulnar fracture with traditional implants is difficult due to the subcutaneous location, comminution, and osteoporosis. We describe an intrafocal pin plate that provides fixation by a locking plate on the distal ulna and intramedullary fixation within the shaft. The low profile and percutaneous technique make this device a useful alternative for treatment of subcapital ulna fractures in the elderly (Fig 2).

▶ This surgical technique article describes a method for fixation of distal ulna fractures. This technique is of use, particularly in distal fracture patterns and in osteopenic/-porotic patients, in whom other techniques may be less desirable. It is a low profile fixation technique that may be particularly of use in this area with limited soft tissue coverage. Contraindications include comminuted distal ulnar head fractures. Associated distal radius fractures are stabilized, then the ulna fracture is approached through a small open incision between the flexor carpi ulnaris and extensor carpi ulnaris. The device is an intramedullary intrafocal pin plate. It is composed of a long curved intramedullary portion that provides stability via 3-point bending, with a distal interlocking portion to stabilize the

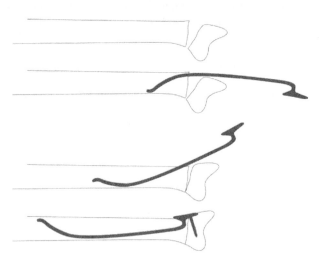

FIGURE 2.—Schematic drawing of fixation of a distal ulna fracture with the intrafocal pin plate. The intramedullary portion is inserted through the fracture site into the proximal fracture fragment, the plate is turned 180° to afford reduction, and the distal plate is positioned on the ulnar border of the distal ulna. The metaphyseal fragment is fixed to the plate with locking screws placed into the ulnar head. (Reprinted from Foster BJ, Bindra RR. Intrafocal pin plate fixation of distal ulna fractures associated with distal radius fractures. *J Hand Surg.* 2012;37A:356-359, Copyright 2012, with permission from the American Society for Surgery of the Hand.)

distal fragment with 1 or 2 locking screws. The device is introduced into the medullary canal proximally through the fracture site, the fracture is reduced, and then locking screws placed through the distal portion of the fracture (Fig 2). The technique was used successfully in 5 patients over the age of 55 years as described by the article.

This technique is interesting and may be useful in select patients in whom distal ulna fractures require stabilization. The article does not describe ease or feasibility of hardware removal, should that become necessary, but that might be of concern to the interested reader who might consider use of this technique.

J. Adams, MD

Chronic Psychological and Functional Sequelae After Emergent Hand Surgery
Richards T, Garvert DW, McDade E, et al (Stanford Univ School of Medicine, CA; VA Palo Alto Health Care System, CA)
J Hand Surg 36A:1663-1668, 2011

Purpose.—Several studies have shown that upper extremity trauma has serious, acute psychological effects after injury. This study's goal was to assess the psychological outcomes, including symptoms of major depression, posttraumatic stress disorder (PTSD), and other psychosocial variables, as well as the Quick Disabilities of the Arm, Shoulder, and Hand (*Quick*DASH) results, after severe hand trauma. We hypothesized that hand trauma would have persistent psychological sequelae long after the physical injury.

Methods.—We performed a cross-sectional survey of 34 patients who had emergency hand surgery at a Level 1 trauma center an average of 16 months (range, 7–32 mo) earlier. The hand disability measure was the *Quick*DASH, and the psychological measures included the Center for Epidemiologic Studies Depression Scale, the Screen for Posttraumatic Stress Symptoms, the Medical Outcomes Study Social Support Survey Form, the Social Constraints Survey (to assess interpersonal stressors), and the Perceived Stress Scale.

Results.—The overall *Quick*DASH score was 27. The mean score for PTSD was 13 (above the clinical threshold for PTSD), and 29% of respondents had high levels of both depression and PTSD. High pain scores on the *Quick*DASH were strongly correlated with both depression and PTSD symptoms.

Conclusions.—This study found high levels of psychological distress in patients after hand trauma. Hand disability was strongly related to pain, depression, and PTSD symptoms. This study shows that the psychological sequelae of hand trauma can persist long after the physical injury.

Type of Study/Level of Evidence.—Therapeutic IV.

▶ The authors investigate the psychosocial sequelae after acute upper extremity trauma in a group of 34 patients. They find a high prevalence of residual pain that correlates with symptoms of depression and posttraumatic stress disorder (PTSD). While I agree with the authors that the psychological consequences of severe upper extremity trauma have been widely neglected in the past and deserve more attention, the findings of this study are severely limited by several methodologic flaws. First, only 104 patients (averaging 5 patients per surgeon per year) met the quite broad inclusion criteria. Unfortunately, in addition to this already low number, only about one-third of patients were available for follow-up, which makes any scientific conclusion questionable. Second, the authors should have characterized the patients better. From the data presented, I have the impression that the patients' medical and social histories are quite heterogeneous. Couldn't there be any patterns of injury or social issues that lead to higher rates of psychological problems? Third, I am missing any work-related information. How many patients were able to return to their original jobs? How many are currently unemployed? This information could have been obtained very easily and might have been very valuable to the reader.

I applaud the authors for bringing this important issue to attention, but I think more reliable scientific data are needed.

K. Megerle, MD

Isolated Diaphyseal Fractures of the Ulna
McAuliffe JA (Broward Health Orthopaedics, Fort Lauderdale, FL)
J Hand Surg 37A:145-147, 2012

Background.—Isolated fractures of the ulnar diaphysis are the only adult forearm injuries for which closed treatment is considered. Acceptable fracture healing and restoration of forearm rotation is often achieved after closed treatment or benign neglect. Although evidence to support thresholds for operative treatment are lacking, it is proposed that surgery is best for fracture displaced by more than half the diameter of bone or angulated by more than 10 degrees.

> *Case Report.*—Woman, 64, injured her left nondominant forearm, then struck it on the edge of a step some time later. Local pain and mild swelling developed, but no wound or pain or tenderness was found at the wrist or elbow. Neurovascular evaluation showed an intact limb. A nondisplaced ulnar diaphysis fracture was found on radiographs taken the day of the second injury. The patient was given a removable wrist splint and told the fracture would heal with minimal protection. After 3 weeks, radiographs showed 50% loss of apposition and 10 degrees of angulation with some callus formation. The patient was concerned about the findings, but strongly preferred to avoid surgery. Despite these changes, displacement and angulation were still within acceptable limits and early callus was identified. A sugar tong splint was used for 2 weeks,

a therapist-fabricated cylindrical splint reaching the length of the forearm for 4 weeks, and a lightweight, over-the-counter wrist splint for 6 weeks. Clinical and radiographic healing was apparent after 11 weeks, and the patient had 80 degrees of pronation and 60 degrees of supination. Eight months later, forearm rotation was identical to the contralateral uninjured limb.

Analysis of Evidence.—A comparison of various nonoperative treatments for isolated diaphyseal fractures of the middle and distal third of the ulnar in adults concluded that no evidence showed immobilization of the elbow to relieve pain or achieve fracture union was better than using casts or braces to immobilize the forearm alone. Nonunion rates are generally low for nonoperative treatments; no consistent differences in times to union correlate with method of immobilization. Range of motion when the fracture heals is slightly better with early mobilization or functional bracing, but the effect may not persist over time. Few injuries involve a displacement exceeding 50% of the ulnar diameter, but these had a higher incidence of nonunion, as did high-energy injuries and injury through an indirect mechanism. Worse anatomic and functional results also occurred with fractures exceeding 10 degrees of angulation when braces were applied. Open reduction and internal fixation were superior to cast immobilization in restoring forearm rotation when fracture angulation exceeds 15 degrees.

Evidence quality suffers from too few randomized trials covering isolated diaphyseal fractures treated with various nonoperative methods. Methodologic flaws, especially in patient allocation, produces a high risk of bias. Loss of patients to follow-up also complicates many studies. Time to union is a relatively unreliable measure, and no studies had validated measures of patient-rated outcome.

Conclusions.—Future research should include a large prospective cohort of patients treated nonoperatively to determine risk factors for nonunion and malunion and the consequences of residual translation or angulation of a diaphyseal ulnar fracture. Cost-effectiveness and arm-specific disability also should be considered.

▶ This article surveys the available evidence for treatment of isolated shaft fractures of the ulna. The authors highlight numerous case series that show acceptable healing rates and good functional recovery following nonoperative treatment of these fractures. Although many of these studies are uncontrolled case series and are compromised by poor clinical follow-up, a spectrum of immobilization techniques has been successfully reported for treatment of these fractures, including casts and custom splints, with or without immobilization of the elbow. As the author states, there is no generalized agreement on the best form of immobilization, but it is generally agreed that isolated ulnar fractures with less than 50% displacement and less than 10° immobilization are amenable to nonoperative management.

The indication for operative treatment, however, has never been clearly defined because no randomized series exist comparing patients treated with surgery with patients treated nonoperatively. In general, widely displaced or shortened fractures should be considered unstable, and operative management seems appropriate. Additionally, patients with ulnar fractures in the setting of multitrauma may benefit from open reduction and internal fixation to facilitate patient mobilization.

P. Murray, MD

2 Hand: Arthritis and Arthroplasty

Current Trends in Nonoperative and Operative Treatment of Trapeziometacarpal Osteoarthritis: A Survey of US Hand Surgeons
Wolf JM, Delaronde S (Univ of Connecticut Health Ctr, Farmington, CT)
J Hand Surg 37A:77-82, 2012

Purpose.—Multiple procedures have been described for trapeziometa-carpal (TM) osteoarthritis with varying levels of evidence support. The purpose of this study was to evaluate current trends in the treatment of TM arthritis by surveying active members of the American Society for Surgery of the Hand.

Methods.—We sent an online questionnaire to the e-mail addresses of 2,326 active members of the American Society for Surgery of the Hand, consisting of 5 treatment and 2 demographic questions. Surgeons were contacted twice by e-mail and provided with a link to a de-identified online survey. We performed statistical analysis of correlations between demographics and treatment preferences using chi-square testing.

Results.—We received responses from 1,156 out of 2,326 hand surgeons, a response rate of 50%. The vast majority of surgeons use corticosteroid injections for TM arthritis, and 719 out of 1,156 perform trapeziectomy with ligament reconstruction and tendon interposition (LRTI) for common Eaton stage III arthritis. For scaphotrapeziotrapezoid (STT) arthritis, approximately half of respondents also perform trapeziectomy/LRTI, followed by STT fusion. For a younger woman with minimal radiographic change and pain, 535 out of 1,142 surgeon respondents would advocate continued conservative treatment, whereas the remainder chose Eaton ligament reconstruction, arthroscopy, and metacarpal osteotomy.

Conclusions.—This survey study presents the current opinions of a group of hand surgeons who responded to an online questionnaire regarding treatment of TM arthritis. The results show that trapeziectomy/LRTI is the treatment of choice by most respondents. The use of trapeziectomy/LRTI in the treatment of STT arthritis has not been studied in depth, but this procedure was chosen by half the respondents. The process of choosing treatment strategies is a question for future study.

Type of Study/Level of Evidence.—Prognostic IV.

▶ This article presents data from an online questionnaire posed to active members of the American Society for Surgery of the Hand regarding treatment approaches for trapeziometacarpal osteoarthritis. The results are not surprising: Most hand surgeons utilize corticosteroid injections for conservative care, with only 4% offering hyaluronic acid injections. About 62% of surgeons report trapeziectomy with ligament reconstruction and tendon interposition (LRTI) as their procedure of choice for Eaton stage III osteoarthritis. Regional differences are also uncovered by this study. For example, LRTI is most commonly performed in the mid-Atlantic (72%) compared with the South (58%) and West (58%).

Current trends in the management of trapeziometacarpal osteoarthritis are highlighted by this study. While the response rate to the online questionnaire was remarkably good at 50%, respondent bias may make it difficult to interpret the data. The questions also limited responses to predefined categories without allowing for open-ended answers.

This study will not alter most surgeons' practices. However, it will reveal whether one is staying consistent with practice trends in one's region and demographic. The manuscript's findings may serve as a starting point for additional studies examining evidence-based medicine's effect on treatment philosophies.

E. K. Shin, MD

Objective Functional Outcomes and Patient Satisfaction After Silicone Metacarpophalangeal Arthroplasty for Rheumatoid Arthritis

Waljee JF, Chung KC (Univ of Michigan Health System, Ann Arbor)
J Hand Surg 37A:47-54, 2012

Purpose.—Patient satisfaction is an essential measure of quality of care for rheumatoid arthritis. Prior research demonstrates that patient satisfaction improves after silicone metacarpophalangeal arthroplasty (SMPA) despite minimal change in hand function. The purpose of this study was to identify the level of objective functional recovery that yields satisfaction after SMPA. We hypothesized that measurable gains in objective hand function after SMPA will discriminate between satisfied and dissatisfied patients.

Methods.—In this prospective, multicenter, cohort study, we observed 46 patients with rheumatoid arthritis and metacarpophalangeal (MCP) joint subluxation for 2 years after reconstructive surgery. We derived satisfaction scores from the Michigan Hand Outcomes Questionnaire, ranging from 0 (least satisfied) to 100 (most satisfied), and dichotomized them using the Cohen large effect size. We measured hand function at baseline and follow-up including strength (grip strength and pinch strength), finger position (extensor lag and ulnar drift), and MCP arc of motion. We constructed receiver operating characteristic curves to identify optimal cutoffs in hand function that correspond with satisfaction.

Results.—At 2 years of follow-up, patients who achieved an extension lag of 30° or less were considered satisfied, which represented a 52% improvement (preoperative lag = 63°). Similarly, patients who gained improvement in ulnar drift from an average of preoperatively 62° to 9° postoperatively were satisfied. Finally, patients who achieved an improvement in MCP arc of motion from an average of 21° to 31° postoperatively were satisfied. No improvements in grip or pinch strength corresponded with postoperative patient satisfaction.

Conclusions.—Patients were satisfied with only modest gains in grip and pinch strength after silicone metacarpophalangeal arthroplasty. However, maintaining finger position, without recurrence of ulnar drift or extensor lag, and MCP arc of motion corresponded with patient satisfaction in the postoperative period.

Type of Study/Level of Evidence.—Therapeutic II (Fig 2).

▶ This study presents statistical data to determine what outcomes yield higher satisfaction scores following silicone metacarpophalangeal arthroplasty (SMPA) in patients diagnosed with rheumatoid arthritis. The authors found that decreased extension lag, decreased ulnar drift, and improved metacarpophalangeal joint motion all correlated highly with satisfied patients. Interestingly, improvements in grip and pinch strength measurements did not correlate with Michigan Hand Outcomes Questionnaire satisfaction scores when measured with receiver operating characteristic curves.

By the time patients make the decision to undergo SMPA for finger deformity and decreased hand function, they would have already developed adaptive mechanisms to complete activities of daily living. This may help to explain why improvements in grip and pinch strength measurements did not lead to more satisfied patients. In the end, it seems that many of these patients are

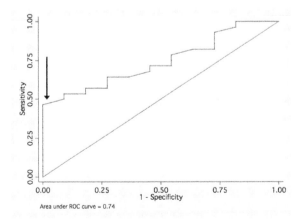

FIGURE 2.—Receiver operating characteristic curve for ulnar drift and patient satisfaction 2 years after SMPA (n = 46). (Reprinted from Waljee JF, Chung KC. Objective functional outcomes and patient satisfaction after silicone metacarpophalangeal arthroplasty for rheumatoid arthritis. *J Hand Surg.* 2012;37A:47-54, Copyright 2012, with permission from the American Society for Surgery of the Hand.)

motivated to improve the appearance of their hands. In this study, ulnar drift improved from 37° to 15° ($P < .001$) and was significantly correlated with patient satisfaction ($R^2 = 0.034$; $P < .001$) (see Fig 2).

While the authors concede that 24 of the 70 originally enrolled patients were lost to follow-up, the results of their study remain consistent with those of other studies examining postoperative expectations and priorities of patients with rheumatoid arthritis. This study will surely improve the ability of providers to communicate realistic and appropriate postoperative goals.

E. K. Shin, MD

Arthroplasty of the Hand: Radiographic Outcomes of Pyrolytic Carbon Proximal Interphalangeal and Metacarpophalangeal Joint Replacements
Petscavage JM, Ha AS, Chew FS (Penn State Hershey Med Ctr, PA; Univ of Washington, Seattle)
AJR Am J Roentgenol 197:1177-1181, 2011

Objective.—The purpose of this study was to describe the radiographic outcomes of pyrolytic carbon implants in the proximal interphalangeal (PIP) and metacarpophalangeal (MCP) joints, determine the most common complications, and assess risk factors associated with complications.

Materials and Methods.—Retrospective review over a 10-year period was performed to identify patients with pyrolytic carbon implants of the PIP or MCP joint. All available radiographs were reviewed and correlated with clinical information. Statistical analysis included calculation of the complication rate, Phi coefficient for variable association with a complication, and Kaplan-Meier survival.

Results.—Forty-seven implants in 43 patients were reviewed. There were 30 PIP and 17 MCP implants. The mean age of the patients was 56 years. The mean radiographic followup was 17.2 months (range, 1–82 months). The indication for arthroplasty included osteoarthritis (55.3%), trauma (27.7%), rheumatoid arthritis (12.8%), and benign neoplasm (4.26%). Fourteen second surgeries were performed: 4 for retrieval and 10 for revision. Radiographic abnormalities included subsidence (31.9%); loosening with dorsal or volar tilt of the stem (34.1%); loosening without tilt (6.38%); periprosthetic fracture (8.51%); and ulnar subluxation of joint (4.26%). There was no statistical association ($r < 0.001$) between 1 mm or less of symmetric lucency around the distal implant with future complications. The sensitivity of radiography for the clinical failure of the implant was 28.6% and specificity, 30.3%.

Conclusion.—Of the 47 pyrolytic carbon PIP and MCP implants, 14 (29.8%) required surgical revision or retrieval, mostly for extensor tendon contractures. Compared with the clinical survival of the implant, radiographic survival was poorer and did not correlate with clinical survival.

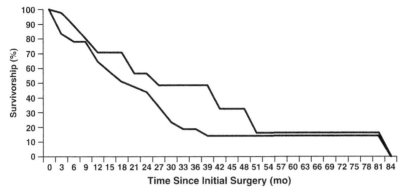

FIGURE 6.—Kaplan-Meier survival analysis curves for pyrolytic carbon proximal interphalangeal or metacarpophalangeal arthroplasty. Upper curve shows clinical survivorship. Lower curve indicates radiographic survivorship (i.e., development of radiographic hardware-associated abnormality). (Reprinted from Petscavage JM, Ha AS, Chew FS. Arthroplasty of the hand: radiographic outcomes of pyrolytic carbon proximal interphalangeal and metacarpophalangeal joint replacements. *AJR Am J Roentgenol.* 2011;197:1177-1181, with permission from the American Journal of Roentgenology.)

Tilt of the proximal stem and subsidence were the more common radiographic complications (Fig 6).

▶ This article in the radiology literature is certainly of interest to hand surgeons as well as radiologists. Radiographic and chart review was undertaken retrospectively of patients who underwent metacarpophalangeal or proximal interphalangeal pyrocarbon arthroplasty. Importantly, radiographic findings did not correlate with clinical findings; periprosthetic loosening, subsidence, or fracture were common, but were not indicative of need for revision or further surgery. Interestingly as well, 71.4% of patients who required revision surgery had normal-appearing radiographs. Nevertheless, the need for additional surgery was common in this series, at 30%, and indications included contracture, pain, or ligament laxity. The authors were all radiologists, which might introduce a confounding factor in review of the charts because of unfamiliarity with the clinical picture. Alternatively and most likely, it represents an unbiased evaluation of the true outcomes of these patients, particularly notable with the high surgical revision rate in this series. Fig 6 provides a sobering view of the implant success: This Kaplan-Meier survival curve demonstrates clinical (upper curve) and radiographic (lower curve) survival in this series. Clinical failure was defined by the authors as the need for retrieval or revision surgery; patients lost to follow-up were censored data. At 1 year, survival was 71%, but by year 3, survival was 48%, and finally, at 42 months, survival was 32%.

J. Adams, MD

Prosthetic hemi-arthroplasty for post-traumatic articular cartilage loss in the proximal interphalangeal joint

Henry M (Hand and Wrist Ctr of Houston, TX)
Hand 6:93-97, 2011

This article discusses the indications, contraindications, and technique for proximal interphalangeal joint prosthetic hemi-arthroplasty in the setting of sub-acute or chronic post-traumatic articular cartilage loss. Two case examples are provided: one for replacement of the head of the proximal phalanx, the other for replacement of the base of the middle phalanx. This procedure serves as a recently available alternative to fusion, silicone total joint replacement, total joint arthroplasty with unlinked surface replacements, volar plate arthroplasty, hemi-condylar osteochondral autograft reconstruction, or free vascularized joint transfer.

▶ This article describes another possible step in the reconstructive ladder for acute and subacute posttraumatic arthritis of the proximal interphalangeal (PIP) joint. After the hyaline cartilage is lost, options for reconstructing it include osteochondral replacement, if only one side of the joint is affected (eg, hemihamate), or vascularized or nonvascularized toe joint transfer. However, a hemihamate can be performed only if there is still hyaline cartilage intact on the head of the proximal phalanx. Toe transfers are morbid and, if vascularized, challenging.

If there is loss of hyaline cartilage but maintenance of subchondral bone at the opposing joint surface, then a hemiarthroplasty can theoretically be performed. The author did so on 2 patients, with very good results: Pain-free range of motion (ROM) was 0° to 90° and 0° to 95° at both 4-year and 18-month follow-ups, respectively. Both patients returned to premorbid activity levels.

The purported advantage of a hemiarthroplasty is better ROM and strength maintenance. However, with only 2 patients and no long-term follow-up, enthusiasm should be guarded. In another study in 2005 from Australia, 8 PIP joints were replaced with a hemiarthroplasty pyrocarbon implant with less favorable results.[1] The ROM in that study at 13 months was 8° to 58°, although the patients were satisfied. More implants will have to be done with a longer follow-up before this can be recommended as a first-line option.

J. Frankenhoff, MD

Reference

1. Couzens G, Hussain N, Gilpin D, Ross M. Pyrocarbon PIPJ and MCPJ hemiarthroplasty. *J Bone Joint Surg Br.* 2005;87-B:328.

Five- to 18-Year Follow-Up for Treatment of Trapeziometacarpal Osteoarthritis: A Prospective Comparison of Excision, Tendon Interposition, and Ligament Reconstruction and Tendon Interposition
Gangopadhyay S, McKenna H, Burke FD, et al (Nottingham Univ Hosps, UK; Royal Derby Hosp, Derby, UK)
J Hand Surg 37A:411-417, 2012

Purpose.—To investigate whether palmaris longus interposition or flexor carpi radialis ligament reconstruction and tendon interposition improve the outcome of trapezial excision for the treatment of basal joint arthritis after a minimum follow-up of 5 years.

Methods.—We randomized 174 thumbs with trapeziometacarpal osteoarthritis into 3 groups to undergo simple trapeziectomy, trapeziectomy with palmaris longus interposition, or trapeziectomy with ligament reconstruction and tendon interposition using 50% of the flexor carpi radialis tendon. A K-wire was passed across the trapezial void and retained for 4 weeks, and a thumb spica was used for 6 weeks in all 3 groups. We reviewed 153 thumbs after a minimum of 5 years (median, 6 y; range, 5−18 y) after surgery with subjective and objective assessments of thumb pain, function, and strength.

Results.—There was no difference in the pain relief achieved in the 3 treatment groups, with good results in 120 (78%) patients. Grip strength and key and tip pinch strengths did not differ among the 3 groups and range of movement of the thumb was similar. Few complications persisted after 5 years, and these were distributed evenly among the 3 groups. Compared with the results at 1 year in the same group of patients, the good pain relief achieved was maintained in the longer term, irrespective of the type of surgery. While improvements in grip strength achieved at 1 year after surgery were preserved, the key and tip pinch strengths deteriorated with time, but the type of surgery did not influence this.

Conclusions.—The outcomes of these 3 variations of trapeziectomy were similar after a minimum follow-up of 5 years. There appears to be no benefit to tendon interposition or ligament reconstruction in the longer term.

Type of Study/Level of Evidence.—Therapeutic I.

▶ This study by Gangopadhyay et al is a follow-up of their original article published in 2004 with a mean follow-up of 6 years. Their conclusions remain the same: There are no clinical differences between trapezial excision, palmaris longus interposition, or flexor carpi radialis ligament reconstruction and tendon interposition.

This is a well-done, powerful study that clearly demonstrates no difference between these 3 surgical procedures. The authors do point out, however, that they are not performing a simple trapeziectomy because they use a K-wire to distract the space for 4 weeks. Given the preponderance of evidence supporting the use of trapezial excision and K-wire distraction, I am going to start performing this procedure in favor of trapezial excision and ligament reconstruction.

Because the authors reexamined the same set of patients, they were able to compare mean 6-year results to mean 1-year results. Good pain relief was maintained, and hand strength was not different between groups at either follow-up period. I found it interesting that only 78% were considered good results; in my experience, rarely are patients not fully pleased with their results after carpometacarpal joint surgery.

A few weaknesses exist. It is unclear why the K-wire was removed at 4 weeks but the cast was removed at 6 weeks. Also, most patients had additional procedures performed, mainly to address metacarpophalangeal joint hyperextension, but the indications for the procedures changed during the study period. Hence, patients had different surgical procedures for similar clinical presentations. This confounding variable would become most notable at longer-term follow-up, as in this study.

L. W. Catalano III, MD

Results of a Method of 4-Corner Arthrodesis Using Headless Compression Screws

Ozyurekoglu T, Turker T (Univ of Louisville, KY)
J Hand Surg 37A:486-492, 2012

Purpose.—To evaluate the functional and radiographic results of a scaphoid excision and four-corner arthrodesis technique using percutaneous headless compression screws.

Methods.—A cohort of 33 patients, mean age 51 (range, 20—72) years, was treated for scapholunate advanced collapse (19), scaphoid nonunion advanced collapse (12), midcarpal instability (1), and Preiser disease (1). After scaphoid excision and removal of cartilage and subchondral bone in the midcarpal joint through a limited arthrotomy, capitolunate fixation was achieved with a percutaneous, transmetacarpal Acutrak screw (Acumed LLC, Hillsboro, OR), and triquetrohamate fixation was done with a percutaneous screw. Scaphoid was used as a bone graft. The average follow-up time was 8 months (n = 32; range, 6—64 mo).

Results.—Union occurred in 31 of 33 wrists (94%). One of the 33 patients had total wrist arthrodesis. Average total active flexion-extension arc was 71° after surgery and 83° before surgery. The postoperative carpal height averaged 0.47 compared to preoperative values of 0.45. The percentage of grip strength significantly improved from 41% before surgery to 80% after surgery. Postoperative mean verbal numerical rating scale pain score was less than 1, statistically better than the preoperative score of 7. Twenty-five of 33 patients were completely pain free. The average postoperative Mayo wrist score was 74, a significant improvement over the preoperative average of 40. Final Disabilities of the Arm, Shoulder, and Hand scores averaged 13 (n = 32; range, 0—49).

Conclusions.—These results were comparable to or better than the results of previously published techniques in terms of fusion rates, alleviation of pain, grip strength, range of motion; Mayo wrist score; and

Disabilities of the Arm, Shoulder, and Hand questionnaire score. The technique exploits the theoretical advantages of strong compression between carpals while avoiding a screw-head sized hole in the lunate articular cartilage and preserving the dorsal capsular ligament attachments to the triquetrum.

Type of Study/Level of Evidence.—Therapeutic IV.

▶ Although an interesting technique, many investigators have described four-bone fusion (FBF) using headless screws. The idea of placing the screws percutaneously is unique but increases the risk of cutaneous nerve injury and may make screw placement more difficult. The screw that is placed antegrade between the triquetrum and the hamate puts the dorsal cutaneous branch of the ulnar nerve at risk, and the authors report dissecting it out if present. The percutaneous idea is also unique in that there is already exposure of the midcarpal joint for the preparation of the fusion, and so extending this incision and performing the hardware placement through the traditional incision could be considered. One benefit of this technique the authors argue is that the capitolunate screw is placed retrograde and not antegrade, which avoids screw placement through the proximal articular surface of the lunate. However, the authors' technique does involve K-wire penetration through this lunate surface. Furthermore, the retrograde screw placement violates the third carpometacarpal joint, so another joint surface is violated with this technique. It is unclear what effect small violations of articular surfaces have or whether they lead to FBF failures, but in FBFs that degenerate at the radiolunate joint, there is no proof that the screw placement, if done antegrade, was not the reason. The triquetrum undoubtedly transmits less load than the lunate, but this technique does violate the triquetral proximal articular surface. Preservation of the dorsal radiocarpal ligament and lunotriquetral ligament for their role in proprioception is a weak argument by the authors because posterior interosseous nerve (PIN) excision is routinely performed in the traditional FBF, and even without PIN excision I have never heard of a Charcot wrist developing after FBF. Limited exposure to preserve blood supply because it may affect union (not argued by authors) may have some validity, but to maintain blood supply to the carpus (authors' point) is not a strong argument.

The most important technical aspects of FBF include reducing the lunate, carefully preparing the arthrodesis sites, placing solid fixation, and placing adequate and good-quality bone graft. The authors present an interesting technique that showed very good union rates as well as comparable outcomes to traditional FBF. However, the limited exposure of the midcarpal joint will compromise lunate reduction and possibly preparation of the arthrodesis. It is unclear to me why they would not also prepare the articular surfaces of the lunate and triquetrum, and the capitate and hamate, to ensure fusion. I would not recommend using the bone graft from the scaphoid alone because it is of a limited amount and not of the best quality. If this technique works for the authors and they are able to obtain union, they should continue to use the technique, but I do not think the benefits of the procedure outweigh the shortcomings and so would not recommend its use.

P. Tang, MD, MPH

3 Hand: Bone and Ligament

Fractures of the Fingers Missed or Misdiagnosed on Poorly Positioned or Poorly Taken Radiographs: A Retrospective Study
Tuncer S, Aksu N, Dilek H, et al (Istanbul Bilim Univ Med Faculty, Turkey; Florence Nightingale Hosp, Istanbul, Turkey)
J Trauma 71:649-655, 2011

Background.—Missed fractures, the most common diagnostic error in emergency departments, are usually the result of a misread radiograph or the failure to obtain a radiograph. However, a poorly positioned or poorly taken radiograph may also result in diagnostic errors. We sought to analyze the frequency of missed or misdiagnosed finger fractures that could be attributed to inadequate radiographs.

Methods.—We reviewed the medical records of the hand surgery divisions of Istanbul Bilim University Medical Faculty Hospital and the Orthopedics Department of Private Florence Nightingale Hospital between January 2008 and March 2010 for patients with fractures of the fingers that had been missed or misdiagnosed on the basis of inadequate radiographs.

Results.—In 182 patients, we identified 7 missed and 7 misdiagnosed fractures of the fingers because of inadequate radiographs. Lack of a true lateral radiographic view of the fingers or a true anteroposterior radiographic view of the thumb was the most frequent reason for diagnostic errors (71%; 10 of 14), leading to missed fractures in six patients and to misdiagnosed fractures in four patients. Superimposition of the fingers on lateral radiographs led to misjudging of displaced proximal phalangeal fractures of the fifth finger in three patients.

Conclusion.—Diagnostic errors attributed to inadequate radiographs are rare. Proper radiographic evaluation of finger trauma requires at least true anteroposterior and lateral views. An oblique view can complement the lateral view but not replace it. Poor quality radiographs or inadequate views should never be accepted or used as a basis for treatment.

▶ This article deals with missed or misdiagnosed fractures of the hand due to improper radiographs. Fourteen misdiagnosed fractures comprise 7.7% of a total of 182 patients in 2 tertiary referral centers. The most common error leading to a wrong diagnosis was the lack of a true lateral view. X-rays of proximal phalangeal fractures, especially of the little finger, were misleading due to super-imposition of fingers.

We are reminded of the importance of the very basic principle to obtain at least a true lateral and an anteroposterior view of proper quality when diagnosing frac-tures. Oblique views in addition to anteroposterior and lateral x-rays can be help-ful in revealing abnormalities and they also increase the confidence of the investigator.[1] Similarly, retrospective monitoring of x-ray readings can improve the standard of care.

Poor-quality radiographs should not be accepted. I do not hesitate to notify the responsible technician of improper x-rays and to ask him to repeat the study for better quality.

M. Choi, MD

Reference

1. De Smet AA, Doherty MP, Norris MA, Hollister MC, Smith DL. Are oblique views needed for trauma radiography of the distal extremities? *AJR Am J Roentgenol.* 1999;172:1561-1565.

Changes in Shape and Length of the Collateral and Accessory Collateral Ligaments of the Metacarpophalangeal Joint During Flexion
Kataoka T, Moritomo H, Miyake J, et al (Osaka Univ, Japan)
J Bone Joint Surg Am 93:1318-1325, 2011

Background.—Although the collateral and accessory collateral ligaments of the metacarpophalangeal joint contribute to the stability of this joint, the functional role of the various portions of these ligaments during flexion is unclear. We investigated changes in the three-dimensional shape and length of the collateral and accessory collateral ligaments during flexion to deter-mine how each portion stabilized the metacarpophalangeal joint.

Methods.—Twelve fingers from three embalmed cadavers were exam-ined. The origin and the insertion point of the dorsal, middle, and volar portions of the radial and the ulnar collateral ligament and of the radial and the ulnar accessory collateral ligament were precisely identified. Micro-computed tomograms were obtained at 10° intervals during passive flexion from 0° to 80°. We created three-dimensional models of the metacarpal, the proximal phalange, and the paths of the twelve ligament portions. Finally, we calculated the change in the shape and length of the path of each liga-ment portion during flexion.

Results.—The region of contact between each collateral ligament and the lateral edge of the metacarpal gradually lengthened during flexion of the joint, and the ligament gradually stretched to pass around the convex radial or ulnar surface of the metacarpal head. In contrast, each accessory collat-eral ligament curved around the volar tubercle of the metacarpal head at all flexion angles. The length of the volar portion of each collateral ligament and the length of the dorsal and middle portions of each accessory collateral ligament underwent little change during flexion. However, the lengths of the dorsal and middle portions of each collateral ligament increased significantly during flexion, and the length of the volar portion of each accessory collateral ligament decreased significantly.

Conclusions.—The collateral and accessory collateral ligaments can each be functionally divided into three portions—dorsal, middle, and volar. The volar portion of each collateral ligament and the dorsal and middle portions of each accessory collateral ligament are nearly isometric, the dorsal and middle portions of each collateral ligament become taut only in flexion, and the volar portion of each accessory collateral ligament becomes taut only in extension.

▶ This is a detailed description of the anatomy of the finger metacarpophalangeal (MCP) joint collateral and accessory collateral ligaments focusing on changes during motion. The conventional wisdom has been that the collateral ligaments are major stabilizers of the MCP joint and that they are relatively straightforward structures—tightening in flexion and relaxing in extension as they curve around the tubercle of the metacarpal head. The findings of this study disprove much of the conventional wisdom and have implications for clinical treatment of a number of pathologies, although rare.

First the authors found that components of both the collateral and accessory collaterals behaved in a nearly isometric manner. Further, these isometric fibers originated dorsal to the center of curvature of the metacarpal head. Second, the accessory collateral ligaments appear to play a much larger role in MCP stability than previously described. Third, while the volar components of the collateral ligaments are actually tight in extension, they do not limit motion in the abduction/adduction plane because it originates more distally, and the collateral does not have to curve around the MC head. Further, the contact areas of the MCP joint appeared to increase in flexion, adding to stability.

While this is a study with a novel technique, if these findings are corroborated, they have implications for repair and reconstruction of the MCP ligaments and for pathologies that lead to volar subluxation of the MCP joints, such as rheumatoid arthritis and systemic lupus erythematous.

P. Blazar, MD

The Stabilizing Effect of the Distal Interosseous Membrane on the Distal Radioulnar Joint in an Ulnar Shortening Procedure: A Biomechanical Study
Arimitsu S, Moritomo H, Kitamura T, et al (Mayo Clinic, Rochester, MN)
J Bone Joint Surg Am 93:2022-2030, 2011

Background.—The importance of the stabilizing effect of the distal interosseous membrane on the distal radioulnar joint, especially in patients with a distal oblique bundle, has been described. The purpose of this study was to evaluate the stability of the distal radioulnar joint after an ulnar shortening osteotomy and to quantify longitudinal resistance to ulnar shortening when the osteotomy was proximal or distal to the ulnar attachment of the distal interosseous membrane. These relationships were characterized for forearms with or without a distal oblique bundle.

Methods.—Ten fresh-frozen cadavers were used. A transverse osteotomy and ulnar shortening was performed proximal (proximal shortening) and distal (distal shortening) to the ulnar attachment of the distal interosseous membrane. Distal radioulnar joint laxity was evaluated as the volar and dorsal displacements of the radius relative to the fixed ulna with 20 N of applied force. Testing was performed under controlled 1-mm increments of ulnar shortening up to 4 mm, with the forearm in neutral alignment, 60° of pronation, and 60° of supination. Resistance to ulnar shortening was quantified as the slope of the load-displacement curve obtained by displacing the distal ulnar segment proximally.

Results.—In proximal shortening, significantly greater stability of the distal radioulnar joint was obtained with even 1 mm of shortening compared with the control, whereas distal shortening demonstrated significant improvement in stability of the distal radioulnar joint only after shortening of ≥4 mm in all rotational positions. Significantly greater stability of the distal radioulnar joint was achieved with proximal shortening than with distal shortening and in specimens with a distal oblique bundle than in those without a distal oblique bundle. The longitudinal resistance to ulnar shortening was significantly greater in proximal shortening than in distal shortening. The stiffness in proximal shortening was not affected by the presence of a distal oblique bundle in the distal interosseous membrane.

Conclusions.—Ulnar shortening with the osteotomy carried out proximal to the attachment of the distal interosseous membrane had a more favorable effect on stability of the distal radioulnar joint compared with distal osteotomy, especially in the presence of a distal oblique bundle.

▶ This article describes a cadaveric study examining distal radioulnar joint (DRUJ) stability following ulnar shortening osteotomy and quantifying longitudinal resistance to ulnar shortening in reference to the ulnar attachment of the distal interosseous membrane. The authors reported that all specimens had a distal portion of interosseous membrane distal to the central and accessory band at an average of 59 mm from the distal ulna. Shortening the ulna proximal to this band yielded greater DRUJ stability than an osteotomy placed distal to it. Furthermore, specimens with a distinct distal oblique bundle within the distal interosseous membrane had greater DRUJ stability and thicker oblique bundles demonstrated by increased resistance to shortening.

This is a well-designed study that helps surgeons determine the optimal position for an ulnar shortening osteotomy: A more proximal position is indeed desired if attempting to improve DRUJ stability. As with most cadaveric studies, however, clinical correlation is required before definitive conclusions can be drawn.

T. D. Rozental, MD

4 Hand: Carpal Tunnel Syndrome

The Sensitivity and Specificity of Ultrasound for the Diagnosis of Carpal Tunnel Syndrome: A Meta-Analysis
Fowler JR, Gaughan JP, Ilyas AM (Temple Univ Hosp, Philadelphia, PA; Temple Univ School of Medicine, Philadelphia, PA)
Clin Orthop Relat Res 469:1089-1094, 2011

Background.—Carpal tunnel syndrome (CTS) is the most commonly diagnosed compression neuropathy of the upper extremity. Current AAOS recommendations are to obtain a confirmatory electrodiagnostic test in patients for whom surgery is being considered. Ultrasound has emerged as an alternative confirmatory test for CTS; however, its potential role is limited by lack of adequate data for sensitivity and specificity relative to electrodiagnostic testing.

Questions/Purposes.—In this meta-analysis we determined the sensitivity and specificity of ultrasound in the diagnosis of CTS.

Methods.—A PubMed/MEDLINE search identified 323 articles for review. After applying exclusion criteria, 19 articles with a total sample size of 3131 wrists were included for meta-analysis. Three groups were created: a composite of all studies, studies using clinical diagnosis as the reference standard, and studies using electrodiagnostic testing as the reference standard.

Results.—The composite sensitivity and specificity of ultrasound for the diagnosis of CTS, using all studies, were 77.6% (95% CI 71.6–83.6%) and 86.8% (95% CI 78.9–94.8%), respectively.

Conclusions.—The wide variations of sensitivities and specificities reported in the literature have prevented meaningful analysis of ultrasound as either a screening or confirmatory tool in the diagnosis of CTS. The sensitivity and specificity of ultrasound in the diagnosis of CTS are 77.6% and 86.8%, respectively. Although ultrasound may not replace electrodiagnostic testing as the most sensitive and specific test for the diagnosis of CTS given the values reported in this meta-analysis, it may be a feasible alternative to electrodiagnostic testing as the first-line confirmatory test.

Level of Evidence.—Level III, systematic review of Level III studies. See Guidelines for Authors for a complete description of levels of evidence.

▶ This meta-analysis investigated the usefulness of ultrasound for the diagnosis of carpal tunnel syndrome (CTS). The composite pooled sensitivity was

77.6% and the specificity 86.8%. The most sensitive and specific sonographic finding in CTS patients is the cross-sectional area of the median nerve at the inlet of the carpal tunnel.

Currently, the gold standard for the diagnosis of CTS is still under discussion. Electrodiagnosis (EDX) is frequently considered a confirmatory test for diagnosis, and many surgeons rely on clinical diagnosis alone. In the authors' opinion, sonography is more advantageous than EDX because they find the latter to be painful, time-consuming, and more expensive. I agree with the authors that EDX is more painful, and I also consider this a major disadvantage. Concerning the duration of the investigation, an ultrasound scan can also be time-consuming. I cannot agree with the cost argument, because at my hospital, EDX is less expensive than sonography. Both diagnostic tools have in common that they are operator-dependent.

More evidence is needed to evaluate the usefulness of ultrasound for the diagnosis of CTS. In my practice, CTS is diagnosed primarily on a clinical basis. Nevertheless, I seek to confirm the diagnosis by EDX. Ultrasound may be able to solve questions with patients who are clinically diagnosed as CTS but test negatively on EDX.

M. Choi, MD

Determinants of Return to Work After Carpal Tunnel Release
Cowan J, Makanji H, Mudgal C, et al (Massachusetts General Hosp, Boston)
J Hand Surg 37A:18-27, 2012

Purpose.—The determinants of time to return to work—a common measure of treatment effectiveness—are incompletely defined. Our primary hypothesis was that employment circumstances are the strongest determinant of earlier return to work. Our secondary hypothesis was that return to work in patients with desk-based jobs is predicted by patient expectations and other psychosocial factors.

Methods.—We enrolled 65 employed patients with limited incision open carpal tunnel release in a prospective cohort study. Patients completed validated measures of depression, coping strategies, pain anxiety, and job burnout. Heavy lifting was not allowed for 1 month after surgery. Return to modified and full work duty was recorded in days. Although not specifically an exclusion criterion, none of the patients had a workers' compensation claim or other source of secondary gain.

Results.—Patients returned to modified duty an average of 11.8 days and full duty at an average of 18.9 days after surgery. Predictors of earlier return to modified duty in multivariate analyses included desk-based work and both the number of days patients expected to take off and the numbers of days they wanted to take off for the entire cohort, with an additional influence from catastrophic thinking in desk-based workers. Predictors of earlier return to full duty in multivariate analyses included desk-based work and number of days patients expected to take off before for the entire cohort, fewer days off desired in non—desk-based workers, fewer days off desired and change in work role in desk-based workers, and lower pain anxiety in part-time workers.

Conclusions.—The most important determinant of return to full duty work after limited incision open carpal tunnel release is job type, but psychological factors such as patient expectations, catastrophic thinking, and anxiety in response to pain also have a role.

Type of Study/Level of Evidence.—Prognostic II.

► This study evaluates the multifactorial nature of a patient's ability to return to work. The authors state that the most important determinant of return to work after a limited incision open carpal tunnel release is job type, but psychological factors such as patient expectations, catastrophic thinking, and anxiety in response to pain also play a role. This study has several strengths. The authors used a prospective design and validated outcome measures. They also used a broad model to assess the potential contributing factors for return to work. The intervention was standardized and the data were collected by an independent observer. Although they had a small sample size, the study was adequately powered. There may be a component of selection bias in this cohort because the patients included reflect only a small subgroup of carpal tunnel patients, and there were also a significant number of patients lost to follow-up (28%). Another potential weakness is that this study is prone to hazards of multiple comparisons; however, the authors focus on the primary study question and clearly state that the other findings represent hypothesis-generating findings only.

Return to work is an endpoint often used in studies that try to advocate for one treatment's superiority over another. However, in my experience, patients in similar occupations undergoing similar operations do not all predictably return to work after the same amount of time. Although some are able to return after a few days, others need a few months before they are ready, without any objective factors to account for this. Factors outside the surgical intervention play a role and must be taken into consideration. Future studies using return to work as an outcome measure should control for job type and also recognize that psychological factors such as patient expectations, catastrophic thinking, and anxiety can play a role.

R. Grewal, MD

Duration of Postoperative Dressing After Mini-Open Carpal Tunnel Release: A Prospective, Randomized Trial
Ritting AW, Leger R, O'Malley MP, et al (Univ of Connecticut, Farmington)
J Hand Surg 37A:3-8, 2012

Purpose.—In this prospective, randomized, controlled study, we hypothesized that there would be no difference in short-term functional, subjective, and blinded wound outcome measures between patients treated after mini-open carpal tunnel release (CTR) with a postoperative bulky dressing for 2 weeks and those with dressing removal and placement of an adhesive strip after 48 to 72 hours.

Methods.—A total of 94 consecutive patients underwent mini-open CTR and placement of a bulky dressing and were randomized to either bandage removal at 48 to 72 hours with placement of an adhesive strip or continuation of the postoperative dressing until initial follow-up at approximately 2 weeks. We evaluated patient demographics, Levine-Katz scores, range of motion, strength, and a blinded assessment of wound healing at approximately 2 weeks and between 6 and 12 weeks. We conducted paired and independent sample *t*-tests to evaluate for statistical significance.

Results.—There was no significant difference in Levine-Katz scores between groups at either the first follow-up or final visit. One patient with a longer dressing duration had evidence of a wound dehiscence.

Conclusions.—Removal of a bulky dressing after mini-open CTR and replacement with an adhesive strip at 48 to 72 hours causes no wound complications and results in equal short-term clinical and subjective outcome measures compared with using a bulky dressing for 2 weeks.

Type of Study/Level of Evidence.—Therapeutic I.

▶ This simple study showed no difference in wound healing with a less-restrictive dressing. While it shows that quite well, it is unclear that wound healing is a truly valuable outcome to measure, as wound healing complications are not typically associated with carpal tunnel release, especially with a limited incision technique.

Most importantly, they failed to assess patient satisfaction with the dressing or the dressing's restriction of activities or return to work. This is the obvious reason a surgeon might offer a less-restrictive dressing, and there are no data in this study to suggest it leads to improved patient function (which it might not) or improved patient satisfaction (which it likely would). This significantly limits the study's value.

Despite these criticisms, I reviewed this article prior to publication and, as I use the same technique as the authors, I began having my patients remove their soft, bulky dressing on postoperative day 2 or 3 and apply an adhesive bandage strip. Additionally, I now allow patients to wash the hand at that time. The addition of washing was based on small groups of noncompliant patients over 10 years using this surgical technique that had admitted to washing their hand without apparent negative effects.

Anecdotally, I have noted a significant improvement in patient satisfaction since I have made this change. I have not had significant wound complications, although I have noted the incisions look "different" with a greater percentage of macerated wounds. Resultantly, I have instructed patients to dry the wounds well prior to applying the bandage strip and to change the strip often. It is important to note the difference between the level-1 evidence presented in the article (which does not support hand washing) and the anecdotal experience I have presented.

T. Hughes, MD

Diagnosis of Cubital Tunnel Syndrome
Hutchison RL, Rayan G (INTEGRIS Baptist Med Ctr, Oklahoma City, OK)
J Hand Surg 36A:1519-1521, 2011

Background.—The diagnosis of cubital tunnel syndrome (CubTS) has depended on a combination of patient history, physical findings, specific provocative maneuvers, and electrophysiologic tests, although some clinicians choose to consider the clinical examination only and others wait for confirmation through electrodiagnostic testing. The most reliable way to confirm the diagnosis of CubTS was evaluated.

> *Case Study.*—Man, 51, complained of intermittent numbness or tingling of the ring and small fingers of the nondominant hand lasting 1 year. Occasionally this anesthesiologist also suffered medial elbow pain radiating to the ulnar side of the hand. Symptoms worsen with activity and have been increasing gradually in frequency and severity, but he has no upper extremity injury or systemic disease. Physical examination shows tenderness in the retrocondylar groove with no ulnar nerve instability, diminished light touch in the ulnar two digits, and weakness of the ulnar innervated intrinsic muscles without atrophy. The clinician believes the symptoms are characteristic of CubTS.

Analysis of Evidence.—Risk factors for ulnar neuropathy at the cubital tunnel may include remote history of elbow fractures, fall with direct trauma to the medial elbow, habitually placing the elbow on a hard surface, repetitive elbow flexion, and systemic disease. Symptoms ascribed to CubTS include activity-induced and nocturnal paresthesias, constant sensory dysfunction in the small and ring fingers, pain in the medial elbow that radiates to the hand, handgrip weakness, and clumsiness. Neither the risk factors nor the symptoms are supported by evidence.

Among the provocative measures used to confirm a CubTS diagnosis are a positive percussion test (Tinel's sign), an elbow flexion test with or without wrist extension and shoulder abduction, elbow flexion combined with direct pressure, and the scratch collapse test. Positive responses to these maneuvers are associated with varying sensitivity, specificity, and positive and negative predictive values, but most are inadequate or inconsistent in sensitivity and specificity.

Nerve conduction studies assess the function of the larger, myelinated, faster-conducting nerve fibers. Commonly used criteria for abnormal conduction at the elbow include conduction velocity less than 50 m/sec, a 10-m/sec difference from the contralateral side, or a 20% reduction in amplitude compared with the contralateral side. Imaging studies include radiographs, magnetic resonance imaging (MRI) scans, and ultrasound. No studies support the use of radiographs or MRI scans to diagnose CubTS, and limited data support the use of ultrasound.

Conclusions.—Because of the difficulties with available measures, it is more accurate to discuss probabilities of CubTS rather than state with absolute certainty the presence or lack of disease. For the patient in question, if percussion and elbow flexion tests are positive with no sign of nerve compression at another level, CubTS would be highly probable. If nonsurgical treatment (anti-inflammatory medications and nocturnal splinting) for 4 weeks does not relieve symptoms, surgical interventions may be needed. Unless there are masses or elbow abnormalities, radiographs, MRIs, and ultrasound will not be needed.

▶ The authors analyze the currently available evidence for the diagnosis of cubital tunnel syndrome. This subject is of significant interest to hand surgeons because it is a relatively common condition for which the best diagnostic and treatment modalities are continually debated. At the outset, they note that some practitioners will rely on electrodiagnostic testing to set the diagnosis, while others will not. Risk factors for the condition have been speculated but not confirmed. One particular risk factor, subluxation of the nerve, is thought by some to predispose to the condition. However, the authors note that in at least 2 studies in adults and 1 in children, there was a small but definite percentage of asymptomatic patients that have subluxing ulnar nerves at the elbow.

When discussing provocative tests, the chief ones analyzed are the percussion (Tinel) test, the elbow flexion test, and the scratch-collapse test. One of the authors (Rayan) conducted a prior study of normal volunteers and documented positive percussion and elbow flexion tests in 10% and 23%, respectively. The authors cite several studies about each of these tests, and the sensitivity, specificity, and positive and negative predictive values are all listed and are all what one would consider reasonable for a noninvasive test. However, the problem with all of these modalities listed is that there is no single true gold standard diagnostic test for cubital tunnel syndrome by which to conclusively compare any other diagnostic tests, including provocative maneuvers.

Electrodiagnostic testing is, as the authors note, commonly relied on to establish the diagnosis of cubital tunnel syndrome. The common criterion used for diagnosis is conduction velocity less than 50 m/sec, a 10-m/sec difference in velocity when compared with the other side, or a 20% amplitude reduction when compared with the other side. While it is tempting to think of electrodiagnostic testing as the gold standard for this condition, the authors note that in certain cases of cubital tunnel syndrome, the nerve conduction study can be normal.

Imaging tests have been analyzed for cubital tunnel syndrome, specifically, magnetic resonance imaging and ultrasound scan. While these tests can detect space-occupying lesions in the cubital tunnel, their utility in diagnosing the condition is still being tested.

In their summary, the authors rightly point out that there is no gold standard for diagnosis of cubital tunnel syndrome; therefore, in their words, "we can only discuss probabilities rather than certainties of disease." In their estimation, improvement in the diagnosis of this condition will come with large-scale epidemiologic studies and development of clinical prediction rules that incorporate multiple diagnostic modalities to establish the probability of cubital tunnel syndrome.

J. Freidrich, MD

5 Hand: Congenital Differences

The Apert Hand—Angiographic Planning of a Single-Stage, 5-Digit Release for All Classes Of Deformity
Harvey I, Brown S, Ayres O, et al (Women's and Children's Hosp, North Adelaide, South Australia)
J Hand Surg 37A:152-158, 2012

Purpose.—To demonstrate the utility of computed tomography angiographic planning of a single-stage, complete release of syndactyly in Apert syndrome.

Methods.—Computed tomography angiograms were performed as a preoperative planning tool in 6 patients. Five came to surgery. All had a single-stage operation for complete release of their syndactyly.

Results.—Five patients, ranging from Upton type 1 to type 3 Apert hand deformities, have had preoperative computed tomography angiography that delineated the vascular anatomy. This allowed planning and execution of a single-stage syndactyly release in all patients. The preoperative imaging identified noteworthy abnormalities in vascular anatomy that were incorporated into surgical planning.

Conclusions.—The protocol presented allows preoperative planning and single-stage operation for complete release of syndactyly in patients with Apert syndrome (Fig 4).

▶ The authors present a means and rationale to perform 1-stage digit separation for Apert's complex syndactyly, which often lacks terminal branches of digital arteries in concert with distal synostoses. The computed tomography (CT) angiography sufficiently showed the anatomy in 5 patients who underwent surgery and retrospectively proved useful to the surgical planning and execution. The CT angiogram requires at least sedation if not anesthesia (not detailed), but it is performed at the same time as craniofacial planning. This 1-stage hand release arguably cuts down on anesthesia and postoperative care as well as patient and family travel. The authors did not comment on whether they successfully created 5 digits in each of these hands, whether they required osteotomy for the thumb clinodactyly, the duration of procedures, or whether the tourniquet was used.

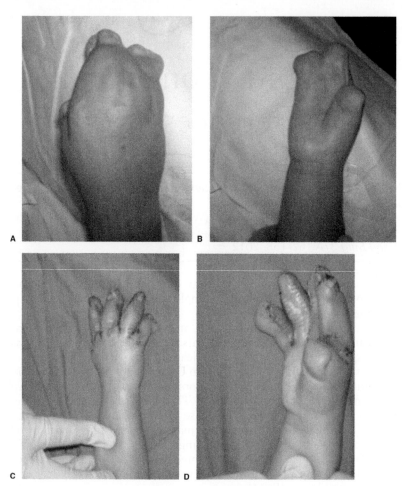

FIGURE 4.—A 5-digit hand created in a single-stage operation. **A, B** Preoperative views. **C, D** Early postoperative views. (Reprinted from Harvey I, Brown S, Ayres O, et al. The apert hand—angiographic planning of a single-stage, 5-digit release for all classes of deformity. *J Hand Surg.* 2012;37:152-158, Copyright 2012, with permission from the American Society for Surgery of the Hand.)

Treatment of the Apert's hand is relatively rare and is typically performed at a center that has a craniofacial program, and those of us who perform these unanimously agree that the hand surgery is tedious and challenging. The most common procedure I perform for Apert's children is bilateral release of 2 web spaces with full-thickness grafting under 1 anesthetic, with 2 surgeons (myself and resident or fellow). Typically 4 to 6 months later I'll proceed with thumb osteotomy and the remaining 2 webs, if the hand accommodates release of 4 fingers. Each procedure takes several hours, requires large full-thickness grafts, suturing in tight places that requires the surgeon to practically stand on his or her head, and it is utterly exhausting. Although the authors' 1-stage procedure cuts the procedural events requiring anesthesia almost in half, the total duration of anesthesia and the comorbidities are unclear. Whether these represent true advantages over staged procedures is also unknown. The mere thought of such a day is exhausting but worthy of consideration (Fig 4).

A. Ladd, MD

6 Hand: Microsurgery and Flaps

A Systematic Review of the Outcomes of Replantation of Distal Digital Amputation
Sebastin SJ, Chung KC (Natl Univ Health System, Singapore; Univ of Michigan Health System, Ann Arbor)
Plast Reconstr Surg 128:723-737, 2011

Background.—The aim of this study was to conduct a systematic review of the English literature on replantation of distal digital amputations to provide the best evidence of survival rates and functional outcomes.

Methods.—A MEDLINE search using "digit," "finger," "thumb," and "replantation" as keywords and limited to humans and English-language articles identified 1297 studies. Studies were included in the review if they (1) present primary data, (2) report five or more single or multiple distal replantations, and (3) present survival rates. Additional data extracted from the studies meeting the inclusion criteria included demographic information, nature and level of amputation, venous outflow technique, nerve repair, recovery of sensibility, range of motion, return to work, and complications.

Results.—Thirty studies representing 2273 distal replantations met the inclusion criteria. The mean survival rate was 86 percent. There was no difference in survival between zone I and zone II replantations (Tamai classification). There was a significant difference in survival between replantation of clean-cut versus the more crushed amputations (crush-cut and crush-avulsion). The repair of a vein improved survival in both zone I and zone II replantation. The mean two-point discrimination was 7 mm ($n = 220$), and 98 percent returned to work ($n = 98$). Complications included pulp atrophy in 14 percent of patients ($n = 639$) and nail deformity in 23 percent ($n = 653$).

Conclusions.—The common perception that distal replantation is associated with little functional gain is not based on scientific evidence. This systematic review showed a high success rate and good functional outcomes following distal digital replantation (Figs 1 and 4).

▶ This article addresses the controversial issue of whether a Tamai Zone 1 and 2 (Fig 1) distal amputation should be replanted. The topic remains controversial, because there are strong opposing views despite the lack of robust studies

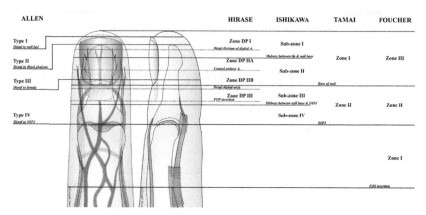

FIGURE 1.—Drawing showing the anatomy of the finger in relation to the Hirase, Ishikawa, Tamai, Foucher, and the commonly used Allen classification of fingertip amputations. *DIPJ*, distal interphalangeal joint; *FDP*, flexor digitorum profundus; *FDS*, flexor digitorum superficialis. (Reprinted from Sebastin SJ, Chung KC. A systematic review of the outcomes of replantation of distal digital amputation. *Plast Reconstr Surg*. 2011;128:723-737, with permission from the American Society of Plastic Surgeons.)

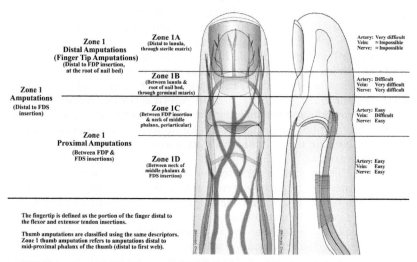

FIGURE 4.—A new classification system for digital amputations distal to the flexor digitorum super-ficialis insertion. *FDP*, flexor digitorum profundus; *FDS*, flexor digitorum superficialis. (Reprinted from Sebastin SJ, Chung KC. A systematic review of the outcomes of replantation of distal digital amputation. *Plast Reconstr Surg*. 2011;128:723-737, with permission from the American Society of Plastic Surgeons.)

comparing the 2 options of replantation versus revision amputation. As shown by the geographic distribution of published work on this area, the practice of distal replantation is done more frequently, and looked on more favorably, in Asia than other regions. A variety of reasons, including physical appearance, maintaining physical integrity, and Confucian moral values, have been cited for the wider practice of replantation in these countries.

In the absence of randomized trials, this work provides a substantial contribution to the scientific literature surrounding this topic. Contrary to commonly held beliefs, their findings show that such surgery can have success rates comparable to more proximal amputations. They also found that patients with replanted digits had a high rate of return to work, as well as good sensibility in the reattached part. A new classification of such amputations to allow better comparison of outcomes was proposed (Fig 4). The authors make a case to develop specialty centers in the United States to do such surgeries.

The limitations of this work include a tendency toward better results because of publication bias and the lack of outcomes information in many of the original studies. As the authors have discussed, more work is required to critically compare the functional, psychological, and economic analysis of revision amputation and distal replantation.

This work bears evidence that replantation in these forms of amputations should be considered where possible.

A. Chong, MD

A Prospective Cohort Study of Fibula Free Flap Donor-Site Morbidity in 157 Consecutive Patients

Momoh AO, Yu P, Skoracki RJ, et al (Univ of Texas M. D. Anderson Cancer Ctr, Houston)
Plast Reconstr Surg 128:714-720, 2011

Background.—Although the fibula free flap is preferred for bony head and neck reconstruction, donor-site morbidity remains a concern. The authors goal was to evaluate potential risk factors for complications and whether the type of wound closure and timing of postoperative ambulation had an effect on the development of short- and long-term morbidities.

Methods.—A prospective cohort study of donor-site morbidity was performed in 157 consecutive patients who underwent fibula free flap reconstruction for head and neck defects.

Results.—Perioperative donor-site complications occurred in 31.2 percent of patients, including skin graft loss (15 percent), cellulitis (10 percent), wound dehiscence (8 percent), and abscess (1 percent). Preoperative chemotherapy ($p = 0.02$) was associated with increased complications. No significant difference in complication rates was observed between primary and skin graft wound closure ($p = 0.59$). The timing of ambulation was not related to the development of complications ($p = 0.41$). Long-term morbidities occurred in 17 percent of patients and included leg weakness (8 percent), ankle instability (4 percent), great toe contracture (9 percent), and decreased ankle mobility (12 percent). The occurrence of perioperative complications, flap type, and closure technique were not significantly associated with long-term morbidities. Functionally, 96 percent of patients returned to their preoperative level of ambulatory activity. Decreases in ambulatory status could all be ascribed to causes other than donor-site morbidity.

TABLE 4.—Long-Term Morbidity in Patients Undergoing Fibula Free Flap Reconstruction
($n = 157$)

Morbidity	No. of Patients (%)*
Leg weakness	12 (8)
Ankle instability	6 (4)
Great toe flexion contracture	14 (9)
Decreased ankle range of motion	3 (2)
Total	26 (17)

*Seven patients experienced more than one long-term morbidity.

Conclusion.—Fibula free flap harvest is associated with a high rate of complications, but the majority of patients have no long-term functional limitations (Table 4).

▶ Although this retrospective analysis focuses on patients who have undergone head/neck cancer reconstruction, the information is important to any upper extremity surgeon who uses free fibula transfers for skeletal reconstruction. Donor site morbidity is a significant concern to patients and their families. This study benefits from the large number of patients included, a large volume reconstructive service, and, what appears to be overall very good follow-up. Similar to other studies on the topic, there are a fair number of donor site complications (dehiscence, infection, and so forth), although the number of significant long-term problems is quite small and fairly subjective. As outlined in Table 4, 17% of patients had long-term (> 1 month) complications, which ranged from weakness to sensation of ankle instability. However, no patients had donor site—related changes causing a decrease from preoperative ambulatory status. Of note, taking a skin paddle with the bone graft did not increase complications, and the authors note that the decision to use skin graft verses primary closure should be made according to the surgeon's subjective intraoperative discretion. The article supports the philosophy that the trade-off of using a free fibula graft for reconstruction is not risk free but that the risks seem acceptable. This is valuable information that will help us counsel patients regarding their treatment options.

J. Isaacs, MD

Vascular complications and microvascular free flap salvage: the role of thrombolytic agents

Chang EI, Mehrara BJ, Festekjian JH, et al (UCLA Med Ctr; Memorial Sloan-Kettering Cancer Ctr, NY)
Microsurgery 31:505-509, 2011

Background.—Vascular thrombosis with flap loss is the most dreaded complication of microvascular free tissue transfer. Thrombolytic agents such as tissue plasminogen activator have been used clinically for free flap salvage in cases of pedicle thrombosis. Yet, there is a paucity of data in the literature validating the benefit of their use.

Methods.—A retrospective review of the breast reconstruction free flap database was performed at a single institution between the years of 1991–2010. The incidence of vascular complications (arterial and/or venous thrombosis) was examined to determine the role of adjuvant thrombolytic therapy in flap salvage. Pathologic examination was used to determine the incidence of fat necrosis after secondary revision procedures.

Results.—Seventy-four cases were identified during the study period. In 41 cases, revision of the anastamoses was performed alone without thrombolytics with 38 cases of successful flap salvage (92.7%). In 33 cases, anastamotic revision was performed with adjuvant thrombolytic therapy, and successful flap salvage occurred in 28of these cases (84.8%). Thrombolysis did not appear to significantly affect flap salvage. Interestingly, only two of the salvaged flaps that had received thrombolysis developed fat necrosis, whereas 11 of the nonthrombolysed flaps developed some amount fat necrosis (7.1% vs. 28.9%, $P < 0.05$).

Conclusions.—The decreased incidence of fat necrosis may be attributable to dissolution of thrombi in the microvasculature with the administration of thrombolytics. Although the use of adjuvant thrombolytic therapy does not appear to impact the rate of flap salvage, their use may have secondary benefits on overall flap outcomes.

▶ Although this article discusses breast reconstruction, it is a fascinating topic to any upper extremity flap surgeon who has experienced a failed free vascularized tissue transfer. The idea that a magic bullet (in this case, thrombolytics) could save a dying flap is obviously exciting. Alas, based on a retrospective review, Chang et al have not really discovered a miracle cure. All of their salvaged flaps required revision of the anastomosis, and they were unable to demonstrate an increased salvage rate when thrombolytics were added to the treatment. Of course, the study was not randomized, so a true evaluation of the effects of the thrombolytics is not possible. In fact, the flaps they used the thrombolytics on seemed to be in worse condition (eg, clot progressing into the flap) than the ones they did not use thrombolytics on. A better test of the thrombolytics would be to randomly assign thrombolytic treatment, regardless of clot propagation. The authors did think that they had less fat necrosis (an indirect measurement of presumed ischemic tissue damage) in the thrombolytic group (although their method of quantifying this was a little vague), suggesting that even when clot propagation was not noted, it may have been present in the microcirculation, which would only be treated in the thrombolytic group. In expanding this observation, the authors point out several theoretical benefits to thrombolytics, including a potential prophylactic effect on rethrombosis. Still, the article leaves many unanswered questions, such as what role Fogarty catheter embolectomy may play, or, as I would be concerned about, the increased risk of bleeding associated with giving thrombolytics to what is basically a large raw tissue surface (the thrombolytics were not given systemically but were "flushed" through the flaps and leaked out the venous system). For my part, I will add thrombolytics to my armamentarium for dealing with thrombosed vessels in flap surgery, although their role, despite this retrospective review, has clearly not yet been defined.

J. Isaacs, MD

Long-term results of finger reconstruction with microvascular toe transfers after trauma

Kotkansalo T, Vilkki S, Elo P (Turku Univ Hosp, Finland; Tampere Univ Hosp, Finland; Med Imaging Centre, Tampere, Finland)
J Plast Reconstr Aesthet Surg 64:1291-1299, 2011

Amputation of all or most of the fingers severely disturbs the gripping function of the hand. The purpose of this study was to evaluate the long-term functional results of finger-amputation patients rehabilitated with microvascular toe transfers.

Fifteen such patients (10 males, median age at injury 26 years (range 5–49 years)) were examined after a median follow-up of 18 years. Eight patients had no fingers spared by the initial trauma and the rest had at least two fingers amputated. The function of the hand was accessed subjectively (questionnaires) and objectively (tests). Further, physical parameters were measured and compared to the other healthy hand.

Patients scored consistently well in the test measuring function (the Sollerman hand function test and the modified Tamai score). Activities of daily living presented on average minor difficulties. Patients regained on average 42% of grip and 84% of key pinch strength compared to the other hand. The average movement of the transfer was 28°. One transfer was lost due to inability to restore permanent circulation. In addition, there were one donor and one recipient site superficial infections.

We conclude that microvascular toe transfer is a reliable way to improve gripping function after amputation of fingers. Patient approval is generally good and the achieved function satisfactory. Two toe transfers should be considered for patients with no fingers left. Work-related injury may be related to decreased occupational capability.

▶ The authors report their long-term results of toe to finger transplantation. Fifteen patients with amputation of 2 or more fingers were included. Similar to previous work by the same team regarding toe to thumb transfers, toe to metacarpal hand, and toe to forearm transfers, hand function was assessed both subjectively and objectively. Three tests—the Sollerman hand function test, the modified Tamai score, and a test designed by the authors based on activities of daily living—were used in combination. The points for all 3 test were used as a sum with the limit for good results set at higher than 172. Details for this decision are not given. None of the patients with a single toe transfer obtained good results in this study. Patients scoring higher than 172 were those who received 2 toe transfers.

Interestingly, all patients of this series went back to work. Five of the patients had moderate arthritis, and 5 had osteopenia on radiographic evaluation. All except 1 were satisfied with the overall result. Average active range of motion was 28°, which is less than reports by Wei et al (51°), Cosunfirat et al (39°), and Foucher and Moss (33°).[1-3]

Toe to finger transfer is a reliable procedure and improves hand function. In view of the authors' results, transfer of 2 toes or double toe transfer may be preferred over a single toe transfer.

M. Choi, MD

References

1. Wei FC, Chen HC, Chuang CC, Noordhoff MS. Simultaneous multiple toe transfers in hand reconstruction. *Plast Reconstr Surg.* 1988;81:366-377.
2. Coskunfirat OK, Wei FC, Lin CH, Chen HC, Lin YT. Simultaneous double second toe transfer for reconstruction of adjacent fingers. *Plast Reconstr Surg.* 2005;115:1064-1069.
3. Foucher G, Moss AL. Microvascular second toe to finger transfer: a statistical analysis of 55 transfers. *Br J Plast Surg.* 1991;44:87-90.

Functional pectoralis minor muscle flap transplantation for reconstruction of thumb opposition: an anatomic study and clinical applications

Zhuang Y-Q, Xiong H-T, Fu Q, et al (Jinan Univ, Guangzhou, People's Republic of China; et al)
Microsurgery 31:365-370, 2011

In this report, we present the results of an anatomic study on the dimensions of the pectoralis minor muscle and its neurovascular supply in 10 adult human cadavers, in attempt to evaluate the feasibility of microsurgical transplantation of a part of the muscle for thumb opposition reconstruction. A series of five patients consequently underwent thenar reconstruction with the pectoralis minor muscle flap from December 2004 to October 2006. The transferred muscle was reinnervated with the third lumbrical branch of the ulnar nerve. Follow-up assessment showed that the patients recovered functional opposition of carpometacarpal joint with 24 degrees of pronation, and a muscle power with M4 to M5. All patients were satisfied with the appearance of reconstructed thenar eminence. We recommend this new technique for thenar and opposition reconstruction in patients who have severe loss of thenar muscles, injury to the median nerve, and wish to improve the appearance of thenar eminence.

▶ This study evaluates functional free muscle transfer of the pectoralis minor muscle for the reconstruction of thumb opposition. The traditional solution for the reconstruction of thumb opposition is tendon transfers. Even though objective data on long-term outcome are sparse, these methods are capable of providing some substantial improvement of hand function by adding a certain degree of thumb opposition. Tendon transfers, however, have the disadvantage in that a certain function is acquired in exchange for a loss of a different function, the latter of which is of course considered less important for a specific setting.[1] By choosing the functional free muscle transfer of the pectoralis minor muscle, the authors avoid any functional loss to the hand. The use of this muscle as a functional free graft is well known from reconstructions for facial paralysis.[2] Harvesting of the pectoralis minor muscle is associated with minimal morbidity. Unlike tendon transfers, this method seems to provide a high degree of thumb opposition without the loss of any other hand function. In addition, esthetics is improved as well.

It would have been more helpful if the authors would have added some more details about which portion of pectoralis minor was used for their reconstruction.

If future long-term results of a larger study population support the positive results of this study, functional free muscle transfer of the pectoralis minor muscle for the reconstruction of thumb opposition could be an excellent choice for the highly motivated young patient.

For patients with systemic diseases or patients with advanced age, tendon transfers remain the treatment of choice.

M. Choi, MD

References

1. Cooney WP, Linscheid RL, An KN. Opposition of the thumb: an anatomic and biomechanical study of tendon transfers. *J Hand Surg Am*. 1984;9:777-786.
2. Harrison DH, Grobbelaar AO. Pectoralis minor muscle transfer for unilateral facial palsy reanimation: an experience of 35 years and 637 cases. *J Plast Reconstr Aesthet Surg*. 2012 Feb 14 [Epub ahead of print].

7 Hand: Peripheral Nerve

Evaluation of the Scratch Collapse Test in Peroneal Nerve Compression

Gillenwater J, Cheng J, Mackinnon SE (Univ of Southern California, Los Angeles, CA; Univ of Texas Southwestern Med Ctr, Dallas; Washington Univ in St Louis, MO)
Plast Reconstr Surg 128:933-939, 2011

Background.—The scratch collapse test is a recently described provocative test for diagnosis of peripheral nerve compression.

Methods.—The scratch collapse test was studied prospectively in 24 consecutive patients with a diagnosis of common peroneal nerve compression neuropathy. The diagnosis was confirmed by history, physical examination, and electrodiagnostic testing. Provocative testing by the scratch collapse test and Tinel's sign was performed.

Results.—The scratch collapse test showed a sensitivity of 0.77 and a specificity of 0.99, while the Tinel's sign showed 0.65 and 0.99, respectively.

Conclusion.—The scratch collapse test is a sensitive and specific provocative test that compares favorably to existing clinical tests and aids in the diagnosis of common peroneal neuropathy.

Clinical Question/Level of Evidence.—Diagnostic, II.

▶ Diagnosing peripheral nerve compression may still be difficult in 2012. In particular, compressions in the lower extremity can be missed when physicians are not familiar with the exact anatomy and pathophysiology of nerves. In many instances, electrodiagnostic studies (EDS) are obtained to confirm or rule the diagnosis. Early nerve compression may not cause an axonal damage severe enough to demonstrate changes with EDS. For that reason, besides an adequate history and thorough physical examination, additional tests such as the Tinel sign have been used. The scratch collapse test (SCT) has shown to be superior to detect nerve compressions in the upper extremity for diagnosing ulnar nerve compression at the elbow. This article reports on comparable results for the peroneal nerve compression in the lower extremity. Comparable to the Tinel sign, the SCT has many advantages compared with EDS: reduced medical costs, higher patients' compliance for repeated tests, and the ability to diagnose early nerve compressions. The disadvantage when to use quantitative sensory testing (QST) is the lack of quantitative data, and "yes-no" result. Especially for early nerve compressions with normal EDS results, the correlation of the SCT with QST should be studied.

The SCT for nerve compressions in the lower extremity will be a valuable additional tool in the armamentarium of the peripheral nerve surgeon.

H. Coert, MD, PhD

Reconstruction of Digital Nerves With Collagen Conduits
Taras JS, Jacoby SM, Lincoski CJ (Thomas Jefferson Univ, Philadelphia, PA; Drexel Univ College of Medicine, Philadelphia, PA; Univ Orthopedics Ctr, State College, PA)
J Hand Surg 36A:1441-1446, 2011

Purpose.—Digital nerve reconstruction with a biodegradable conduit offers the advantage of providing nerve reconstruction while providing a desirable environment for nerve regeneration. Many conduit materials have been investigated, but there have been few reports of human clinical trials of purified type I bovine collagen conduits.

Methods.—We report a prospective study of 22 isolated digital nerve lacerations in 19 patients reconstructed with a bioabsorbable collagen conduit. The average nerve gap measured 12 mm. An independent observer performed the postoperative evaluation, noting the return of protective sensation, static 2-point discrimination, and moving 2-point discrimination, and recording the patient's pain level using a visual analog scale. Minimal follow-up was 12 months and mean follow-up was 20 months after surgery.

Results.—All patients recovered protective sensation. The mean moving 2-point discrimination and static 2-point discrimination measured 5.0 and 5.2 mm, respectively, for those with measurable recovery at final follow-up visit. Excellent results were achieved in 13 of 22 digits, good results in 3 of 22 digits, and fair results in 6 of 22 digits, and there were no poor results. Reported pain scores at the last postoperative visit were measured universally as 0 on the visual analog scale.

Conclusions.—Our data suggest that collagen conduits offer an effective method of reconstruction for digital nerve lacerations. This study confirms that collagen conduits reliably provide a repair that restores nerve function for nerve gaps measuring less than 2 cm.

▶ This is a carefully conducted prospective study that evaluates the use of collagen nerve conduits in digital nerve reconstruction. In these patients, because nerve gaps did not exceed 2 cm and did not involve crush injury, they presented as typical indications for this kind of synthetic conduits. Not surprisingly, the authors obtained rather good outcomes. The results attest to the effectiveness of synthetic conduits under optimal clinical conditions and add to the hand surgery literature further confirmation of the values of synthetic conduits for rather short nerve gaps. However, this study is weak compared with previously published controlled prospective studies, in that it does not discuss whether this method is superior or inferior to the use of other materials—actually a major subject of debate and current investigation. I also note that the nerve gaps in this report are 2 mm or less; it is unclear whether use of synthetic conduits for a gap between 2 and 3 cm is suggested and considered appropriate. Nerve conduits—autogenous or synthetic—are currently indicated for a gap up to 3 cm.

Injection of saline into the conduit is proposed by the authors to prevent clots; no nerve slices were inserted, likely because the gap was short. In a larger series, comparing synthetic conduits to autogenous vein grafting, Rinker and Liau[1] reported that the 2 techniques produced basically equal sensory recovery in digital nerves but noted 2 extrusions of synthetic conduits that required secondary removal. In my practice, I would harvest a vein from the forearm for a case of a digital nerve defect of 2 cm, and cut a slice of nerve from its proximal nerve stump and place it in the middle of the vein conduit to aid extension of axons over the gap. I believe that a synthetic conduit is equally workable and have used it in some cases, but the higher cost and the introduction of a foreign material often tip the balance in my choice of treatment, favoring autogenous tissues in most cases. Thus far, the literature has offered limited information on complications of synthetic conduits and salvage treatment for failed cases (particularly when the gap length is large—chances of recovery likely worsen as the gap becomes greater). In addition, I understand that different synthetic conduits are now available; I am eager to read future reports comparing outcomes of these conduits (and of nerve allografts) and to learn effective measures to tackle the problem of failed cases or lengthy defects.

J. B. Tang, MD, PhD

Reference

1. Rinker B, Liau JY. A prospective randomized study comparing woven polyglycolic acid and autogenous vein conduits for reconstruction of digital nerve gaps. *J Hand Surg Am.* 2011;36:775-781.

Comparisons of Outcomes from Repair of Median Nerve and Ulnar Nerve Defect with Nerve Graft and Tubulization: A Meta-Analysis
Yang M, Rawson JL, Zhang EW, et al (Univ of Mississippi Med Ctr, Jackson; et al)
J Reconstr Microsurg 27:451-460, 2011

In this study, an updated meta-analysis of all published human studies was presented to evaluate the recovery of the median and the ulnar nerves in the forearm after defect repair by nerve conduit and autologous nerve graft. Up to June of 2010, search for English language articles was conducted to collect publications on the outcome of median or ulnar nerve defect repair. A total of 33 studies and 1531 cases were included in this study. Patient information was extracted from these publications and the postoperative outcome was analyzed using meta-analysis. There was no significant difference in the postoperative recovery between the median and the ulnar nerves (odds ratio = 0.98). Sensory nerves were found to achieve a more satisfactory recovery after nerve defect repair than motor nerves ($p < 0.05$). Median nerve can also achieve more satisfactory recovery in both sensory and motor function than ulnar nerve ($p < 0.05$). There was no statistical difference between tubulization and autologous nerve graft in repairing defects less than 5 cm. Based on the results of this study, a median nerve with sensory impairment was associated with improved postoperative prognosis, while an ulnar nerve with motor nerve damage was prone to a worse prognosis. Tubulization can be a good alternative in the reconstruction of small defects.

▶ I don't understand how articles like this get published. After reading the article 4 times, I'm still not entirely sure how the authors analyzed their data. Even the abstract does not make sense. "No statistical difference in the postoperative recovery between the median and ulnar nerves," yet the median nerve is able to achieve better motor recovery and better sensory recovery than the ulnar nerve. How does this make sense? There have been several meta-analyses published in the past few years that seem to be changing the way we think about major nerve repairs,[1] although I think the primary change in mentality is in the reporting of M4 versus M3 as satisfactory (which historically has been the case). With this 1 (albeit big) change in data interpretation, we now accept that only about 50% of major nerve repairs will result in satisfactory functional recovery. In this meta-analysis, the authors rehash data that have already been reported but try to put a new twist on them—they take issue with the statistical analysis used on previous meta-analyses (saying their technique is better) and claim novelty by including tubulization studies. Although the majority of the article is directed at comparisons of ulnar versus median nerve recovery (again, I cannot follow how they performed this analysis), the eye-catching emphasis of the title, abstract, and conclusion is on the comparison with conduit repairs. They conclude that there is no difference in outcomes between conduit and autologous graft repairs for defects less than 5 cm. I was able to identify 3 studies mentioned in their analysis with conduit repairs greater than 3 cm. Braga-Silva[2] concluded that the results were unsatisfactory greater than 3 cm; Stanec and Stanec[3] concluded that their results were unsatisfactory greater than 4 cm, and Rosson et al[4] (a study with only 6 patients with an average gap of 2.9 cm) did not repair a gap greater than 4 cm. How then do the authors feel they can publish a conclusion in which they claim to analyze 1531 patients (in which there is literally a handful of conduit repairs greater than 3 cm—none of which offer convincing evidence that this is a good idea) and find that conduit repairs up to 5 cm are equivalent? This article is irresponsible at best and dangerous at worse, and I would suggest that any reader tempted to repair 5 cm gaps in major peripheral nerves with conduits, based on this article, read the original studies as well as the recently published Moore et al[5] in which the poor results associated with this approach to median and ulna nerves are emphasized.

J. Isaacs, MD

References

1. Ruijs AC, Jaquet JB, Kalmijn S, Giele H, Hovius SE. Median and ulnar nerve injuries: a meta-analysis of predictors of motor and sensory recovery after modern microsurgical nerve repair. *Plast Reconstr Surg.* 2005;116:484-494.
2. Braga-Silva J. The use of silicone tubing in the late repair of the median and ulnar nerves in the forearm. *J Hand Surg Br.* 1999;24:703-706.
3. Stanec S, Stanec Z. Reconstruction of upper-extremity peripheral-nerve injuries with ePTFE conduits. *J Reconstr Microsurg.* 1998;14:227-232.
4. Rosson GD, Williams EH, Dellon AL. Motor nerve regeneration across a conduit. *Microsurgery.* 2009;29:107-114.
5. Moore AM, Kasukurthi R, Magill CK, Farhadi HF, Borschel GH, Mackinnon SE. Limitations of conduits in peripheral nerve repairs. *Hand (N Y).* 2009;4:180-186.

Comparisons of Outcomes from Repair of Median Nerve and Ulnar Nerve Defect with Nerve Graft and Tubulization: A Meta-Analysis

Yang M, Rawson JL, Zhang EW, et al (Univ of Mississippi Med Ctr, Jackson, CA)
J Reconstr Microsurg 27:451-460, 2011

In this study, an updated meta-analysis of all published human studies was presented to evaluate the recovery of the median and the ulnar nerves in the forearm after defect repair by nerve conduit and autologous nerve graft. Up to June of 2010, search for English language articles was conducted to collect publications on the outcome of median or ulnar nerve defect repair. A total of 33 studies and 1531 cases were included in this study. Patient information was extracted from these publications and the postoperative outcome was analyzed using meta-analysis. There was no significant difference in the postoperative recovery between the median and the ulnar nerves (odds ratio = 0.98). Sensory nerves were found to achieve a more satisfactory recovery after nerve defect repair than motor nerves ($P < 0.05$). Median nerve can also achieve more satisfactory recovery in both sensory and motor function than ulnar nerve ($P < 0.05$). There was no statistical difference between tubulization and autologous nerve graft in repairing defects less than 5 cm. Based on the results of this study, a median nerve with sensory impairment was associated with improved postoperative prognosis, while an ulnar nerve with motor nerve damage was prone to a worse prognosis. Tubulization can be a good alternative in the reconstruction of small defects.

▶ This study confirms via a meta-analysis that which has been shown experimentally on numerous occasions, ie, nerve conduits work over small distances. The authors collated all known articles on the subject, written in the English language, where data were recoverable.

As such, the limitations of the analysis are recognized by the author, namely, the differential recoverable data between studies on grafts or conduits, the lack of included randomized controlled trials, and the exclusion of non—English-language publications.

This study suggests that there is no significant difference in nerve repair via either method for defects of less than 5 cm for median or ulnar nerve. The authors, however, rightly inject a note of caution by commenting that most studies suggest tubulization is only recommended for defects of 3 cm or less.

This meta-analysis is unlikely to change any existing peripheral nerve injury practice, but it does have interesting points to make about the relative quality of sensory and motor recovery for median and ulnar-grafted defects.

In my practice, most median and ulnar defects seen are longer than 3 cm, and autologous nerve grafting remains our current standard, utilizing sural nerve or medial cutaneous nerve of the forearm.

M. Fox, MD

8 Hand: Tendon

Evaluation of Tumor Necrosis Factor α Blockade on Early Tendon-to-Bone Healing in a Rat Rotator Cuff Repair Model

Gulotta LV, Kovacevic D, Cordasco F, et al (Hosp for Special Surgery, NY)
Arthroscopy 27:1351-1357, 2011

Purpose.—The purpose was to determine whether systemic tumor necrosis factor α (TNF-α) blockade can improve rotator cuff healing in a rat model.

Methods.—One hundred twenty Lewis rats underwent unilateral detachment and repair of the supraspinatus. Rats were randomized into 2 groups. The experimental group received injections of pegylated soluble tumor necrosis factor receptor type I (3.0 mg/kg every other day for 3 doses). The control group received saline solution on the same dosing schedule. At 2, 4, and 8 weeks, 20 animals in each group were killed (4 for histologic assessment and 16 for biomechanical testing). Outcomes included qualitative histologic assessment to determine new fibrocartilage formation and collagen fiber organization. Immunohistochemical staining was performed to localize TNF-α, ED1 and ED2 macrophages, and tartrate-resistant acidic phosphatase. Biomechanical testing was performed to determine the ultimate load to failure, stiffness, cross-sectional area, and ultimate stress to failure.

Results.—Qualitative assessments of histology showed that the experimental group had more cartilage formation at 4 weeks but not at 2 or 8 weeks. There was less TNF-α staining in the experimental group at 4 and 8 weeks, and there were fewer ED1 macrophages at 4 weeks compared with controls. The ultimate load to failure was greater in the experimental group compared with controls at 2 weeks (13.3 ± 2.6 N v 11.2 ± 2.7 N, $P = .05$) and at 4 weeks (21.7 ± 4.6 N v 18.5 ± 2.1 N, $P = .04$). The experimental group also had a higher stiffness at 2 weeks (7.2 ± 2.3 N/mm v 5.8 ± 1.4 N/mm, $P = .04$) and at 4 weeks (10.5 ± 2.7 N/mm v 8.4 ± 1.7 N/mm, $P = .01$). There were no differences in any biomechanical variable at 8 weeks.

Conclusions.—TNF-α blockade can improve the biomechanical strength of tendon-bone healing in a rat rotator cuff model at early time points, which corresponded with modest qualitative improvements in histology. However, these differences were not maintained at 8 weeks.

Clinical Relevance.—TNF-α blockade may influence rotator cuff tendon healing.

▶ Increasing the healing strength of the tendon-bone junction is a relatively little-attended area of investigation. The authors sought to block tumor necrosis factor—α (hence decreasing inflammatory responses) to modulate tendon-bone healing. It is interesting to note that the increase in strength was statistically significant at weeks 2 and 4 after surgical repair and the blockage, but not at week 8. This is understandable—the treatment increases the strength at the earlier postsurgical period—because such blockage at several postsurgical days might have an early effect through suppressing inflammation. However, the strength difference between the treated and control tendons at weeks 2 or 4 were actually quite small (less than 20%). This begs the question of whether such a small increase is biologically meaningful, despite being statistically significant. To decrease rupture of the repair, a biological modulation should be able to substantially increase the strength. I believe an increase of at least 30% to 50% is necessary. Of course, it is not possible to know how an increase in animal models translates to clinically relevant treatment.

Modulation of inflammatory changes appears not sufficient to produce large increases in strength, but it may well be a part of compound molecular modulation in the future. Because this study was performed in a rat model, future investigations using large animals are necessary. It will also be necessary to compare the effects of a number of methods and their combination in 1 study setting.

I have used gene therapy in end-to-end tendon repair and have not been able to extend it to biological augmentation of tendon-bone healing. The tendon-bone junction is a fertile area for research efforts. Multiple methods can be tested. Healing events at cellular, molecular, or histologic levels can be modulated. Yet, achieving substantial gain (eg, 50% or more) in mechanical strength remains the goal. Increasing the strength by great amplitude can be exponentially more difficult than achieving only a small strength gain, and our journey is arduous toward the goal.

J. B. Tang, MD

A Retrospective Review to Determine the Long-term Efficacy of Orthotic Devices for Trigger Finger
Valdes K (Hand Works Therapy, Sarasota, FL)
J Hand Ther 25:89-96, 2012

Purpose.—To evaluate the use of orthotic devices (splints) in an attempt to resolve trigger finger.

Methods.—Data were extracted from 46 charts during a five-year period from January 2005 to December 2010. At ten weeks, patients were seen for follow-up assessment of pain and stage of stenosing tenosynovitis (SST). One-year follow-up was performed to determine if the patients required further surgical intervention or steroid injection. The data were analyzed to determine the efficacy of orthosis intervention.

Results.—Mean pain score preorthotic is 5.63 and postorthotic is 1.20. Mean SST score preorthotic is 3.93 and postorthotic is 1.21. There was an 87% (40 patients) success rate with the orthotic intervention; 4.3% (two patients) had surgery and 8.5% (four patients) received a steroid injection in the year after orthotic application.

Conclusion.—This study demonstrated the efficacy of orthoses for the reduction of pain and SST score for patients who have trigger finger (Fig 4).

▶ This retrospective study adds to the existing body of evidence that supports the use of orthotic devices in the management of trigger finger. Although not a large study, it was well controlled in that all the participants in this study were treated by the same certified hand therapist (CHT). The CHT fabricated the static orthotic devices using 1 of 2 different designs. If a single digit was involved, the CHT fabricated a circumferential finger-based orthosis to block proximal interphalangeal joint motion. In subjects with multiple digits that triggered, the CHT fabricated a hand-based orthosis to restrict metacarpophalangeal (MP) flexion. Both splints were designed to restrict composite digit flexion while allowing for function of the hand. Along with orthotic wear, the subjects were instructed to remove the orthosis 3 times a day to complete specific passive-range-of-motion and active-range-of-motion exercises issued by the CHT. Excellent results were achieved, with 40 of the 46 subjects requiring no further treatment interventions (Fig 4).

Hand therapists have historically used various orthotic devices for conservative treatment of trigger finger. I have used a hand-based MP flexion block orthosis for over 20 years noting positive results when there is good patient compliance. More recently I have used a dorsal interphalangeal blocking orthosis for the thumb, as it allows for function while preventing composite flexion.

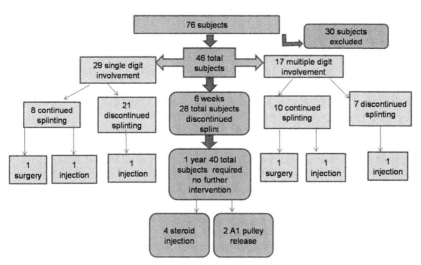

FIGURE 4.—Patient flow chart. (Reprinted from Valdes K. A retrospective review to determine the long-term efficacy of orthotic devices for trigger finger. *J Hand Ther.* 2012;25:89-96, with permission from Hanley & Belfus, an imprint of Elsevier Inc.)

I appreciate that this article provides additional evidence supporting the use of orthoses as well as practical instructions for the fabrication and schedule of wear for the orthoses used in the study. Since many of our patients prefer to avoid injections and/or surgical intervention, orthotic use should continue to be one of our first treatment options. Suggestions for continued research include a larger sample size as well as a comparison of the efficacy of the different types of orthotic devices used.

S. J. Clark, OTR/L, CHT

Complications After Flexor Tendon Repair: A Systematic Review and Meta-Analysis

Dy CJ, Hernandez-Soria A, Ma Y, et al (Hosp for Special Surgery, NY)
J Hand Surg 37A:543-551.e1, 2012

Purpose.—Although outcomes after flexor tendon repair have reportedly improved with modern treatment, complications are common. The purpose of this study was to determine the incidence of these complications and the potential contributory factors within the published literature.

Methods.—We performed a systematic review of the available literature to identify publications in which patients with flexor tendon ruptures were surgically treated. We extracted demographics, zone of injury, core suture technique (only modified Kessler or a combination of techniques), use of epitendinous suture, and date of publication (before or after January 1, 2000). We excluded articles if they did not report information on reoperation, rupture, or adhesions. We used unadjusted pooled meta-analysis to report the incidence of complications, and meta-regression to describe the potential contributory factors for each complication while controlling for age, gender, and zone of injury.

Results.—Unadjusted meta-analysis revealed rates of re-operation of 6%, rupture of 4%, and adhesions of 4%. Meta-regression analysis of 29 studies showed that core suture technique or use of an epitendinous suture does not influence rupture. However, the presence of an epitendinous suture decreases re-operation by 84%. Adhesion development is 57% lower when the modified Kessler technique is used. The incidence of complications did not vary with publication date.

Conclusions.—The published literature supports use of the modified Kessler repair technique with an epitendinous suture to minimize complications. Although complication rates are low, our data suggest that there has been no definitive improvement in reported complications before and after 2000.

▶ This article is significant because the authors perform a thorough review of the literature and meta-analysis to report the incidence of complications after flexor tendon repair, a surgery well known to hand surgeons and one with generally less than ideal outcomes. Even with reported improvements in flexor tendon repair technique and rehabilitation protocols, the published incidence of complications was not well known until this analysis was performed.

Strengths of this study are the thorough review of the published literature and statistical analysis of the studies finally chosen for the meta-analysis. Weaknesses of the study, as also stated by the authors, are the lack of patient-centered outcomes and the heterogeneity in repair techniques and rehabilitation protocols postrepair among the studies. Also, because surgeons are not usually inclined to publish their complications as often as their successful results, it is impossible to know the true incidence of complications after flexor tendon repair. I would surmise that it is in fact higher than the 4% to 6% stated in this article.

This study reports, as well as possible based on the published literature, the incidence of complications following flexor tendon repair and finds that it is similar before and after 2000. The conclusion I found most interesting was that the modified Kessler repair with epitendinous suture was the technique that had the fewest complications; other repair techniques have been touted to be stronger and better but perhaps have greater complications.

Although I believe my incidence of rerupture following flexor tendon repair is quite low and therefore consistent with this study's finding, I have to admit that my rates of reoperation (usually for tenolysis) and adhesions are definitely higher than the 6% and 4%, respectively, reported in this study. My preferred technique for flexor tendon repair is also a modified Kessler repair with epitendinous suture, and I was pleased to learn that this is supported by the literature.

S. S. Shin, MD, MMSc

9 Dupuytren's Contracture

Preliminary Soft-Tissue Distraction versus Checkrein Ligament Release after Fasciectomy in the Treatment of Dupuytren Proximal Interphalangeal Joint Contractures
Craft RO, Smith AA, Coakley B, et al (Mayo Clinic, Scottsdale, AZ)
Plast Reconstr Surg 128:1107-1113, 2011

Background.—Checkrein ligament release for treatment of proximal interphalangeal joint Dupuytren contractures does not address the short-ened arteries or deficient skin. The Digit Widget uses soft-tissue distraction to overcome these issues. This study compares checkrein ligament release after fasciectomy versus preliminary soft-tissue distraction, followed by operative release, for treatment of proximal interphalangeal joint Dupuy-tren contractures.

Methods.—The authors compared operative and postoperative character-istics of patients treated with either fasciectomy plus checkrein ligament release or Digit Widget distraction between 2001 and 2008. Seventeen patients (20 digits) underwent ligament release (mean contracture, 55.9 degrees); six of these 20 were reoperations. Thirteen patients (17 digits) under-went distraction (mean contracture, 67.6 degrees); 10 of 17 were reoperations.

Results.—The 20 digits treated with fasciectomy plus ligament release had an average extension improvement of 31.4 degrees (range, −4 to 70 degrees). Digits treated with distraction had an average extension improvement of 53.4 degrees (range, 30 to 75 degrees) ($p < 0.001$ versus ligament release). Three digits treated with distraction improved to full proximal interphalan-geal extension. Initial contractures of 60 degrees or less treated by ligament release ($n = 12$) or distraction ($n = 7$) improved by means of 28.8 degrees and 47.7 degrees, respectively ($p = 0.048$). Contractures greater than 60 degrees treated by ligament release ($n = 8$) or distraction ($n = 10$) improved by means of 35.3 degrees and 57.3 degrees, respectively ($p = 0.02$).

Conclusion.—Soft-tissue distraction followed by operative release showed greater correction than Dupuytren fasciectomy plus checkrein ligament release.

Clinical Question/Level of Evidence.—Therapeutic, III.

▶ Treating severe proximal interphalangeal (PIP) joint Dupuytren's contractures continues to be challenging, especially in patients with recurrent disease. Not uncommonly following fasciectomy, even after all diseased fascia is excised, there will be residual PIP contracture. In these patients, capsuloligamentous release has been recommended by some investigators, although in a prospective study in patients with PIP contracture greater than 60°, Beyermann et al[1] found that residual contracture was the same regardless of whether a capsuloligamentous release was performed.

The authors of this article seek to determine whether a slow, progressive soft-tissue distraction, prior to operative release, improves outcomes compared with simultaneous fasciectomy and capsuloligamentous release. Distraction was obtained through use of the "Digit Widget" device, which attaches through 2 pins into the middle phalanx of the affected digit and a cuff worn on the hand (Fig 3 in the original article). Rubber bands are used to maintain a constant extension torque on the PIP joint, with average period of distraction being 6 weeks. Although the number of patients in the study was small, there was a statistically significant improvement of contracture in the Digit Widget group (17 digits) of 54.7° compared with 27.7° in the simultaneous release group (20 digits). And while at final follow-up 3 patients in the simultaneous group had a worsening of contracture, all patients in the Digit Widget cohort improved, even in patients undergoing revision surgery and in those with contractures greater than 60°.

Although randomized, prospective trials comparing fasciectomy alone, fasciectomy with capsuloligamentous release, and distraction followed by fasciectomy are still needed, the authors have shown a distinct advantage in the staged approach to severe PIP contractures in both primary and recurrent Dupuytren's disease. One major failure of the article is the lack of reporting patient's final flexion. Stiffness is a known complication of fasciectomy, with some patients struggling to regain full flexion. It would be important to know if the patients who had constant PIP extension over an average of 6 weeks, followed by surgery, had a delay or inability to regain full flexion.

F. T. D. Kaplan, MD

Reference

1. Beyermann K, Prommersberger KJ, Jacobs C, Lanz UB. Severe contracture of the proximal interphalangeal joint in Dupuytren's disease: does capsuloligamentous release improve outcome? *J Hand Surg Br.* 2004;29:240-243.

Cost-Effectiveness of Open Partial Fasciectomy, Needle Aponeurotomy, and Collagenase Injection for Dupuytren Contracture
Chen NC, Shauver MJ, Chung KC (Univ of Michigan Med School, Ann Arbor)
J Hand Surg 36A:1826-1834, 2011

Purpose.—We undertook a cost-utility analysis to compare traditional fasciectomy for Dupuytren with 2 new treatments, needle aponeurotomy and collagenase injection.

Methods.—We constructed an expected-value decision analysis model with an arm representing each treatment. A survey was administered to a cohort of 50 consecutive subjects to determine utilities of different interventions. We conducted multiple sensitivity analyses to assess the impact of varying the rate of disease recurrence in each arm of the analysis as well as the cost of the collagenase injection. The threshold for a cost-effective treatment is based on the traditional willingness-to-pay of $50,000 per quality-adjusted life years (QALY) gained.

Results.—The cost of open partial fasciectomy was $820,114 per QALY gained over no treatment. The cost of needle aponeurotomy was $96,474 per QALY gained versus no treatment. When we performed a sensitivity analysis and set the success rate at 100%, the cost of needle aponeurotomy was $49,631. When needle aponeurotomy was performed without surgical center or anesthesia costs and with reduced hand therapy, the cost was $36,570. When a complete collagenase injection series was priced at $250, the cost was $31,856 per QALY gained. When the injection series was priced at $945, the cost was $49,995 per QALY gained. At the market price of $5,400 per injection, the cost was $166,268 per QALY gained.

Conclusions.—In the current model, open partial fasciectomy is not cost-effective. Needle aponeurotomy is cost-effective if the success rate is high. Collagenase injection is cost-effective when priced under $945.

Type of Study/Level of Evidence.—Economic and Decision Analysis II.

▶ This study provides a well-conducted cost-benefit analysis for the treatment options for Dupuytren's disease. The overall conclusion is that none of the currently available treatments for Dupuytren's disease are cost effective given average recurrence rates for each of these treatment modalities.

The high cost per quality-adjusted life year (QALY) is based primarily on the low utility assigned to the improvements obtained with surgery and the limited disability assigned to the disease itself. While the author's techniques are well thought out and thorough, this seems to be the variable that may have the greatest effect on the cost-effectiveness. The authors assign utility by creating a survey of unaffected healthy volunteers. As we all know, people are much more willing to accept deformity and disability more for others than for themselves. A spouse in an examination room is more willing to accept an injection for their partner than the patient is themselves, as the spouse doesn't have to experience the pain of the injection.

If this survey artificially lowers the level of disability of the disease, the resultant improvement with treatment would go up with a more accurate survey. Therefore, the cost per QALY would decrease. Perhaps administering this survey to patients with the described Dupuytren's deformity could help put into perspective a more accurate reflection of the true disability.

Another item mentioned by the authors worth noting is that cost-effectiveness is of little value if the treatment is ineffective. Given the data used for this study (15% recurrence, no nerve injuries, 0.3% rate of chronic regional pain syndrome) in regard to collagenase injection, this may be a much more effective treatment than the others studied. Therefore, the cost-effectiveness needs to be weighed against the clinical effectiveness.

T. Hughes, MD

10 Carpus

Effect of Partial Wrist Denervation on Wrist Kinesthesia: Wrist Denervation Does Not Impair Proprioception
Gay A, Harbst K, Hansen DK, et al (Mayo Clinic, Rochester, MN)
J Hand Surg 36A:1774-1779, 2011

Purpose.—To evaluate the potential effect of partial wrist denervation on wrist kinesthesia, we hypothesized that anesthetizing the anterior interosseous nerve and the posterior interosseous nerve does not impair the kinesthesia.

Methods.—We performed a double-blinded, prospective, randomized study on 80 healthy volunteers (20–54 y old) to compare the ability to detect active and passive wrist movement in 2 conditions. The test group received an anesthetic block of the anterior and posterior interosseous nerves, and the control group subjects received an injection of saline. The kinesthesia of the 2 groups was then tested in 2 conditions by measuring the error in an active and passive wrist repositioning task. Results were analyzed using a repeated measures analysis of variance.

Results.—In both active and passive conditions, there was no difference in the repositioning errors between the test group and the control group.

Conclusions.—Our results show that kinesthesia is not impaired by blocking the anterior and posterior interosseous nerves. These findings are consistent for both active and passive motion. The study gives strong evidence that partial denervation does not impair wrist kinesthesia. However, because only kinesthesia was studied, we cannot conclude that partial denervation is a totally safe procedure for all aspects of proprioception.

Type of Study/Level of Evidence.—Therapeutic I.

▶ The authors of this article present a high-quality, well-developed randomized study examining the effect of simulated partial wrist denervation on wrist proprioception. Although the study concludes that kinesthesia is not impaired by blocking the anterior and posterior interosseous, results should be interpreted with caution. Kinesthesia represents a single aspect of proprioception, namely, the ability to identify position and motion sense. There are many other aspects of proprioception that may be affected by denervation that this study does not address. The important finding here is that the articular kinesthetic inputs via the anterior and posterior interosseous nerves act as contributors to joint position and sense, in conjunction with muscular and cutaneous inputs, and not as the sole contributors. In the absence of the articular innervation, the other inputs appear to compensate so that the kinesthetic sense is not lost. This finding supports the use of partial denervation for pain relief without compromising the kinesthetic component of proprioception.

A. Wolff, OTR, CHT

Results of 189 wrist replacements: A report from the Norwegian Arthroplasty Register
Krukhaug Y, Lie SA, Havelin LI, et al (Haukeland Univ Hosp, Bergen, Norway; et al)
Acta Orthop 82:405-409, 2011

Background and Purpose.—There is very little literature on the long-term outcome of wrist replacements. The Norwegian Arthroplasty Register has registered wrist replacements since 1994. We report on the total wrist replacements and their revision rates over a 16-year period.

Material and Methods.—189 patients with 189 primary wrist replacements (90 Biax prostheses (80 of which were cementless), 23 cementless Elos prostheses, and 76 cementless Gibbon prostheses), operated during the period 1994–2009 were identified in the Norwegian Arthroplasty Register. Prosthesis survival was analyzed using Cox regression analyses. The 3 implant designs were compared and time trends were analyzed.

Results.—The 5-year survival was 78% (95% CI: 70–85) and the 10-year survival was 71% (CI: 59–80). Prosthesis survival was 85% (CI: 78–93) at 5 years for the Biax prosthesis, 77% (CI: 30–90) at 4 years for the Gibbon prosthesis, and 57% (CI: 33–81) at 5 years for the Elos prosthesis. There was no statistically significant influence of age, diagnosis, or year of operation on the risk of revision, but females had a higher revision rate than males (RR = 3, CI: 1–7). The number of wrist replacements performed due to osteoarthritis increased with time, but no such change was apparent for inflammatory arthritis.

Interpretation.—The survival of the total wrist arthroplasties studied was similar to that in other studies of wrist arthroplasties, but it was still not as good as that for most total knee and hip arthroplasties. However, a failed wrist arthroplasty still leaves the option of a well-functioning arthrodesis (Table 2).

▶ Total wrist arthroplasty (TWA) is less popular than other forms of total joint arthroplasty. The many types of prostheses used and the limited number of TWA operations performed by many surgeons make statistical analysis for the outcomes of TWA difficult. Many surgeons may believe that the long-term outcomes of TWA are catastrophic, although the short-term ones might be excellent.[1,2] Although TWA can provide patients with a functional range of wrist movement, it is still followed by a high revision rate. Loosening of the prostheses, pain, deep infections, and incorrect fixation of the prostheses (incorrect axis) are the main reasons for revision of a TWA (Table 2). Patients having had total hip or knee arthroplasties obtain almost complete pain relief

TABLE 2.—Reasons for Revision (more than one reason could be given)

Brand	Biax	Elos	Gibbon	Total
Loosening of proximal component	3	2		5
Loosening of distal component	8	8	5	21
Dislocation	2	—	—	2
Instability	3	—	—	3
Axis problems	7	—	1	8
Deep infection	1	—	3	4
Pain	7	1	2	10
Wear of liner	1	—	—	1
Total number of revisions	18	10	11	39

after the operations. Pain was still a reason for revision in patients with TWA, although pain was not the only cause for revision (Table 2). Other articles also reported cases with complex regional pain syndrome after TWA.[3] Coverage of the wrist joint by thin soft tissue predisposes patients with a TWA to infection. Loosening of the prostheses is the most common reason for TWA revision. It might be true that fixation of the prostheses is difficult in deformed and osteoporotic carpal bones affected by rheumatoid arthritis. This study revealed no significant difference in the revision rate between those patients with inflammatory diseases and those without them, indicating that the TWA prostheses that had been used had mechanical and structural problems. A recent cadaveric study has revealed that the mechanical axes of the wrist are oriented obliquely to the anatomical axes and that radial extension to ulnar flexion ("dart thrower's wrist motion") is motion around the mechanical axis of the wrist.[4] The dart thrower's wrist motion might be a key concept for manufacturing new TWA prostheses, which would reduce the revision rate caused by implant loosening.

R. Kakinoki, MD, PhD

References

1. Ward CM, Kuhl T, Adams BD. Five to ten-year outcomes of the Universal total wrist arthroplasty in patients with rheumatoid arthritis. *J Bone Joint Surg Am.* 2011;93:914-919.
2. Radmer S, Andresen R, Sparmann M. Total wrist arthroplasty in patients with rheumatoid arthritis. *J Hand Surg Am.* 2003;28:789-794.
3. Strunk S, Bracker W. Wrist joint arthroplasty: results after 41 prostheses. *Handchir Mikrochir Plast Chir.* 2009;41:141-147.
4. Crisco JJ, Heard WMR, Rich RR, Paller DJ, Wolfe SW. The mechanical axes of the wrist are oriented obliquely to the anatomical axes. *J Bone Joint Surg Am.* 2011; 93:169-177.

Nonoperative Treatment for Acute Scaphoid Fractures: A Systematic Review and Meta-Analysis of Randomized Controlled Trials

Doornberg JN, Buijze GA, Ham SJ, et al (Academic Med Centre, Amsterdam, the Netherlands; Onze Lieve Vrouwe Gasthuis, Amsterdam, the Netherlands; et al)
J Trauma 71:1073-1081, 2011

Background.—Recommendations for cast immobilization of acute scaphoid fractures vary substantially. We reviewed data from randomized controlled trials comparing nonoperative treatment methods for acute scaphoid fractures to determine the best available evidence.

Methods.—A systematic search of the medical literature from 1966 to 2010 was performed. Two authors independently screened titles and abstracts, reviewed articles, assessed methodological quality according to the Grading of Recommendations Assessment Development and Evaluation system, and extracted data. The primary outcome parameter was nonunion. Data were pooled using random-effects models with standard mean differences for continuous and risk ratios for dichotomous variables, respectively. Heterogeneity across studies was assessed with calculation of the I^2 statistic.

Results.—The search resulted in five potentially eligible trials of which four met our inclusion criteria. In total, 523 patients were included in four trials including two evaluating below-elbow casting versus above-elbow casting; one trial comparing below-elbow casting including the thumb versus excluding the thumb; and one trial comparing fractures with a below-elbow cast with the wrist in 20-degrees flexion to 20-degrees extension, with both types excluding the thumb. There were no significant differences in union rate, pain, grip strength, time to union, or osteonecrosis for the various nonoperative treatment methods.

Conclusions.—There is no evidence from randomized controlled trials on physician-based or patient-based outcome to favor any nonoperative treatment method for acute scaphoid fractures.

▶ Controversies in the treatment of scaphoid fractures by cast immobilization include joints that should be immobilized in the cast (including or excluding the elbow joint or the thumb metacarpophalangeal joint) and the immobilization period. Scaphoid fractures typically require a longer period of immobilization than other fractures, such as the distal radius, ulna, metacarpals, and phalanges. Even nondisplaced scaphoid fractures that appear to be achieving union after 6 to 8 weeks of cast immobilization sometimes develop a nonunion. Minimally displaced or undisplaced scaphoid fractures can be treated successfully by percutaneous fixation using cannulated headless compression screws. A recent trend for the treatment of scaphoid fractures is surgery rather than cast immobilization, even though the fracture might be undisplaced or minimally displaced. An interesting article about the treatment of nondisplaced scaphoid wrist fractures was published recently from Austria.[1] The authors divided patients with acute nondisplaced scaphoid wrist fractures randomly into 2 groups, one treated by screw fixation and the other by cast immobilization. The patients treated by screw fixation obtained more rapid bone union and returned to work earlier than those treated by cast immobilization. Although the medical costs are different in each country, surgery in Austria was less expensive than cast immobilization. This was because of increased compensation costs because of the long time off work and costs for hand therapy to improve joint stiffness after long-term immobilization. It is true that surgical treatment is associated with several risks such as infection and nonunion. The nonunion rate of scaphoid fractures treated by screw fixation is reported to be 4% to 6%,[2,3] whereas nonunions occur in 5% to 10% of patients treated by cast immobilization. Internal screw fixation might be more beneficial than cast immobilization in the treatment of acute scaphoid fractures.

R. Kakinoki, MD, PhD

References

1. Arora R, Gschwentner M, Krappinger D, Lutz M, Blauth M, Gabl M. Fixation of nondisplaced scaphoid fractures: making treatment cost effective. Prospective controlled trial. *Arch Orthop Trauma Surg.* 2007;127:39-46.
2. Patillo DP, Khazzam M, Robertson MW, Gainor BJ. Outcome of percutaneous screw fixation of scaphoid fractures. *J Surg Orthop Adv.* 2010;19:114-120.
3. Low CK, Ang BT. Herbert screw fixation of scaphoid fractures. *Hand Surg.* 1999; 4:63-66.

Occult fractures of the scaphoid: the role of ultrasonography in the emergency department
Platon A, Poletti P-A, Van Aaken J, et al (Univ Hosp of Geneva, Switzerland; et al)
Skeletal Radiol 40:869-875, 2011

Objective.—To evaluate ultrasonography (US) performed by an emergency radiologist in patients with clinical suspicion of scaphoid fracture and normal radiographs.

Materials and Methods.—Sixty-two consecutive adult patients admitted to our emergency department with clinical suspicion of scaphoid fracture and normal radiographs underwent US examination of the scaphoid prior to wrist computed tomography (CT), within 3 days following wrist trauma. US examination was performed by a board-certified emergency radiologist, non-specialized in musculoskeletal imaging, using the linear probe (5-13 MHz) of the standard sonographic equipment of the emergency department. The radiologist evaluate for the presence of a cortical interruption of the scaphoid along with a radio-carpal or scaphotrapezium-trapezoid effusion. A CT of the wrist (reference standard) was performed in every patient, immediately after ultrasonography. Fractures were classified into two groups according to their potential for complication: group 1 (high potential, proximal or waist), group 2 (low-potential, distal or tubercle).

Results.—A scaphoid fracture was demonstrated by CT in 13 (21%) patients: eight (62%) of them belonged to group 1 (three in the proximal

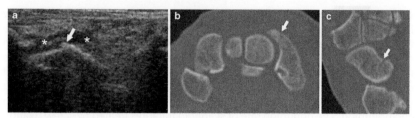

FIGURE 1.—A 36-year-old man admitted after wrist trauma, with positive clinical signs for scaphoid fracture and normal radiographs. **a** US of the scaphoid in the longitudinal plane shows cortical discontinuity (*arrow*), along with radio-carpal effusion and surrounding hematoma (*asterisk*), suggestive of scaphoid fracture. **b** Axial CT image depicts the fracture as a radiolucent line (*arrow*), traversing the scaphoid. **c** Sagittal-oblique multiplanar reformation CT image demonstrates the proximal location of the scaphoid fracture (*arrow*). (Reprinted from Platon A, Poletti P-A, Van Aaken J, et al. Occult fractures of the scaphoid: the role of ultrasonography in the emergency department. *Skeletal Radiol.* 2011;40:869-875, with permission from ISS.)

pole, five in the waist), five (38%) to group 2 (three in the distal part, two in the tubercle). US was 92% sensitive (12/13) in demonstrating a scaphoid fracture. It was 100% sensitive (8/8) in demonstrating a fracture with a high potential of complication (group 1).

Conclusions.—Our data show that, in emergency settings, US can be used for the triage to CT in patients with clinical suspicion of scaphoid fracture and normal radiographs (Fig 1).

▶ This study examines the efficacy of ultrasonography (US) technology in diagnosing occult fractures of the scaphoid, using computed tomography (CT) as the reference standard. Clearly, the authors were interested in the ability of US to diagnose scaphoid injuries in the emergency department and not in a subspecialist's office. Patients were suspected of having a possible scaphoid fracture and were included in the study if they demonstrated wrist pain on axial loading of the thumb ray and tenderness to palpation at the anatomic snuffbox.

The authors note that US examination correctly predicted the presence of a scaphoid fracture in 12 (92%) of the 13 patients with a CT-proven fracture (Fig 1). Moreover, US examination was particularly sensitive in detecting fractures that were deemed to have a "high potential for complications": namely, fractures localized to the proximal or middle third of the scaphoid. In these cases, US use was 100% sensitive in detecting these injuries. The negative predictive values or the capacity of the test in predicting that a patient with a negative US of the scaphoid does not truly have a fracture, were 97% for all scaphoid fractures and 100% in the high-risk fractures.

However, the authors concede that the false-positive rate was relatively high, which is expected when concomitant injuries could obfuscate the primary diagnosis. The character of the fracture line might also be difficult to delineate with US evaluation alone. For these reasons, US examination may be a useful adjunct to diagnosing scaphoid injuries in the emergency department. In a subspecialist's office, however, supplemental imaging modalities such as CT or magnetic resonance imaging are strongly recommended to help appreciate the full extent and character of the fracture and to guide treatment decisions.

E. K. Shin, MD

Comparison of CT and MRI for Diagnosis of Suspected Scaphoid Fractures

Mallee W, Doornberg JN, Ring D, et al (Academic Med Ctr of Amsterdam, The Netherlands; Massachusetts General Hosp, Boston)
J Bone Joint Surg Am 93:20-28, 2011

Background.—There is no consensus on the optimum imaging method to use to confirm the diagnosis of true scaphoid fractures among patients with suspected scaphoid fractures. This study tested the null hypothesis that computed tomography (CT) and magnetic resonance imaging (MRI) have the same diagnostic performance characteristics for the diagnosis of scaphoid fractures.

Methods.—Thirty-four consecutive patients with a suspected scaphoid fracture (tenderness of the scaphoid and normal radiographic findings after a fall on the outstretched hand) underwent CT and MRI within ten days after a wrist injury. The reference standard for a true fracture of the scaphoid was six-week follow-up radiographs in four views. A panel including surgeons and radiologists came to a consensus diagnosis for each type of imaging. The images were considered in a randomly ordered, blinded fashion, independent of the other types of imaging. We calculated sensitivity, specificity, and accuracy as well as positive and negative predictive values.

Results.—The reference standard revealed six true fractures of the scaphoid (prevalence, 18%). CT demonstrated a fracture in five patients (15%), with one false-positive, two false-negative, and four true-positive results. MRI demonstrated a fracture in seven patients (21%), with three false-positive, two false-negative, and four true-positive results. The sensitivity, specificity, and accuracy were 67%, 96%, and 91%, respectively, for CT and 67%, 89%, and 85%, respectively, for MRI. According to the McNemar test for paired binary data, these differences were not significant. The positive predictive value with use of the Bayes formula was 0.76 for CT and 0.54 for MRI. The negative predictive value was 0.94 for CT and 0.93 for MRI.

Conclusions.—CT and MRI had comparable diagnostic characteristics. Both were better at excluding scaphoid fractures than they were at confirming them, and both were subject to false-positive and false-negative interpretations. The best reference standard is debatable, but it is now unclear whether or not bone edema on MRI and small unicortical lines on CT represent a true fracture.

▶ This study is a prospective analysis that compared the use of CT and MRI for the diagnosis of the so-called occult scaphoid fracture. The phenomenon of a patient with radial-sided wrist pain and anatomic snuffbox tenderness after a fall on an outstretched hand is a common one, and these patients undergo wrist immobilization as a precaution. Although cast immobilization is thought to be risk-free, the authors point out that it can be associated with a substantial loss of productivity.

To be included in the study, a patient had to have had radial-sided wrist pain and anatomic snuffbox tenderness after a fall on an outstretched hand. All patients underwent both CT and MRI an average of 3.6 days after injury. The patients then returned 6 to 7 weeks after injury for plain radiographs. These radiographs were used as the reference standard for comparison of the CT and MRI. The images were shown to a panel of hand surgeons (who were blinded to patient identities and their other radiographs), and the panelists had to determine whether there was a fracture. CT detected 4 of 6 fractures later found on reference radiographs, and MRI detected the same number. The statistical analyses for both tests were remarkably similar, and both showed better specificity than sensitivity.

One interesting phenomenon that arose from the study was that of "bone edema," as seen on MRI, and whether that signified a fracture. There were a few cases in the study where edema was seen, but a clear fracture line was not detected. If bone edema had not been considered a fracture, the sensitivity of the test would have been lower, but the specificity and accuracy would have been slightly higher. Ultimately, one is left to wonder if bone edema alone on MRI is sufficient to diagnose a scaphoid fracture.

An issue that comes to light after reading the study is whether 6-week radiographs are an appropriate reference standard. The authors conclude that they likely are not, and they further conclude that latent class analysis would be a better method to analyze CT and MRI in the absence of a true gold standard.

In the end, one can conclude from the study that CT and MRI are, at this time, appropriate secondary tests to evaluate for a suspected scaphoid fracture. Because of the lower costs associated with CT, this could be considered a preferred diagnostic modality in this clinical setting.

J. Isaacs, MD

Comparison of Radiographic Stress Views for Scapholunate Dynamic Instability in a Cadaver Model

Lee SK, Desai H, Silver B, et al (New York Univ School of Medicine)
J Hand Surg 36A:1149-1157, 2011

Purpose.—Many different stress views for the diagnosis of scapholunate (SL) instability have been described in the literature. The purpose of this study is to compare these stress views and determine which view has the greatest utility for demonstrating SL gap radiographically.

Methods.—We performed a literature search for articles describing SL radiographic stress views. We created SL instability in 9 cadaveric wrists by ligamentous sectioning and imaged each specimen using all radiographic views found in the literature. These included the "clenched pencil" view, clenched fist views in varying positions, and traction views. Scapholunate gaps were measured using digital calipers.

Results.—We found 8 different SL radiographic stress views specifically described in the literature. In order to further characterize the best stress views, we studied additional parameters, including varied ulnar deviation and degree of obliquity. The clenched pencil view resulted in the most consistent views with the widest SL gaps. With clenched fist views, SL gap trended to a peak at 30° of ulnar deviation.

Conclusions.—The clenched pencil view was the best stress view to demonstrate dynamic SL instability. It also allows for a contralateral comparison on 1 radiograph. We recommend this view when evaluating for SL pathology.

Clinical Relevance.—This assessment of relative diagnostic utility might assist clinicians in the creation and use of protocols for the diagnosis of dynamic SL instability.

▶ The authors have reported on radiographic evaluation of scapholunate (SL) instability in a cadaver model. Following a literature review, they performed a comparative study of published techniques with the goal of determining which view is most useful for diagnosis of dynamic SL instability.

The authors serially sectioned the wrist ligaments to create an SL instability pattern and then imaged the 9 cadaver wrists with the 8 described views: posteroanterior (PA) clenched fist, PA clenched fist in radial deviation, PA finger traction pronation, PA thumb traction, anteroposterior (AP) clenched fist, AP clenched fist radial deviation, AP clenched fist ulnar deviation, and clenched pencil view.

They found the clenched pencil view, followed by the AP clenched fist in ulnar deviation, to be the most consistent and widest SL gap. The clenched pencil view has an advantage of imaging the contralateral wrist for comparison.

Radiographic views can vary, and it can be challenging to obtain a reproducible image. This technique can be an additional tool to consistently image the wrist for dynamic SL instability.

This will not replace other diagnostic modalities, such as MRI or wrist arthroscopy, although it will minimize variability and should be considered a screening radiograph for patients with suspected SL instability.

W. Hammert, MD

Correlation of Histopathology With Magnetic Resonance Imaging in Kienböck Disease

Ogawa T, Nishiura Y, Hara Y, et al (Kikkoman General Hosp, Noda, Chiba, Japan; Univ of Tsukuba, Ibaraki, Japan)
J Hand Surg 37A:83-89, 2012

Purpose.—Diagnosis and treatment remain controversial for Kienböck disease. A few reports have correlated magnetic resonance imaging (MRI), which is essential for early diagnosis, and histopathology of Kienböck biopsy specimens, but histopathological correlations of whole lunate bones or histological slices compared with MRI images are lacking. The purpose of this study was to compare presurgical MRI scans with corresponding histological slices of Kienböck-diseased lunates.

Methods.—We excised whole lunates at the time of surgery from 6 patients with Kienböck disease (stage IIIB) undergoing tendon-ball replacement or a Graner procedure. We stained paraffin-embedded, coronally sectioned specimens with hematoxylin-eosin and compared them with presurgical coronal scans using MRI with a 47-mm microscopy surface coil.

Results.—Toward the center of the lunates, the signal intensity in the proton density—weighted images was reduced, whereas the dorsal and palmar sides of the lunates exhibited no changes in intensity. In correlation, histopathological findings revealed strongly disrupted trabeculae toward the center of the lunates and intact trabeculae in the dorsal side of the lunates. Likewise, the necrotic and vitalized bone exhibited low and high signal intensities, respectively, in the proton density—weighted images; however, in the fast-field echo images, there were no correlations with histopathological observations.

Conclusions.—Proton density—weighted MRIs but not fast-field echo images using a 47-mm microscopy coil reflected the extent and localization of the necrotic area in Kienböck-diseased lunates, as evidenced by comparison with histological analyses of the lunate specimens.

Clinical Relevance.—Proton density—weighted MRIs accurately reflect the vascular status of the lunate and may help plan treatment on a case-by-case basis.

▶ The authors correlate the histopathologic appearance of the excised lunate with preoperative magnetic resonance imaging (MRI) studies in 6 patients with advanced (stage IIIB) Kienböck disease. I found this article interesting, but quite difficult to read, because a large amount of information is presented in a rather disorganized fashion. In general, correlations between MRI and histopathology of the lunate have been performed before for Kienböck disease, so the main finding of this article is not really surprising. The authors were, however, able to demonstrate granulation tissue and blood vessels in all sections that were described as necrotic. They have, therefore, demonstrated that even radiographic evidence of degeneration and edema does not preclude osseous perfusion. It would have been of great value to include gadolinium-enhanced MRI scans to assess possible blood flow in these vessels. These scans may be the most important information when determining the best treatment strategy, not only for Kienböck disease but for any condition in which viability of the bone is questionable, such as scaphoid nonunion.

K. Megerle, MD

Scaphoid Fractures in Children and Adolescents: Contemporary Injury Patterns and Factors Influencing Time to Union
Gholson JJ, Bae DS, Zurakowski D, et al (Children's Hosp Boston, MA)
J Bone Joint Surg Am 93:1210-1219, 2011

Background.—Historically, scaphoid fractures in children and adolescents have predominantly involved the distal pole, requiring neither surgical care nor extended follow-up. Changing patient characteristics, however, appear to be altering fracture epidemiology and treatment. The purpose of this investigation was to characterize contemporary fracture patterns in children and adolescents and to identify factors influencing time to healing following both nonoperative and operative treatment.

Methods.—A retrospective analysis of 351 scaphoid fractures that had been treated from 1995 to 2010 was performed to characterize fracture patterns. The mean patient age was 14.6 years (range, seven to eighteen years). Complete clinical and radiographic follow-up data were available for 312 fractures (89%), with 222 fractures presenting acutely and ninety not acutely. Union rates following casting or surgical treatment were determined, and Cox regression analysis was utilized to identify factors influencing both the union rate and the time to union.

Results.—Overall, 248 fractures (71%) occurred at the scaphoid waist, eighty-one (23%) occurred at the distal pole, and twenty-two (6%) occurred at the proximal pole. Male sex, high-energy mechanisms of injury, closed physes, and high body-mass index were associated with fractures of the waist or proximal pole. Treatment of acute fractures with casting alone resulted in a 90% union rate. Lower union rates were seen in association with the use of casting alone for the treatment of chronic fractures, displaced fractures, and proximal fractures. Longer time to union was seen in association with older fractures, displaced fractures, proximal fractures, and fractures in patients with osteonecrosis. The union rate following surgery was 96.5% (109 of 113). Increased time to union was seen in association with open physes, fracture displacement,

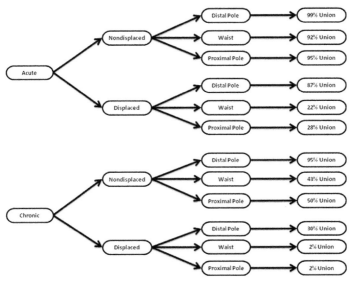

FIGURE 4.—Multivariate logistic regression based on maximum likelihood estimation was used to develop an algorithm for predicting the union rate with cast treatment. Displacement, more proximal location, and chronic presentation each decreased the probability of achieving union with casting. (Reprinted from Gholson JJ, Bae DS, Zurakowski D, et al. Scaphoid fractures in children and adolescents: contemporary injury patterns and factors influencing time to union. *J Bone Joint Surg Am.* 2011;93:1210-1219, with permission from the Journal of Bone and Joint Surgery, Incorporated.)

proximal fracture, the type of screw used for surgical fixation, and the use of bone graft at the time of surgery.

Discussion.—With changes in patient characteristics and activities, scaphoid fracture patterns in children and adolescents are now similar to the published patterns in adults. While 90% of acute nondisplaced fractures heal with nonoperative treatment, three months of cast immobilization or more may be required for more proximal injuries. Almost one-third of pediatric patients with scaphoid fractures will present late with chronic nonunions; in these instances, surgical reduction and internal fixation should be considered the primary treatment option (Fig 4).

▶ Scaphoid fractures in children have been thought to be less problematic than fractures in adults largely because of the historical assumption that most injuries occurred at the distal pole. The scaphoid is not completely ossified until about age 15, with ossification following vascularization in a distal-to-proximal direction. Open physes have also been thought to confer greater healing potential. This study highlights a trend in all pediatric fractures toward more adult-type injuries and adult-type complications. As expected, high union rates were seen with casting for nondisplaced fractures at all locations on the scaphoid. However, other than chronic nondisplaced distal pole fractures, union rates were poor in chronic fractures with casting alone. For those of us who have been treating pediatric scaphoid fractures as if they were adult injuries, these findings should come as no surprise. The rise in adult-type injuries in children and adolescents should be alarming to all of us who treat these injuries. The days of reflexive casting of most chronic pediatric scaphoid fractures[1] should be behind us.

D. A. Zlotolow, MD

Reference

1. Stanciu C, Dumont A. Changing patterns of scaphoid fractures in adolescents. *Can J Surg.* 1994;37:214-216.

Ununited Fracture of the Proximal Pole of the Scaphoid With Avascular Necrosis

Kakar S, Shin AY (Mayo Clinic, Rochester, MN)
J Hand Surg 36A:1522-1524, 2011

Background.—Avascular necrosis (AVN) of the proximal pole occurs in about 3% of all scaphoid fractures. Delay in diagnosis and treatment, proximal fracture, over 1 mm of displacement, and carpal malalignment may contribute to this complication. For proximal pole nonunions, vascular bone grafts are recommended, especially for those with osteonecrosis, but nonvascularized bone grafts are sometimes used.

Case Report.—Man, 25, had radial-sided wrist pain for 8 months after falling off a skateboard. The patient had tenderness of the anatomical snuffbox and discomfort with radial and ulnar deviation of the wrist. Radiographs, computed tomography (CT), and magnetic resonance imaging (MRI) revealed a nondisplaced nonunited fracture of the proximal pole of the scaphoid but no arthrosis. AVN was diagnosed.

Management Options.—Among the nonvascularized bone graft options to manage scaphoid nonunion are iliac crest bone grafts and distal radius bone grafts. High rates of union have been reported with corticocancellous iliac crest bone grafts in the excavated scaphoid. Lower success rates accompany the use of distal radius bone grafts.

Vascularized bone grafts for uniting the scaphoid include the 1,2 intercompartmental praretinacular artery (ICSRA). The presence of AVN is associated with a low rate of union, as is the presence of early arthritic changes, the performance of previous bone grafting procedures, and the presence of humpback deformity of the scaphoid and dorsal intercalated segment instability. Patients treated with a vascularized graft plus either a screw or Kirschner wire fixation have higher rates of union compared to those treated with a nonvascularized graft and screw fixation.

Conclusions.—The dorsal approach, with care taken to protect the 1,2 ICSRA, is preferred for patients with nondisplaced or minimally displaced proximal scaphoid nonunion with AVN of the proximal pole and no humpback deformity or carpal collapse. Fibrous tissue is curetted, with lack of punctate bleeding on tourniquet deflation indicating AVN. If there is no AVN, internal fixation can be used alone or with nonvascularized bone grafts. If AVN is present, the 1,2 ICSRA is fixed with a headless screw. Kirschner wires are used when the proximal pole cannot accommodate a screw. The 1,2 ICSRA graft is situated in a dorsal bony trough crossing the fracture site. The patient is immobilized in a long arm thumb spica cast for 6 weeks, then a short arm thumb spica cast is applied until union. Kirschner wires are not removed until union is verified by CT scan. Immobilization is continued for another month and a second CT scan done if union has not occurred after 12 weeks.

▶ This article represents an evidence-based medicine publication in the *Journal of Hand Surgery*. The authors attempt to answer whether vascularized bone grafting and open reduction with internal fixation are helpful in patients with a nondisplaced scaphoid nonunion and avascular necrosis of the proximal pole. Multiple studies have touted the benefits of nonvascularized bone grafts for the treatment of these injuries. The results appear to be fair when bone graft is harvested from the iliac crest or the distal radius.

Vascularized bone grafts have also been described to treat scaphoid nonunions, most commonly from the 1,2 intercompartmental supraretinacular artery (ICSRA). Again, the results appear to be fair and somewhat inconsistent depending on the series.

The authors correctly point out that our data to date consist of retrospective uncontrolled case series with short follow-up, inconsistent identification of nonunions, and heterogeneity in the method of internal fixation. Prospective, randomized, controlled trials with long-term follow-up are needed to determine the best approach to these vexing problems.

My approach to scaphoid nonunions is similar to that presented by the authors: Through a dorsal approach, the nonunion site is carefully curetted to remove all fibrous tissues. Once the tourniquet is deflated, punctate bleeding is assessed at the proximal pole of the scaphoid. With intact vascularity, scaphoid internal fixation is performed with cancellous bone graft harvested from the distal radius. Otherwise, I prefer to use the 1,2-ICSRA vascularized bone graft to supplement bone healing. A substantial trough needs to be made about the scaphoid's dorsal aspect and across the nonunion site to inset the vascularized bone graft.

E. K. Shin, MD

Scaphoid Excision and Midcarpal Arthrodesis: The Effect of Triquetral Excision—A Biomechanical Study

Cohen MS, Werner FW, Sutton LG, et al (Rush Univ Med Ctr, Chicago, IL; SUNY Upstate Med Univ, Syracuse, NY)

J Hand Surg 37A:493-499, 2012

Purpose.—To evaluate the biomechanical alterations that occur after traditional scaphoid excision and midcarpal arthrodesis with and without excision of the triquetrum. The hypothesis of this study was that removal of the triquetrum increases the radiolunate contact pressure.

Methods.—We cyclically moved 10 fresh cadaver wrists using a wrist joint motion simulator while measuring the contact pressures between the proximal carpal row and the distal radius and ulna using a dynamic pressure sensor. We acquired data in the intact wrist, after a midcarpal arthrodesis with the scaphoid excised, and then again with the triquetrum removed, which is also known as a capitolunate arthrodesis.

Results.—The peak pressures in the radiolunate fossa significantly increased with either of the midcarpal arthrodeses compared with the intact wrist during each of the 3 dynamic wrist motions. In comparing the 2 midcarpal arthrodeses, the peak pressure in the ulnocarpal fossa significantly decreased after the triquetrum was removed during wrist radioulnar deviation and in the static ulnarly deviated position. After arthrodesis, we could identify no differences during any motion or static wrist position in the peak radiolunate pressures with or without the triquetrum.

Conclusions.—We found that scaphoid excision and 4-corner arthrodesis shifts loads to the radiolunate joint. Isolated capitolunate arthrodesis with excision of the scaphoid and triquetrum further alters carpal kinematics and loading patterns.

Clinical Relevance.—These findings raise concern about routine excision of the triquetrum when performing a midcarpal arthrodesis.

▶ This article deals with an interesting topic. In 1935, Navarro described his column theory, subsequently modified by Taleisnik (1978): the carpal bones are arranged into 3 columns: (1) the central column (lunate, capitate, and hamate), (2) the lateral column (scaphoid, trapezium, and trapezoid), and (3) the medial or rotational column (triquetrum and pisiform).

Eliminating 1 or 2 of these columns will alter load bearing in the radiocarpal joint: One would assume that the load bearing would increase. Surprisingly, the results of this study do not show a difference in dynamic and static weight bearing in the lunate fossa when the triquetrum is excised after a 4-corner fusion. This outcome may be explained by the relative high standard deviation.

The dorsal capsule may have an important role in stabilizing the intrinsic and extrinsic intercarpal and radiocarpal ligaments. This was not reconstructed in this experiment and may influence the load bearing.

In the test setup, no mention is made on the position of the lunate or on whether a reduction of the position of the lunate had been done after excision of the scaphoid. It is not clear if the authors verified the position of the lunate in relation to the lunate fossa on PA in lateral views.

Each wrist served as its own control, avoiding variation between specimens.

The article does not end with a take-home message: What should we learn from this study? What should be done differently?

It would also be interesting to learn why the contact pressure was not higher as expected by the column theory and better understand the clinical observation that radio lunate osteoarthritis occurs after scaphoid and triquetrum excision. Weber (1980) described 2 columns: the load-bearing column (capitate, trapezoid, scaphoid, and lunate) and the control column (triquetrum and hamate). Of key importance is the helicoidal joint between the triquetrum and hamate. This contradicts with the findings in this article.

H. Coert, MD, PhD

Does scaphoid bone bruising lead to occult fracture? A prospective study of 50 patients
Thavarajah D, Syed T, Shah Y, et al (The Royal Berkshire Hosp, London road, UK; Peterborough and Stamford NHS Foundation Trust, UK; et al)
Injury 42:1303-1306, 2011

Introduction.—Bone bruising of the scaphoid is a term reported when magnetic resonance imaging (MRI) is carried out for scaphoid injury. The aim of our study was twofold: to see if bone bruising alone without fracture of the scaphoid bone seen on initial MRI, in a clinically symptomatic (tender) patient at 10–14 days, progressed to fracture, and to define how this entity of bone bruising should be managed.

Methods.—This was a prospective study looking at 170 patients with scaphoid injuries, of which 50 had bone bruising without fracture. These were followed up for at least 8 weeks to ascertain whether or not they had developed a fracture. They were assessed for continuity or resolution of their symptoms by way of clinical examination and/or a further MRI and X-ray (scaphoid views).

Results.—Of the 170 scaphoid injuries identified, there were 120 scaphoid fractures seen on scaphoid view radiographs. The remaining 50 were clinically symptomatic and had MRI scaphoid imaging, which demonstrated various grades of bone bruising. All were treated in a scaphoid plaster, and re-examined at 8 weeks. There were four patients who remained symptomatic, for whom MRI scans were performed, which revealed all four with resolving scaphoid bone bruising, and one with a scaphoid fracture (*p* value = 0.0386). Incidentally, 2 further weeks of immobilisation resolved the symptoms of those four patients. The one patient with a fracture was offered further treatment for the risk of progressing to a nonunion.

Conclusion.—Bone bruising detected on MRI without fracture is an important entity, and can lead to occult fracture (2%). It can take anywhere up to 8 weeks to declare. Treatment for bone bruising should be with a scaphoid cast and follow-up X-ray.

▶ MRI is frequently used as an evaluation tool in the setting of suspected scaphoid fractures. However, not infrequently, bony edema without overt fracture, or a "bone bruise," may be noted. The fate of this condition and the clinical implications are unknown. Currently, patients are most often offered immobilization and are followed over time. It is unclear, however, what the risk is of these "bone bruises" progressing to a fracture, and if immobilization, other than for comfort, is truly necessary.

The authors of this article report on the natural history of MRI "bone bruise." In this series, the authors followed patients who underwent MRI for suspected scaphoid fracture and who had bone bruise without fracture noted on MRI. Patients were immobilized then reexamined at 8 weeks. Only 4 of 54 were still symptomatic, and repeat MRI in those 4 revealed only 1 patient to have a scaphoid fracture. The remaining 3 patients were successfully treated with further immobilization of 2 weeks. Although the study does report on the natural history of the MRI diagnosis of "bone bruise" (ie, most heal uneventfully after a period of immobilization of 8 to 10 weeks, although there appears to be some risk of progression to fracture), it might have been more interesting if the study reevaluated the patients with repeat MRI at various time frames to determine when bone bruising resolves. Likewise, the duration of immobilization in this series was essentially the same as for an uncomplicated minimally displaced fracture diagnosed on plain films. It would be interesting to determine whether symptoms resolved in a majority of patients after some lesser period of immobilization, thus determining if it is safe to mobilize sooner.

J. Adams, MD

The total scaphoid titanium arthroplasty: A 15-year experience

Spingardi O, Rossello MI (Ospedale San Paolo, Savona, Italy)
Hand 6:179-184, 2011

Scaphoid nonunion followed by necrosis of bone segments is a common pathologic condition for the hand surgeon, and the difficulty of its management is well known. The total titanium scaphoid replacement, although not well-described in the literature, in our experience represents a reasonable choice in the treatment of this condition. Strict patient selection is necessary to achieve good clinical results. The titanium avoids the silicone synovitis, a well-described complication of silastic implants. Furthermore, this technique permits other surgical steps in case of failure (Table 1).

▶ One of the authors of this study (O.S.) was on the development team for Wright's titanium scaphoid implant and has since used it exclusively for select scaphoid nonunions. This article summarizes that 15-year experience. During that time, he placed 113 implants, but had a follow-up of more than 6 months (mean follow-up of 46 months) for only 75 patients (66%).

Patients chosen did not have arthritis or any signs of carpal collapse. Of note, the patients had failed prior conservative or surgical management of their scaphoid nonunions, including Matti-Russe grafting, screw fixation, or vascularized bone grafting.

The results for range of motion (ROM) and grip strength were similar to those found for proximal row carpectomy (PRC) or 4-corner fusion by Kiefhaber.[1] See Table 1. Overall, the patients were satisfied. The authors found that 5 of the 75 patients had mechanical failure (as defined by volar rotation of the implant and dorsal intercalated segment disability on plain films). However, only 2 patients were symptomatic enough to undergo reoperation. They did not note any problems related to the titanium implants, such as those seen in silicone implants (carpal resorption cysts or intolerance to the material). It is important to keep in mind, however, that 34% of the patients were lost to follow-up.

In general, scaphoid replacement seems like a reasonable alternative to PRC or a 4-corner fusion in the pre—scaphoid nonunion advanced collapse (SNAC) wrist that has failed vascularized bone grafting (VBG). In the ideal situation, a successful VBG maintains ROM of the wrist and grip strength in comparison with the contralateral side. In the article by Waitayawinyu et al,[2] the union rate was 93%. However, results from VBG are not always that successful. A meta-analysis found a union rate of 88% with VBG in the presence of avascular necrosis (AVN).[3] Chang et al,[4] in an article describing their experience with 50 patients

TABLE 1.—The Clinical Findings

	Excellent Results (20 pts)	Satisfactory Results (36 pts)	Poor Results (19 pts)
Active ROM	Extension 85° Flexion 80°	Extension 50° Flexion 60°	Extension ≤40° Flexion ≤40°
Grip strength	80–95%	60–80%	≤60%

using the 1, 2-intercompartmental supraretinacular artery grafts for SNAC, concluded that the graft might not be ideal for women, smokers, patients with humpback deformity, or those with AVN of the proximal pole. The replacement would obviate the need for healing of bone in the presence of AVN or for the smoker. The use of the replacement in this setting makes more sense than the original use of the implant as described by Swanson et al[5] in their 1997 article, which described their 10-year experience with 102 titanium scaphoid implants. In this study, the criteria included an early scapholunate advanced collapse wrist, and the investigators performed a concomitant partial wrist fusion in 41% of the patients. The benefit of the implant in those cases is not clear. The ultimate ROM in the study by Swanson et al is the same as that for a salvage procedure, bringing to question the benefit of adding an artificial scaphoid to the procedure.

As the authors of this article state, the procedure in this setting does not "burn any bridges," and a salvage procedure can always be performed if the arthroplasty fails. That being said, it is a small study and the follow-up was not great. Before I would incorporate this in my practice, I would want to see a larger study with better follow-up.

J. Frankenhoff, MD

References

1. Kiefhaber TR. Management of scapholunate advanced collapse pattern of degenerative arthritis of the wrist. *J Hand Surg.* 2009;34A:1527-1530.
2. Waitayawinyu T, McCallister WV, Katolik LI, Schlenker JD, Trumble TE. Outcome after vascularized bone grafting of scaphoid nonunions with avascular necrosis. *J Hand Surg Am.* 2009;34:387-394.
3. Merrell GA, Wolfe SW, Slade JF III. Treatment of scaphoid nonunions: quantitative meta-analysis of the literature. *J Hand Surg Am.* 2002;27:685-691.
4. Chang MA, Bishop AT, Moran SL, Shin AY. The outcomes and complications of 1,2-intercompartmental supraretinacular artery pedicled vascularized bone grafting of scaphoid nonunions. *J Hand Surg.* 2006;31A:387-396.
5. Swanson AB, de Groot Swanson G, DeHeer DH, et al. Carpal bone titanium implant arthroplasty 10 years' experience. *Clin Orthop Relat Res.* 1997;342:46-58.

A Comparison of 2 Methods for Scaphoid Central Screw Placement From a Volar Approach

Meermans G, Verstreken F (Monica Hosp, Deurne, Belgium)
J Hand Surg 36A:1669-1674, 2011

Purpose.—We studied 2 methods used for screw placement through a volar approach for fixation of scaphoid fractures.

Methods.—We performed measurements on 20 computed tomography scans of unfractured scaphoids. A central virtual guidewire was computed in 10 scaphoids with the wrist in neutral or in extension and ulnar deviation. Second, we compared the central guidewire and a guidewire representing a volar approach to the scaphoid avoiding the trapezium.

Results.—The central guidewire passed through the trapezium in all cases with the wrist either in neutral or in extension and ulnar deviation. There was a statistically significant difference only in the sagittal plane.

When the central guidewire was compared with a guidewire placed through a standard volar approach, the latter was more eccentric in the distal and waist portions.

Conclusions.—We showed that central placement throughout the scaphoid with a standard volar approach is not feasible without partially resecting, manipulating, or drilling through the trapezium.

Clinical Relevance.—Our data suggest that a volar transtrapezial approach can be an alternative for optimum central placement in volar percutaneous fixation of scaphoid fractures.

▶ The authors use computed tomography scans of healthy wrists to investigate the ideal placement of compression screws from a volar approach. They find that perfect alignment of the screw is not possible without considerable manipulation of the trapezium. Although the authors choose a rather theoretical approach, I found this article very interesting. Even if the authors' findings may not have a direct impact on clinical practice, this study highlights that minimally invasive scaphoid surgery is not trivial but may be very challenging even for the experienced surgeon. As the authors point out, it should be kept in mind that conservative treatment is a valid treatment option for scaphoid fractures and may even be superior to surgery in selected cases. Suboptimal screw alignment probably may be tolerated to a certain extent if good reduction and adequate compression is achieved.

K. Megerle, MD

Displaced fracture of the waist of the scaphoid
Dias JJ, Singh HP (Univ Hosps of Leicester NHS Trust, UK)
J Bone Joint Surg Br 93-B:1433-1439, 2011

A displaced fracture of the scaphoid is one in which the fragments have moved from their anatomical position or there is movement between them when stressed by physiological loads. Displacement is seen in about 20% of fractures of the waist of the scaphoid, as shown by translation, a gap, angulation or rotation. A CT scan in the true longitudinal axis of the scaphoid demonstrates the shape of the bone and displacement of the fracture more accurately than do plain radiographs. Displaced fractures can be treated in a plaster cast, accepting the risk of malunion and nonunion. Surgically the displacement can be reduced, checked radiologically, arthroscopically or visually, and stabilised with headless screws or wires. However, rates of union and deformity are unknown. Mild malunion is well tolerated, but the long-term outcome of a displaced fracture that healed in malalignment has not been established.

This paper summarises aspects of the assessment, treatment and outcome of displaced fractures of the waist of the scaphoid.

▶ This is an outstanding review focusing on the current treatment of displaced scaphoid fractures. The authors have done an excellent job summarizing some of the most important aspects that need to be considered when dealing with these injuries. After some years of very aggressive surgical treatment, conservative management seems now to be emerging again as a valuable and sometimes even superior treatment option. The authors provide a great overview of the available evidence for both options. In addition, they provide some interesting technical tips for reducing displaced fractures.

I agree with the authors that a preoperative computed tomography scan in the true longitudinal axis of the scaphoid is the most important imaging study when choosing the correct treatment strategy for the individual patient. In my opinion, it should be performed in all patients with scaphoid fractures, but especially for those for whom conservative treatment is considered. Displaced or comminuted, that is, unstable fractures, usually require operative management, because the contact area between the 2 fragments is often too small for robust healing to occur. Intraoperatively, correction of excessive dorsal rotation of the lunate is a very important radiographic sign that helps to confirm correct reduction.

I recommend this article not only to all residents, but also experienced surgeons interested in scaphoid fracture care.

K. Megerle, MD

A Comparison of 2 Methods for Scaphoid Central Screw Placement From a Volar Approach
Meermans G, Verstreken F (Monica Hosp, Deurne, Belgium)
J Hand Surg 36A:1669-1674, 2011

Purpose.—We studied 2 methods used for screw placement through a volar approach for fixation of scaphoid fractures.

Methods.—We performed measurements on 20 computed tomography scans of unfractured scaphoids. A central virtual guidewire was computed in 10 scaphoids with the wrist in neutral or in extension and ulnar deviation. Second, we compared the central guidewire and a guidewire representing a volar approach to the scaphoid avoiding the trapezium.

Results.—The central guidewire passed through the trapezium in all cases with the wrist either in neutral or in extension and ulnar deviation. There was a statistically significant difference only in the sagittal plane. When the central guidewire was compared with a guidewire placed through a standard volar approach, the latter was more eccentric in the distal and waist portions.

Conclusions.—We showed that central placement throughout the scaphoid with a standard volar approach is not feasible without partially resecting, manipulating, or drilling through the trapezium.

Clinical Relevance.—Our data suggest that a volar transtrapezial approach can be an alternative for optimum central placement in volar percutaneous fixation of scaphoid fractures.

▶ This is a well-performed and well-written study that should guide surgeons' treatment of scaphoid fractures.

As many previous studies have documented, it is critical to place the screw as centrally as possible to achieve maximum fracture fixation and minimize the risk of screw failure. In my experience, as this study clearly demonstrates, volarly placed screws tend to be volar to the central axis, both distally and at the scaphoid waist. This may lead to nonunion and/or screw failure.

The data using a virtually placed K-wire transtrapezially along the central axis of the scaphoid reveals that the central axis can be accurately and reliably achieved with this method. I have no experience with this but am concerned about the significant iatrogenic injury imparted to the scaphotrapezial (ST) joint using this technique.

Using a volar approach, to place the guide as dorsal as possible in the distal scaphoid, the trapezium must be partially resected or displaced dorsally. This study determined that an average of 5 to 6 mm of volar trapezium (in the sagittal plane) must be excised to reach the central axis of the distal pole. Conceptually, this seems like an excessive amount of bone resection that may lead to ST joint instability or premature ST joint arthritis.

Given these concerns, I prefer to place screws dorsally (either percutaneously or open) in all proximal pole fractures and most scaphoid waist fractures. I am certain that I am able to place a screw along the central axis using a dorsal approach.

The major weakness of this study, as the authors point out, is that there are no clinical or biomechanical data to demonstrate differences between central and eccentric screws at the scaphoid waist and distal pole (prior studies have focused on proximal pole screw location only).

L. W. Catalano III, MD

A biomechanical study on variation of compressive force along the Acutrak 2 screw
Sugathan HK, Kilpatrick M, Joyce TJ, et al (Queen Elizabeth Hosp, Gateshead, UK; Newcastle Univ, Newcastle upon Tyne, UK)
Injury 43:205-208, 2012

Introduction.—Acutrak 2 screws are commonly used for scaphoid fracture fixation. To our knowledge, the variation in compressive force along the screw has not been investigated before. The objectives of our study were to measure variance in compression along the length of the standard Acutrak 2 screw, to identify the region of the screw which produces the greatest compression and to discuss the clinical relevance of this to the placement of the screw for scaphoid fractures.

Materials and Methods.—A laboratory model was set up to test the compressive force at 2 mm intervals along the screw, using solid polyurethane foam (Sawbone) blocks of varying width. The Acutrak 2 screws were introduced in the standard method. Forces were measured using a custom-made load cell washer introduced between the Sawbone blocks and were plotted as a graph along the whole length of the screw.

Results.—Maximum compression was at the mid-point of the screw. Overall compressive forces were higher in the proximal half of the screw by 19% when compared with the distal half. Minimum compression was seen at 4 mm or less from either end of the screw.

Conclusions.—There is variation in compression along the length of the standard Acutrak 2 screw and the maximum compression was obtained at the mid-point of the screw. From this study, we would recommend when using an Acutrak 2 screw for internal fixation of scaphoid fractures, to attain maximum compressive force, place the fracture at the mid-point of the Acutrak screw. If this is not possible, then place the fracture towards the proximal half of the screw.

▶ The authors designed and performed a well thought-out study to evaluate the compressive properties of the Acutrak 2 screw. These independent studies are important to validate the claims of companies about their products. The protocol can be easily used to study other headless compression screws, and I would encourage authors to do so. These authors make some valuable recommendations, including placing the fracture at the midpoint of the screw or, if not possible, to place it closer to the proximal half of the screw. Furthermore, the minimum compressive force is seen for bone fragments of 4 mm or less. These recommendations have clinical significance to surgeons and add important information to orthopedics.

P. Tang, MD, MPH

Modified Carpal Stretch Test as a Screening Test for Detection of Scapholunate Interosseous Ligament Injuries Associated with Distal Radial Fractures

Kwon BC, Choi S-J, Song S-Y, et al (Hallym Univ Sacred Heart Hosp, Gyeonggi-do, South Korea)
J Bone Joint Surg Am 93:855-862, 2011

Background.—Intra-articular distal radial fractures are frequently accompanied by a scapholunate interosseous ligament injury, which may adversely affect the outcomes. Arthroscopy may not be appropriate as a first-line evaluation method to diagnose these injuries because of time, expense, and availability issues. The purpose of this study was to evaluate the effectiveness of the modified carpal stretch test for screening for scapholunate interosseous ligament injuries in patients with an intra-articular distal radial fracture.

Methods.—The carpal stretch test is a radiographic evaluation in which disruption of the smooth arc of the proximal carpal row joint line indicates a lack of integrity of the scapholunate interosseous ligament. We modified the original carpal stretch test and prospectively performed the modified test on forty-eight patients with a total of forty-nine unstable intraarticular distal radial fractures. With the patient under anesthesia, the injured wrist was evaluated with the modified carpal stretch test with fluoroscopy. The wrist was then examined arthroscopically to classify the scapholunate interosseous ligament injury. Three observers independently determined whether there was disruption of the proximal carpal row joint line (Gilula's arc II), used as an indicator of a grade-III or IV scapholunate interosseous ligament tear, on fluoroscopic images. The fluoroscopic results were compared with the arthroscopic findings.

Results.—The average sensitivity of the modified carpal stretch test was 78%, the average specificity was 72%, the average positive predictive value was 60%, the average negative predictive value was 87%, and the average accuracy was 74%. The intraclass correlation coefficient (ICC) for interobserver agreement was 0.73, and the ICCs for intraobserver agreement were 0.86, 0.68, and 0.84 for the three observers.

Conclusions.—The modified carpal stretch test was useful to rule out grade-III or IV scapholunate interosseous ligament tears associated with intra-articular distal radial fractures, but it was not as useful to confirm the presence of a tear. This test may reduce the necessity for arthroscopic assessment to identify scapholunate interosseous ligament injuries following distal radial fractures and may improve the rates of detection of important carpal ligament injuries accompanying intra-articular distal radial fractures.

▶ The authors of this study tested whether the carpal stretch test (radiographic disruption of the proximal carpal row with wrist distraction) was a reliable indicator of scapholunate injury following distal radius fractures. Patients with intra-articular injuries who met operative criteria were prospectively enrolled and underwent the stretch test under anesthesia on the injured and uninjured extremity. All patients subsequently underwent wrist arthroscopy. The test had a sensitivity of 78% and a specificity of 72% in detecting grade III or IV scapholunate injuries. The average positive predictive value was 60%, the average negative predictive value was 87%, and the average accuracy was 74%. The test is therefore most useful in ruling out a scapholunate injury in the presence of a distal radius fracture.

The advantage of the described stretch test is that it is inexpensive and easy to perform in the operating room. Its limitations, however, lie in that measurements are subjective and the amount of traction applied can be difficult to standardize. Furthermore, we have limited information as to which scapholunate injuries require treatment in the setting of a distal radius fracture and, perhaps more importantly, what the optimal treatment method should be. As such, the authors' conclusion that the stretch test should be used as a screening tool to determine which patients require arthroscopy for assessment and treatment of ligamentous injuries should be interpreted with caution.

T. D. Rozental, MD

Delays and Poor Management of Scaphoid Fractures: Factors Contributing to Nonunion

Wong K, von Schroeder HP (Univ of Toronto Hand Program, Ontario, Canada)
J Hand Surg 36A:1471-1474, 2011

Purpose.—Scaphoid fracture nonunion remains prevalent, and it was our purpose to examine the initial care, fracture site, and patient gender and age to determine factors contributing to fracture nonunion.

Methods.—The charts of 96 consecutive patients with 99 scaphoid fracture nonunions were reviewed for demographic information, and contact was made with 85 patients (with 88 scaphoid nonunions) to determine the pattern of presentation and initial treatment, if any.

Results.—Of the 88 scaphoid nonunions, 78 were in men, and 46 were sports injuries; 7 patients had no recollection of an injury. Twenty were proximal pole fractures. For 57 fractures, patients sought care following their injury, but only 42 were diagnosed with scaphoid fractures and received appropriate treatment, although one did not follow up in the clinic. Fifteen patients with nonunions did not receive radiographic investigations or did not have an identifiable fracture on initial x-rays and received no further follow-up or treatment. For 27 nonunions, medical attention was sought but was delayed, with an average time of 57 days between injury and initial assessment. For 31 fractures, medical attention was not sought for the acute injury but presented later following a re-injury (17 nonunions) or with progressive pain or stiffness (13 nonunions).

Conclusions.—The high rates of delayed presentation and incomplete evaluation and treatment suggest a strong need for better patient and doctor education on the subject of scaphoid injuries and nonunions particularly because the initial injury is, unfortunately, sometimes perceived as trivial. Nonunions do occur despite appropriate immobilization. Proximal pole fractures and fractures that show inadequate progression toward union while being treated in a cast should be considered for surgical intervention based on the high number of such cases identified in this study.

▶ The retrospective review of scaphoid nonunions does provide some epidemiologic insight to the etiology of scaphoid nonunion. There is still, as of 2004 when this study started collecting patients, a need for better vigilance in diagnosing scaphoid fractures. It will be hard to effect a change in the group of patients that don't seek medical care (∼35%). However, for those that sought attention, 15 (17%) fell through the cracks by either not having radiographs taken or by not being treated clinically for the injury with appropriate splinting and follow-up.

Perhaps as disturbing, and not commented on during the discussion, are the 42 nonunions that were diagnosed and treated appropriately. That means that still close to half of the nonunions studied were immobilized appropriately and didn't heal. Even with extreme vigilance, this group cannot be eliminated completely. Of course, there is no denominator in this study (how many other scaphoid fractures were diagnosed and treated successfully), and that information would have been more useful looking at the group that did receive appropriate care.

In my practice I speak to patients of being aggressive in the diagnosis, not the treatment of scaphoid fractures. This includes short-term immobilization when needed or additional studies (magnetic resonance imaging) to confirm or rule out the suspected. I do feel the rate of union for nondisplaced, difficult-to-diagnose scaphoid fractures is relatively low when treated early, and so the most important step is to avoid missing the diagnosis initially.

T. Hughes, MD

Gadolinium-enhanced preoperative MRI scans as a prognostic parameter in scaphoid nonunion
Megerle K, Worg H, Christopoulos G, et al (Inst for Diagnostic and Interventional Radiology Bad Neustadt/Saale and Handcenter Ravensburg Germany)
J Hand Surg Eur Vol 36E:23-28, 2011

The purpose of this prospective study was to correlate preoperative gadolinium-enhanced MRI scans with intraoperative bleeding of the proximal fragment and postoperative union in a series of consecutive patients with established scaphoid nonunions. In 60 patients (6 females, 54 males) with a mean age of 29 years, scaphoid perfusion was judged preoperatively as normal, impaired or absent using a gadolinium-enhanced MRI scan. Scaphoid reconstruction was performed using a nonvascularized bone graft and screw fixation. Perfusion of the proximal fragment was assessed intraoperatively in 49 of 60 patients; compromised or absent vascularity was predicted with a specificity of 90% by contrast-enhanced MRI. However, there was no significant correlation between preoperative MRI assessment of vascularity and subsequent union of the scaphoid.

▶ The authors of this study have used contrast-enhanced preoperative MRI scans to assess vascularity of the proximal pole in scaphoid fractures, as determined by intraoperative bleeding, and to determine if this correlates to postoperative union. They provide data on two difficult clinical problems: preoperative determination of decreased perfusion or avascular necrosis of the proximal pole in scaphoid nonunions and whether scaphoids with decreased or absent perfusion can heal with nonvascularized bone grafts.

They present data of 60 of 95 eligible patients over a 3-year period at least 6 months following injury. MRI classification was normal, and impaired or absent perfusion to the proximal pole and intraoperative assessment of bleeding was completed in 49 of 60 wrists. Perfusion based on MRI scans was read as impaired in 15 wrists and absent in 11 wrists. When compared to clinical bleeding, MRI scans were found to have high specificity (0.9) and low sensitivity (0.7).

Fifty-four of 60 scaphoids healed with nonvascularized bone grafting and compression screw, but 4 of 6 nonunions showed decreased or absent perfusion on preoperative MRI. Proximal pole fractures and absence of clinical bleeding were statistically significant for persistent nonunion.

These authors did not describe the strength of the magnet or whether a dedicated wrist coil was used, but this study still provides useful information. In addition, it demonstrated that decreased perfusion of wrist fractures can heal with nonvascularized bone grafts. The decision on the use of vascularized bone grafts is still controversial.

W. Hammert, MD

11 Distal Radius

Complications of Low-Profile Dorsal Versus Volar Locking Plates in the Distal Radius: A Comparative Study
Yu YR, Makhni MC, Tabrizi S, et al (Beth Israel Deaconess Med Ctr and the Harvard Med School, Boston, MA)
J Hand Surg 36A:1135-1141, 2011

Purpose.—Dorsal plating of distal radius fractures with traditional 2.5-mm-thick plates is associated with extensor tendon complications. Consequently, volar locking plates have gained widespread acceptance. A new generation of 1.2- to 1.5-mm, low-profile dorsal plates was designed to minimize tendon irritation. This study examines the complication rates of low-profile dorsal plates compared with volar locking plates.

Methods.—We identified patients with distal radius fractures treated between September 2002 and June 2006 by low-profile dorsal or volar locking plates. Information pertaining to 7 categories of complications (hardware discomfort and pain, tendon irritation/rupture, failure of reduction, infection, complex regional pain syndrome, stiffness, and neuropathy/hypersensitivity) was collected. Complications were defined as any postoperative plating complications requiring additional surgical intervention, whereas those that only caused patient discomfort were considered secondary problems.

Results.—We included 100 patients, comprising 104 plating cases (57 dorsal, 47 volar), in this study. Overall length of follow-up was 44 ± 21 months (range, 12–80 mo). A total of 18 patients (8 dorsal, 10 volar) experienced complications, whereas 47 (25 dorsal, 22 volar) had secondary reports. Three dorsal and 4 volar patients had complete plate removals. Three dorsal and no volar plates had screw removals only. One volar plate (no dorsal plates) had a major tendon rupture (flexor pollicis longus); 3 dorsal and 3 volar plates resulted in tendon irritation complications, and 4 dorsal and 3 volar plates had secondary problems from tendon irritation. None of the above measures approached statistical significance. Volar cases were associated with significantly more neuropathic complications than dorsal cases.

Conclusions.—Dorsal low-profile plates are not associated with significantly more tendon irritation or rupture complications. However, volar plating is associated with a higher rate of neuropathic complications.

Type of Study/Level of Evidence.—Therapeutic III.

▶ The pendulum right now swings to the end favoring volar locked plating for fixation of all unstable distal radius fractures. The technique is so familiar to our residents; an external fixator is so foreign. Even less familiar are dorsal plates, and this single-institution study debunks some of the myths associated with them. A lower profile dorsal plating system had fewer serious complications. Tendon irritation was similar in both groups; the one tendon rupture was associated with a volar plate. All neurologic complications requiring intervention (3 carpal tunnel releases and 1 ulnar tunnel release) occurred in the volar plate group. This study supports those who favor the pendulum's swing toward versatile options, including dorsal plating and less invasive techniques that match the severity and fracture pattern, as well as the comfort level of the surgeon.

A. Ladd, MD

Trends in Wrist Fractures in Children and Adolescents, 1997–2009
de Putter CE, van Beeck EF, Looman CWN, et al (Erasmus MC Rotterdam, The Netherlands; Consumer Safety Inst, Amsterdam, The Netherlands)
J Hand Surg 36A:1810-1815, 2011

Purpose.—Distal radius and carpal fractures in children and adolescents represent approximately 25% of all pediatric fractures. Incidence rates and causes of these fractures change over time owing to changes in activities and risk factors. The purpose of this study was to examine recent population-based trends in incidence and causes of wrist fractures in children and adolescents.

Methods.—We obtained data from the Dutch Injury Surveillance System of emergency department visits of 15 geographically distributed hospitals, and from the National Hospital Discharge Registry. This included a representative sample of outpatients and inpatients, respectively. We calculated incidence rates of wrist fractures per 100,000 person-years for each year between 1997 and 2009. Using Poisson's regression, we analyzed trends for children and adolescents 5 to 9, 10 to 14, and 15 to 19 years of age separately for boys and girls.

Results.—During the study period, incidence rates increased significantly in boys and girls 5 to 9 and 10 to 14 years of age, with the strongest increase in the age group 10 to 14 years. The observed increases were mainly due to increased incidence rates during soccer and gymnastics at school.

Conclusions.—This population-based study revealed a substantial sports-related increase in the incidence rate of wrist fractures in boys and girls aged 5 to 9 and 10 to 14 years in the period 1997 to 2009 (Figs 1 and 2).

▶ Because this is a population-based study that examined 12% of the population of The Netherlands, the trends the authors witnessed may not be found elsewhere. They saw a rise in injuries from soccer and school gymnastics and an overall rise in sports-related injuries in children aged 5 to 14 (Figs 1 and 2). Nonetheless, their data may represent changing activity levels in that population that may also be occurring in the United States. Many of today's children participate in competitive sports at a younger age, while at the same time others increasingly participate in

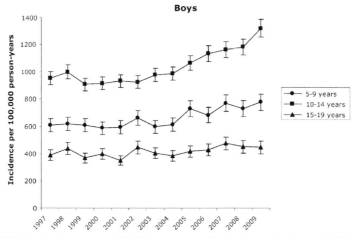

FIGURE 1.—Incidence rate (per 100,000 person-years) of wrist fractures in the period 1997 to 2009, for boys aged 5 to 9, 10 to 14 and 15 to 19 years; error bars indicate 95% confidence intervals. (Reprinted from de Putter CE, van Beeck EF, Looman CWN, et al. Trends in wrist fractures in children and adolescents, 1997–2009. *J Hand Surg.* 2011;36A:1810-1815, with permission from the American Society for Surgery of the Hand.)

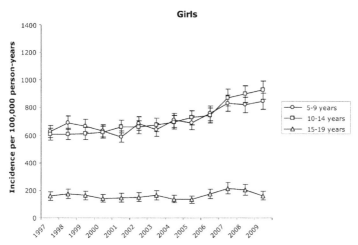

FIGURE 2.—Incidence rate (per 100,000 person-years) of wrist fractures in the period 1997 to 2009, for girls aged 5 to 9, 10 to 14, and 15 to 19 years; error bars indicate 95% confidence intervals. (Reprinted from de Putter CE, van Beeck EF, Looman CWN, et al. Trends in wrist fractures in children and adolescents, 1997–2009. *J Hand Surg.* 2011;36A:1810-1815, Copyright 2011, with permission from the American Society for Surgery of the Hand.)

sedentary activities such as television or video games. Our children may be becoming weekend warriors, with similar consequences as those found in adults.

D. A. Zlotolow, MD

The Effect of Distal Radius Locking Plates on Articular Contact Pressures

Walker MH, Kim H, Hsieh AH, et al (Univ of Maryland, Baltimore; Univ of Maryland, College Park; Univ of Maryland School of Medicine, Baltimore)
J Hand Surg 36A:1303-1309, 2011

Purpose.—Fractures of the distal radius are among the most common injuries treated in hand surgery practice, and distal radius locking plates have become an increasingly popular method of fixation. Despite widespread use of this technology, it is unknown whether the subchondral placement of locking screws affects the loading profile of the distal radius. Our study was designed to determine whether subchondral locking screws change the articular contact pressures in the distal radius.

Methods.—Twelve cadaveric forearms underwent a previously described axial loading protocol in a materials testing machine. We used an intra-articular, real-time computerized force sensor to measure peak contact pressure, total pressure, and contact area in the distal radius. Internal validation of sensor placement and reproducibility was conducted. Each specimen was tested before fixation (control), after application of a palmar distal radius locking plate, and after simulation of a metaphyseal fracture.

Results.—We identified no statistically significant differences in maximum pressure, total pressure, and contact area among control, plated, and plated and fractured specimens. However, the contact footprint—represented by squared differences in force across the sensor—were significantly different between the control group and both plated groups.

Conclusions.—The technique for measuring contact pressures produces highly repeatable values. Distal radius locking plates with subchondral hardware placement do not seem to significantly change articular contact pressures.

Clinical Relevance.—Although locking screws placed in subchondral bone of the distal radius for fracture fixation may alter the stress distribution across the radiocarpal joint, we found no evidence that peak stresses across the joint were changed. Therefore, it seems unlikely that periarticular locking screws contribute to long-term arthrosis after fixation of extra-articular distal radius fractures.

▶ The mechanical effects of placement of subchondral screws have been suggested as a possible cause of articular degeneration. The concern arises because the stiffness of metallic screws differs markedly from that of subchondral bone and articular cartilage. Charlton et al[1] found that in the tibiotalar joint, marked increases in forces were seen directly over locked implants. As distal radius volar locking plates are among the most commonly implanted locking fracture fixation devices,[2] a comparable phenomenon in the wrist would argue for hardware removal when required and against placing subchondral locking implants in general.

Walker et al investigated this concern with 12 cadaver specimens with digital pressure sensors applied to intact specimens, after a Synthes volar locking plate was applied and with a simulated extra-articular fracture. An attempt was made to place the implants within 2 mm of subchondral bone as has been shown to lead to more stable constructs in vitro. The only significant difference found was between the fracture model and the plated but intact bone specimen. Presumably in the clinical situation, this difference is transient (over a matter of weeks as the fracture unites).

Degenerative changes in patients after distal radius fractures are a significant concern, and the current conventional wisdom is that operative reduction decreases the incidence of this problem. Given the concern raised regarding locking implants, which have revolutionized the treatment of distal radius fractures, the finding that pressures were only likely to be transiently changed is comforting. Our community can continue to try and investigate and solve the other causes of articular degeneration following distal radius fractures, including articular step and gaps, ligament injury, carpal instability, and direct chondral injury.

P. Blazar, MD

References

1. Charlton M, Costello R, Mooney JF, Podeszwa DA. Ankle joint biomechanics following transepiphyseal screw fixation of the distal tibia. *J Pediatr Orthop.* 2005;25:635-640.
2. Drobetz H, Bryant AL, Pokorny T, Spitaler R, Leixnering M, Jupiter JB. Volar fixed-angle plating of distal radius extension fractures: influence of plate position on secondary loss of reduction—a biomechanic study in a cadaveric model. *J Hand Surg.* 2006;31A:615-622.

Variations in the Use of Internal Fixation for Distal Radial Fracture in the United States Medicare Population

Chung KC, Shauver MJ, Yin H, et al (Univ of Michigan, Ann Arbor)
J Bone Joint Surg Am 93:2154-2162, 2011

Background.—Distal radial fractures affect an estimated 80,000 elderly Americans each year. Although the use of internal fixation for the treatment of distal radial fractures is becoming increasingly common, there have been no population-based studies to explore the dissemination of this technique. The aims of our study were to determine the current use of internal fixation for the treatment of distal radial fractures in the Medicare population and to examine regional variations and other factors that influence use of this treatment. We hypothesized that internal fixation of distal radial fractures would be used less commonly in male and black populations compared with other populations because the prevalence of osteoporosis is lower in these populations, and that use of internal fixation would be correlated with the percentage of the patients who were treated by a hand surgeon in a particular region.

Methods.—We performed an analysis of complete 2007 Medicare data to determine the percentage of distal radial fractures that were treated with internal fixation in each hospital referral region. We then analyzed the association of patient and physician factors with the type of fracture treatment received, both nationally and within each hospital referral region.

Results.—We identified 85,924 Medicare beneficiaries with a closed distal radial fracture who met the inclusion criteria, and 17.0% of these patients were treated with internal fixation. Fractures were significantly less likely to be treated with internal fixation in men than in women (odds ratio, 0.84; 95% confidence interval, 0.80 to 0.89) and in black patients than in white patients (odds ratio, 0.74; 95% confidence interval, 0.65 to 0.85). Patients were more likely to be treated with internal fixation rather than with another treatment if they were treated by a hand surgeon than if they were treated by an orthopaedic surgeon who was not a hand surgeon (odds ratio, 2.49; 95% confidence interval, 2.29 to 2.70). Use of internal fixation ranged from 4.6% to 42.1% (nearly a ten-fold difference) among hospital referral regions. The percentage of patients treated with internal fixation within a hospital referral region was positively correlated with the percentage of patients in that region who were treated by a hand surgeon (correlation coefficient, 0.34; p < 0.0001).

Conclusions.—The use of internal fixation for the treatment of a distal radial fracture differs widely among geographical regions and patient populations. Such variations highlight the need for improved comparative-effectiveness data to guide the treatment of this fracture.

▶ This article investigates the treatment of distal radius fractures in elderly Americans using the Medicare database from 2007. More than 85 000 distal radius fractures were found and internal fixation was used as the treatment for 17% of this group. Variation in the use of internal fixation was noted by region, and patients treated by hand surgeons were more likely to be treated with internal fixation. The use of internal fixation was also noted to be higher in women compared with men, and white patients compared with black patients.

This study clearly demonstrates in a large population that among other trends in treatment of distal radius fractures previously documented by Chung et al, patients treated by hand surgeons were more likely to receive internal fixation. Although thought-provoking, this is not an unexpected finding. The authors point out that hand surgeons may be referred the more complex fracture patterns, likely for their expertise in the use of newer techniques of internal fixation. Furthermore, the phenomenon of differently trained surgeons treating the same condition with different techniques is not unexpected and has been documented for decades.[1] Specific to distal radius fractures, the advent of fragment-specific fixation and distal radius locking plates have been discussed extensively in the hand surgery community, and much of the literature is written by self-described hand surgeons. Using the references specifically related to distal radius fractures from this article, by my count 10 of 12 articles are authored by hand surgeons.

The question of whether the increased use of internal fixation results in superior outcomes for patients in this population remains unanswered. There is clearly some additional cost to the use of internal fixation, and in the absence of comparative outcomes data that address this issue, it is likely that providers will be subject to the criticism of adopting more expensive, newer technology without documented improvement for patients. This issue can clearly only be resolved by additional high-quality studies specifically addressing the issue of distal radius fractures in this population.

P. Blazar, MD

Reference

1. Irwin ZN, Hilibrand A, Gustavel M, et al. Variation in surgical decision making for degenerative spinal disorders. Part I: lumbar spine. *Spine (Phila Pa 1976)*. 2005;30:2208-2213.

A Prospective Randomized Trial Comparing Nonoperative Treatment with Volar Locking Plate Fixation for Displaced and Unstable Distal Radial Fractures in Patients Sixty-five Years of Age and Older
Arora R, Lutz M, Deml C, et al (Med Univ Innsbruck, Austria)
J Bone Joint Surg Am 93:2146-2153, 2011

Background.—Despite the recent trend toward the internal fixation of distal radial fractures in older patients, the currently available literature lacks adequate randomized trials examining whether open reduction and internal fixation (ORIF) with a volar locking plate is superior to nonoperative (cast) treatment. The purpose of the present randomized clinical trial was to compare the outcomes of two methods that were used for the treatment of displaced and unstable distal radial fractures in patients sixty-five years of age or older: (1) ORIF with use of a volar locking plate and (2) closed reduction and plaster immobilization (casting).

Methods.—A prospective randomized study was performed. Seventy-three patients with a displaced and unstable distal radial fracture were randomized to ORIF with a volar locking plate (n = 36) or closed reduction and cast immobilization (n = 37). The outcome was measured on the basis of the Patient-Rated Wrist Evaluation (PRWE) score; the Disabilities of the Arm, Shoulder and Hand (DASH) score; the pain level; the range of wrist motion; the rate of complications; and radiographic measurements including dorsal radial tilt, radial inclination, and ulnar variance.

Results.—There were no significant differences between the groups in terms of the range of motion or the level of pain during the entire follow-up period (p > 0.05). Patients in the operative treatment group had lower DASH and PRWE scores, indicating better wrist function, in the early postoperative time period (p < 0.05), but there were no significant differences between the groups at six and twelve months. Grip strength was significantly better at all times in the operative treatment group (p < 0.05). Dorsal radial tilt, radial inclination, and radial shortening were significantly better in the operative treatment group than in the nonoperative treatment group at the time of the latest follow-up (p < 0.05). The number of complications was significantly higher in the operative treatment group (thirteen compared with five, p < 0.05).

Conclusions.—At the twelve-month follow-up examination, the range of motion, the level of pain, and the PRWE and DASH scores were not different between the operative and nonoperative treatment groups. Patients in the operative treatment group had better grip strength through the entire time period. Achieving anatomical reconstruction did not convey any improvement in terms of the range of motion or the ability to perform daily living activities in our cohorts.

▶ As surgeons, we generally offer surgery to our patients so they can achieve the best outcomes; however, this study reports there is no evidence to suggest that operative fixation of distal radius fractures in patients aged 65 years and more achieves this. In this study, the operative group had a higher complication rate without any significant long-term advantages in pain resolution, function, or cosmesis. The authors should be commended on conducting a high-quality, randomized controlled trial on such a relevant topic. They used valid outcome measures and had an appropriate sample size and low dropout rate. The results of this study force us to reflect on our management of distal radius fractures in this age group. The indications for open reduction and internal fixation (ORIF) of distal radius fractures in this population need to be clarified.

Although many articles report that low-demand elderly patients tolerate deformity well, the unanswered question is whether an active patient older than 65 years will have similar results. This study suggests that they may, as these subjects were all living independently and were not considered low demand. However, there was no formal assessment of their activity levels and physical demands and a very wide age range (65-89 years) was included.

In my experience, most patients in this age group tolerate malunion quite well. However, I have difficulty advising patients in this age group who have high expectations and high physical demands whether they would be able to tolerate a malunion. How malunion will affect the active elderly patient who is still playing tennis and golf regularly remains unanswered in my mind. Future studies must clarify the role of ORIF in this population, and our definition of acceptable and unacceptable alignment needs to be re-examined, as it may be different for younger patients.

R. Grewal, MD

A Prospective Randomized Controlled Trial Comparing Occupational Therapy with Independent Exercises After Volar Plate Fixation of a Fracture of the Distal Part of the Radius
Souer JS, Buijze G, Ring D (Massachusetts General Hosp, Boston)
J Bone Joint Surg Am 93:1761-1766, 2011

Background.—The effect of formal occupational therapy on recovery after open reduction and volar plate fixation of a fracture of the distal part of the radius is uncertain. We hypothesized that there would be no difference in wrist function and arm-specific disability six months after open reduction and volar plate fixation of a distal radial fracture between patients who receive formal occupational therapy and those with instructions for independent exercises.

Methods.—Ninety-four patients with an unstable distal radial fracture treated with open reduction and volar locking plate fixation were enrolled in a prospective randomized controlled trial comparing exercises done under the supervision of an occupational therapist with surgeon-directed independent exercises. The primary study question addressed combined wrist flexion and extension six months after surgery Secondary study questions addressed wrist motion, grip strength, Gartland and Werley scores, Mayo wrist scores, and DASH (Disabilities of the Arm, Shoulder and Hand) scores at three months and six months after surgery.

Results.—There was a significant difference in the mean arc of wrist flexion and extension six months after surgery (118° versus 129°), favoring patients prescribed independent exercises. Three months after surgery, there was a significant difference in mean pinch strength (80% versus 90%), mean grip strength (66% versus 81%), and mean Gartland and Werley scores, favoring patients prescribed independent exercises. At six months, there was a significant difference in mean wrist extension (55° versus 62°), ulnar deviation (82% versus 93%), mean supination (84° versus 90°), mean grip strength (81% versus 92%), and mean Mayo score, favoring patients prescribed independent exercises. There were no differences in arm-specific disability (DASH score) at any time point.

Conclusions.—Prescription of formal occupational therapy does not improve the average motion or disability score after volar locking plate fixation of a fracture of the distal part of the radius.

▶ This article has generated much discussion among the hand-therapy profession. Of obvious concern is that this study indicates that formal occupational therapy does not improve outcome post—volar plate fixation of a distal radius fracture. If interpreted literally, there is a concern that therapy services may not be considered as necessary for reimbursement. The usual practice at our clinic is to provide the patient with a custom wrist orthosis at the first postoperative visit followed by formal therapy to address edema reduction, scar management, recovery of range of motion (ROM), strengthening, and return of upper extremity function. Without this intervention, a protective posture is assumed that can lead to stiffness, pain, and loss of function. This study would have the reader believe that an independent exercise program could easily take the place of therapy. I have many questions concerning this study, which include the following: noninvolvement of therapists in the study design; treating therapists were not aware that their patients were involved in a study; the authors do not indicate whether the occupational therapists were certified hand therapists; it is unclear whether the therapists used the same exercise program that was given to the surgeon-directed independent exercise group; and whether patients perceive the surgeon's instructions as being more valid than a therapist's. In addition, the authors stated that all patients were examined and measured by a research assistant, although the research assistant was not blinded to assignment. This has the potential of biased measurements. The ROM and strength measurements were statistically greater in the independent exercise group, but there was no statistical difference at any time in upper extremity function as measured by the Disabilities of the Arm, Shoulder and Hand questionnaire. I believe that formal hand therapy should continue to be a part of the surgical recovery plan and appreciate the authors' statement that the benefits of therapy may be an "improved trajectory of recovery and a relatively low-cost method of preventing infrequent but very costly poor outcomes."

Although I am dismayed with the implications of this study, I do agree with the authors' comments about the unexpected advantages to independent exercise that merit additional study. The 2 potential explanations are that patients benefit from a more active and self-reliant exercise program and that therapists may be overly cautious when treating these patients. It was clearly stated in the article that the surgeons used a "sport model" when directing the patients, encouraging patients to perceive pain as a natural part of recovery. This study may be a wakeup call to therapists to provide strong home programs and to adopt the athletic model of rehabilitation to increase our effectiveness.

S. J. Clark, OTR/L, CHT

Prospective Study of Distal Radial Fractures Treated with an Intramedullary Nail
Nishiwaki M, Tazaki K, Shimizu H, et al (Ogikubo Hosp, Tokyo, Japan; Thomas Jefferson Univ Hosp, Philadelphia, PA)
J Bone Joint Surg Am 93:1436-1441, 2011

Background.—Intramedullary nailing for the treatment of unstable distal radial fractures is reported to provide stable fixation with minimal soft-tissue complications, but there is a paucity of data documenting the results of this technique. The purpose of this study was to prospectively determine the functional outcomes of treatment of unstable distal radial fractures with an intramedullary nail.

Methods.—Patients aged fifty years and older with a dorsally displaced unstable distal radial fracture—an extra-articular or simple intra-articular fracture—that was amenable to closed or percutaneous reduction were offered treatment with intramedullary nail fixation (MICRONAIL). Thirty-one patients were enrolled in the study, and twenty-nine patients with a mean age of sixty-seven years (range, fifty-one to eighty-five years) were available for one-year follow-up. According to the AO classification, there was one type-A2, twenty-four type-A3, and four type-C2 distal radial fractures. The patients were evaluated at six weeks, three months, six months, and one year after surgery. Outcome measures included standard radiographic parameters, active wrist range of motion, grip strength, a modified Mayo wrist score, and the Disabilities of the Arm, Shoulder and Hand (DASH) questionnaire.

Results.—At the final one-year follow-up evaluation, the active range of motion of the injured wrist relative to that on the uninjured side averaged

95% of flexion, 95% of extension, 93% of ulnar deviation, 91% of radial deviation, 99% of pronation, and 99% of supination. The mean grip strength was 96% of that on the uninjured side. According to the modified Mayo wrist score, there were twenty excellent and nine good results. The mean DASH score was 4.8 points. The final radiographic measurements demonstrated, on average, 25° of radial inclination, 11° of volar tilt, 10 mm of radial length, and +1 mm of ulnar variance. Loss of reduction occurred in two patients. One patient developed transient superficial radial sensory neuritis, which resolved within two months.

Conclusions.—Intramedullary nailing can be a safe and effective treatment with minimal complications for dorsally displaced unstable extra-articular or simple intra-articular distal radial fractures.

▶ This study is significant in that it is a prospective study evaluating the functional outcomes of patients whose distal radial fractures were treated with a specific intramedullary nail device (MICRONAIL). The volar distal radius plate has become the most widely used device for repairing distal radius fractures; however, this study aims to support the use of an intramedullary device for the repair of certain distal radial fracture types.

Strengths of this study are its prospective nature, the intervals at which outcomes were measured, and the fact that only extraarticular and simple intra-articular dorsal displaced distal radial fractures were included in the study. However, the latter is also a weakness in the device, in that it is not recommended for more complex fracture types. A weakness of the study is the lack of randomization to different treatment methods.

The findings of this study seem to support its use as a surgical treatment option for the fracture types it is indicated for—that is, extra-articular and simple intraarticular dorsally displaced distal radial fractures. It is a minimally invasive device that allows for early active motion, like other internal fixation options. Range of motion and grip strength findings at their follow-up points were similar to those in related studies where a volar distal radius plate was used.

I do not have any personal experience with this device. I have been very satisfied with the distal radius volar plate, which provides me with the flexibility to treat a broad spectrum of distal radius fracture types. This intramedullary device seems easy enough to use, but I believe it is a device "looking for an indication." In this study, I was surprised to see that only 1 patient developed transient superficial radial sensory neuritis. Given the location and size of the implant to be placed, just adjacent to the tip of the radial styloid, I would have expected a greater incidence of this particular complication. In the end, I don't foresee myself using this implant for my patients, but it is yet another option in the orthopedist's armamentarium for the repair of simple distal radius fractures.

S. S. Shin, MD, MMSc

Current and Future National Costs to Medicare for the Treatment of Distal Radius Fracture in the Elderly

Shauver MJ, Yin H, Banerjee M, et al (Univ of Michigan Health System, Ann Arbor; Univ of Michigan School of Public Health, Ann Arbor)
J Hand Surg 36A:1282-1287, 2011

Purpose.—Distal radius fractures (DRFs) are the second most common fracture experienced by elderly individuals. In 2005, 16% of DRFs in the Medicare population were being treated with internal fixation, up from 3% in 1997. This shift in treatment strategy can have substantial financial impact on Medicare and the health care system in general. The specific aims of this project were to quantify the current and future Medicare expenditures attributable to DRF and to compare Medicare payments for the 4 treatment options for elderly DRF.

Methods.—We analyzed the 100% 2007 Medicare dataset for annual DRF-attributable spending. Payments were obtained for claims that were identified as attributable to DRF by International Classification of Diseases, 9th Revision, Clinical Modification codes for DRF in conjunction with a Current Procedural Technology code for relevant treatment or service. We projected annual payments based on increasing internal fixation treatment. All payments are reported in 2007 U.S. dollars.

Results.—In 2007, Medicare made $170 million in DRF-attributable payments. If the usage of internal fixation were to reach 50%, DRF-attributable payments could be nearly $240 million. The mean attributable payment made for each patient in 2007 was $1,983. Most of this is due to facility and staffing cost for the treatment procedure.

Conclusions.—This analysis provides an accurate quantification of Medicare DRF-attributable expenditure. Use of 100% Medicare data allows for the summation of actual patient experience rather than modeling or estimation. The burden of DRF is going to grow as the U.S. population ages and as internal fixation becomes more widely used. The Medicare payment data can help in allocating resources nationally to address the increasing disease burden of DRF.

▶ The authors provide an analysis of Medicare expenditures associated with the treatment of distal radius fractures in the elderly. By searching Medicare databases for appropriate ICD-9 and Current Procedural Technology codes, the authors reported that Medicare made $170 million in payments related to the treatment of distal radius fractures. Demographic data revealed that the majority of patients were female (85%) and that most fractures were treated by closed means (74%). Internal fixation was responsible for the greatest costs associated with these injuries.

This study is important in that it allows us to quantify direct costs associated with a common osteoporotic fracture. With a growing elderly population and the increasing popularity of internal fixation, costs are likely to reach new heights over the next few years. Detailed knowledge of the impact of distal radius fractures on health care expenditures is essential in fostering more research on the optimal management and treatment for these injuries.

T. D. Rozental, MD

Comparison of Intra-Articular Simple Compression and Extra-Articular Distal Radial Fractures
Souer JS, the LCP Distal Radius Study Group (Massachusetts General Hosp, Boston; et al)
J Bone Joint Surg Am 93:2093-2099, 2011

Background.—The impact of a single well-reduced or stable intra-articular fracture oriented in the sagittal plane on the outcome of internal fixation of a distal radial fracture is uncertain. We tested the hypothesis that wrist motion and function scores would not differ between patients with an extra-articular fracture and those with a single sagittal intra-articular fracture following open fracture reduction and internal fixation with use of a volar locking plate.

Methods.—Thirty-seven patients with a single sagittal intra-articular fracture of the distal aspect of the radius and seventy-four age and sex-matched patients with an extra-articular distal radial fracture were retrospectively analyzed with use of data gathered in a cohort study of plate and screw fixation of distal radial fractures. A volar locking plate was used in all patients. The two cohorts were analyzed for differences in motion, grip strength, pain, and Gartland and Werley, DASH (Disabilities of the Arm, Shoulder and Hand), and SF-36 (Short Form-36) scores six, twelve, and twenty-four months after surgery. Differences between the cohorts and differences within each cohort over time were determined with use of regression analysis and the likelihood ratio test.

Results.—Patients with a single sagittal intra-articular fracture and those an extra-articular fracture did not differ significantly with respect to motion, grip strength, Gartland and Werley score, or DASH score at any time point. However, there was a trend toward less pronation (95% compared with 98% of that in the contralateral arm) and less grip strength (76% compared with 81% of that in the contralateral arm) at six months and toward a smaller flexion-extension arc (118°compared with 128°) at one year after surgery in patients with a single sagittal intra-articular fracture.

Conclusions.—Open reduction and volar locking plate and screw fixation of extra-articular fractures and of simple intra-articular fractures of the distal aspect of the radius are associated with comparable impairment and disability within two years of surgery.

▶ The authors present a retrospective study comparing outcomes for stable, well-reduced single sagittal intra-articular distal radius fractures with those for extra-articular fractures after open reduction and internal fixation (ORIF). Outcomes assessed included the Gartland and Werley scoring system, the DASH score, and the SF-36 score. The authors did not demonstrate any significant differences in range of motion or outcome scores between the 2 groups despite a greater likelihood of radiographic posttraumatic arthritis in the intra-articular group. The study challenges the belief that posttraumatic arthritis is associated with worse outcomes.

The study's strength lies in its rigorous design and breadth of outcome assessment scores. As noted by the authors, however, it is difficult to conclude whether radiocarpal arthrosis had no effect on outcome or whether this effect was too small to measure. Furthermore, the results were not stratified by age, and the follow-up period was relatively short. Nevertheless, the study provides important information for the treating physician, allowing us to counsel patients that well-reduced intra-articular injuries treated with ORIF seem to have as good a prognosis as their extra-articular counterparts.

T. D. Rozental, MD

The Relationship Between ASSH Membership and the Treatment of Distal Radius Fracture in the United States Medicare population
Chung KC, Shauver MJ, Yin H (The Univ of Michigan Health System, Ann Arbor)
J Hand Surg 36A:1288-1293, 2011

Purpose.—Internal fixation for distal radius fractures (DRFs) in the elderly has increased from 3% in 1997 to 17% in 2007. This increase has been uneven across regions of the United States. There is some evidence that patients treated by hand surgeons receive internal fixation at an increased rate and that hand surgeons might be driving the increased usage in regions where their presence is greatest. The specific aim of this study was to explore this relationship by analyzing Medicare beneficiaries treated by members of the American Society for Surgery of the Hand (ASSH).

Methods.—Surgeons who were members of ASSH in 2007 were matched with surgeons treating Medicare beneficiaries for DRFs in the same year. We then fit a series of multilevel models to estimate the proportion of total variance in internal fixation usage explained by ASSH membership status, patient demographic data, patient comorbidity, and/or type of fracture diagnosed.

Results.—Beneficiaries treated by ASSH members received internal fixation significantly more often than beneficiaries who were treated by surgeons who were not ASSH members. ASSH member status accounts for 12% of the total variance in internal fixation utilization.

Conclusions.—Medicare beneficiaries who were treated by ASSH member surgeons receive internal fixation at a significantly higher rate than do patients of other physicians. When there is uncertainty about the optimal treatment for a condition, there is the possibility for specialty-related disparities. This specialty effect contributes to the national variations in the treatment of DRFs in the Medicare population.

▶ This study presents a well thought out investigation into the trends in internal fixation of distal radius fractures. It uses complicated statistics to prove its point.

Based on the experience of these authors and their previous work, the statistical methods are sound. However, without a significant background in statistics, the reader will have difficulty assessing the validity of their conclusions; they will just have to take the author's word that these statistical tests are appropriate.

There are several interesting conclusions worth mentioning. Certainly, the increase in internal fixation for distal radius fractures is worth noting, and there is still much work necessary to determine the effects and value of this trend. As the authors point out, there is a need for more level 1 data to support the use of internal fixation for distal radius fractures as well as data to guide its use.

Also interesting is the discovery of the inaccuracy of the Centers for Medicare and Medicaid Services (CMS) specialty designation for its providers. It does call into question other demographic data used in this and other studies, and it does question the accuracy of the CMS system overall.

The article does brush over what I think explains the most likely cause for the difference in treatment by hand surgeons, which is the complexity of injury seen by most hand surgeons. The majority of patients I see in my office referred from a typical emergency room are treated nonoperatively. However, the majority of those I see as inpatients (at a level-1 trauma center) or referred from another orthopedic surgeon are treated with internal fixation. This is more likely to be true for hand surgeons than other nonspecialists.

T. Hughes, MD

Open Fractures of the Distal Radius: The Effects of Delayed Debridement and Immediate Internal Fixation on Infection Rates and the Need for Secondary Procedures

Kurylo JC, Axelrad TW, Tornetta P III, et al (Boston Univ Med Ctr, MA)
J Hand Surg 36A:1131-1134, 2011

Purpose.—There are few clinical data evaluating the outcome of surgery for open distal radius fractures based on treatment method. Specifically, the major contributing factors to infection are largely unknown. The purpose of this study is to determine the effect of early versus delayed debridement and the choice of initial external versus internal fixation on infection rates and the need for secondary procedures.

Methods.—Thirty-two patients with open distal radius fractures were identified from a database. Ten debridements were early (<6 h after hospital admission), and 22 debridements were delayed (>6 h after hospital admission). There were 10 treating surgeons for the 32 patients in this study. Based on the attending surgeon's preference and experience, 20 fractures were treated with external fixation, 7 with plating, and 5 with planned staged conversion from external fixation to plating. The cohort included 19 grade I, 11 grade II, and 3 grade IIIA open injuries.

Results.—There were no infections, regardless of the time to debridement or the use of immediate plating. Other complications requiring secondary procedures occurred more frequently in patients treated with a planned staged conversion from external fixation to plating than in the patients treated with either external fixation or plating.

Conclusions.—We did not encounter infections for grade I and grade II open distal radius fractures, and infections do not appear to be related to either the time to debridement or the initial type of fracture fixation. Plating might be safe at the initial debridement, but temporary external fixation with a staged conversion to plating increases the risk of complications, which necessitates corrective secondary procedures.

Type of Study/Level of Evidence.—Therapeutic III.

▶ The authors have presented a retrospective review of open distal radius fractures treated at their institution over a 6-year period. They evaluated the time from presentation to operative debridement and the type of fixation (internal vs external vs external converted to internal). In their series, there were no infections or nonunions, and the complication rate was low, with the greatest number of complications occurring in those initially treated with external fixation and converted to internal fixation.

Although the numbers are not large (32 patients), this is a good series and demonstrates that in Gustilo and Anderson types I and II injuries to the distal radius, emergent debridement is not necessary to prevent infection or nonunion, and delay until the following morning or later the same day seems appropriate (average time to debridement was over 20 hours in 22 of 32 patients). There is a trend toward this concept for long bone fractures in the lower extremity, and this article provides data for distal radius injuries.

Antibiotics were administered before or upon arrival to the hospital and continued 24 hours postoperatively. They were unable to determine the time following fracture, so time from administration to antibiotic administration is greater than reported.

This also supports the concept that definitive fixation should be performed at the initial treatment, as conversion from external fixation to internal fixation resulted in a greater number of soft tissue complications. They only had 2 patients with grade III open fractures, so these data may not be applicable to more severe open injuries.

This study has the same limitations as all level IV studies, but due to the infrequency with which these injuries occur, a prospective randomized trial is unlikely.

W. Hammert, MD

A Prospective Randomized Controlled Trial Comparing Occupational Therapy with Independent Exercises After Volar Plate Fixation of a Fracture of the Distal Part of the Radius
Souer JS, Buijze G, Ring D (Massachusetts General Hosp, Boston)
J Bone Joint Surg Am 93:1761-1766, 2011

Background.—The effect of formal occupational therapy on recovery after open reduction and volar plate fixation of a fracture of the distal part of the radius is uncertain. We hypothesized that there would be no difference in wrist function and arm-specific disability six months after open reduction and volar plate fixation of a distal radial fracture between patients who receive formal occupational therapy and those with instructions for independent exercises.

Methods.—Ninety-four patients with an unstable distal radial fracture treated with open reduction and volar locking plate fixation were enrolled in a prospective randomized controlled trial comparing exercises done under the supervision of an occupational therapist with surgeon-directed independent exercises. The primary study question addressed combined wrist flexion and extension six months after surgery Secondary study questions addressed wrist motion, grip strength, Gartland and Werley scores, Mayo wrist scores, and DASH (Disabilities of the Arm, Shoulder and Hand) scores at three months and six months after surgery.

Results.—There was a significant difference in the mean arc of wrist flexion and extension six months after surgery (118° versus 129°), favoring patients prescribed independent exercises. Three months after surgery, there was a significant difference in mean pinch strength (80% versus 90%), mean grip strength (66% versus 81%), and mean Gartland and Werley scores, favoring patients prescribed independent exercises. At six months, there was a significant difference in mean wrist extension (55° versus 62°), ulnar deviation (82% versus 93%), mean supination (84° versus 90°), mean grip strength (81% versus 92%), and mean Mayo score, favoring patients prescribed independent exercises. There were no differences in arm-specific disability (DASH score) at any time point.

Conclusions.—Prescription of formal occupational therapy does not improve the average motion or disability score after volar locking plate fixation of a fracture of the distal part of the radius.

▶ Souer and colleagues present their work to answer the following question: is formal therapy better than independent exercises following volar plating of distal radius fracture? The study was well designed and adequately powered to answer this question. The ability to execute a prospective randomized clinical trial is difficult, and the authors have contributed to the unfortunately small body of level 1 evidence and demonstrated that comparable results can be obtained with an independent exercise program.

Although the conclusions are justified from their data, the authors point out that while statistically significant differences were found, these may not be clinically significant. In addition, the specific therapy program was at the discretion of the therapist, and there may be a greater variability in these programs. Some therapy units provide one-on-one therapy and demonstrate manual stretching, while others rely more on the use of machines and have less one-on-one instruction.

Of equal importance may be the amount of time the surgeon spends teaching the patient the independent exercises, and although this may vary from patient to patient, this time is likely more than that required for the typical postoperative appointment.

The take-home message from this article is that a prolonged formal therapy program is not necessary following volar plating of distal radius fractures and that a therapy program can be individualized based on patients' understanding of the program, often allowing the therapist to focus on tendon injuries and other conditions for which a formal therapy program is beneficial.

W. Hammert, MD

Radius Fracture Repair Using Volumetrically Expanding Polyurethane Bone Cement

Boxberger JI, Adams DJ, Diaz-Doran V, et al (Doctors Res Group, Inc, Southbury, CT; Univ of Connecticut Health Ctr, Farmington, CT)
J Hand Surg 36A:1294-1302, 2011

Purpose.—New repair techniques for fragility fractures such as those of the distal radius require biomechanical justification. This study was conducted to investigate a technique using an expanding polymer bone cement to provide strength to a fracture repair.

Methods.—Distal and proximal ends were isolated from 6 pairs of human radii (mean age 65). Transverse osteotomies were made near the head of each specimen. Paired specimens were repaired using 2 materials of differing polymer chemistries: polyurethane versus polymethylmethacrylate. Repaired specimens were subjected to failure tests in a cantilever beam configuration (distal, n = 6 per treatment) or pure tension (proximal, n = 5 per treatment). Cement penetration tests were conducted using a uniform open-cell model of cancellous bone. Baseline mechanical properties of the polyurethane cement were determined according to ASTM standards.

Results.—Distal radii repaired with polyurethane bone cement withstood average shear stress 2.9 times as high as polymethylmethacrylate (0.91 vs 0.31 MPa). Peak tensile bending stress was 2.5 times as high in polyurethane (2.57 vs 1.02 MPa). Under pure tension, polyurethane-repaired samples failed at 0.83 MPa versus 0.74 MPa for polymethylmethacrylate. The polyurethane cement expanded to penetrate 49% farther into the trabeculae. The polyurethane cement had mean compressive yield stress of 20.3 MPa, compressive modulus of 754 MPa, ultimate tensile stress of 18.5 MPa, and tensile elastic modulus of 723 MPa.

Conclusions.—The biomechanical strength data indicate the potential of an expanding bone cement as a candidate strategy for fracture repair. Further evaluation might provide evidence for such an alternative repair strategy for fragility fractures, including those of the distal radius.

▶ The authors present yet another example of bone fixation borrowed from the oral and maxillofacial industry.[1] We see increasing need and use for bone fillers that act as cements, adhesives, and mortars; this particular material, a polyurethane resin, has potential attributes of each. This innovative study examines the use of the cement that they've deemed "Kryptonite" in comparison to polymethylmethacrylate cement to address metaphyseal defects of the distal and proximal radius. The preferential fill within trabecular bone, thus demonstrating interstitial adherence, likely explains the improved shear and tensile strength and suggests its potential utility for future fracture use. Polyurethane is a ubiquitous material used throughout industry in all facets—from automotive to textiles to medicine—and increasing interest in ecologically derived sources may come in handy as it relates to novel fixation techniques in our discipline.

A. Ladd, MD

Reference

1. Weber SC, Chapman MW. Adhesives in orthopaedic surgery. A review of the literature and in vitro bonding strengths of bone-bonding agents. *Clin Orthop Relat Res*. 1984;191:249-261.

Immobilization in Supination Versus Neutral Following Surgical Treatment of Galeazzi Fracture-Dislocations in Adults: Case Series

Park MJ, Pappas N, Steinberg DR, et al (Univ of Pennsylvania, Philadelphia; Vanderbilt Orthopaedic Inst, Nashville, TN)
J Hand Surg 37A:528-531, 2012

Purpose.—The goal of this study was to investigate whether immobilization in supination is necessary to prevent recurrent distal radioulnar joint (DRUJ) instability in patients older than 18 years with a Galeazzi fracture-dislocation and a stable DRUJ following open reduction and internal fixation of the radius.

Methods.—We performed a retrospective chart review of 10 consecutive patients who were immobilized in either supination or a neutral position following surgical treatment of a Galeazzi fracture-dislocation in which the DRUJ was noted to be stable immediately after fixation of the radius. Group 1 consisted of 5 patients who were immobilized in supination for a period of 4 weeks, and group 2 consisted of 5 patients who were immobilized in neutral for 2 weeks, followed by functional bracing.

Results.—Patients were followed up for an average of 68 months (range, 26–124 mo) after surgery. No significant difference was noted between the 2 groups with respect to age, medical comorbidities (no noteworthy medical comorbidities in either group), or hand dominance. None of the patients in either group demonstrated DRUJ instability during the follow-up period or required any additional surgery. At the latest follow-up, patients in the 2 groups had comparable forearm motion.

Conclusions.—The results of the current study suggest that following open reduction and internal fixation of the radius in patients with Galeazzi fracture-dislocations and with stable DRUJs, immobilization in supination for 4 weeks does not have an advantage over immobilization in neutral for a shorter period.

▶ This article seems to conclude the intuitive: that splinting the forearm in supination is unnecessary when the distal radial ulnar joint (DRUJ) is stable after open reduction and internal fixation (ORIF) of the radial shaft fracture. After all, if the DRUJ is stable, why address it?

By comparing 5 patients splinted in supination for 4 weeks with 5 patients splinted in neutral for 2 weeks, the authors demonstrated that there were no differences in DRUJ instability or forearm range of motion at a mean follow-up of 68 months.

This study has many significant weaknesses. First, the study is underpowered and not randomized. Comparing 2 groups of 5 patients each prevents the authors from determining definitive conclusions. Second, the examiners at follow-up were the treating surgeons, thus potentially introducing significant bias into the study.

Third, the authors do not state how pronosupination was measured and imply that the different surgeons may have measured the range of motion differently. Last, the authors twice mention "surgeon to surgeon differences in technique" but do not clearly explain the differences or how these could affect their results.

In my practice, I see no need to address an already stable DRUJ after ORIF. Therefore, I use a protective splint for 10 to 14 days only and then start range of motion after the splint is removed.

L. W. Catalano III, MD

The Surgical Treatment of Unstable Distal Radius Fractures by Angle Stable Implants: A Multicenter Prospective Study

Matschke S, the LCP Study Group (Berufsgenossenschaftliche Unfallklinik Ludwigshafen—Unfallchirurgische Klinik an der Universität Heidelberg, Germany; et al)
J Orthop Trauma 25:312-317, 2011

Objectives.—The goal of this study is to document the 2-year outcome after surgical treatment of distal radius fractures using an angle stable implant.

Design.—Prospective case-series.

Setting.—Multicenter study in nine trauma units with recruitment between December 2001 and May 2003.

Patients.—One hundred eight patients with the same number of distal radius fractures.

Intervention.—Open reduction and internal fixation with the LCP DR 3.5 mm (Synthes GmbH, Oberdorf, Switzerland).

Main Outcome Measurements.—Disabilities of the Arm, Shoulder and Hand, Gartland and Werley, SF-36 scores, radiologic assessment, and return to work status at 2 years.

Results.—At 2 years, the mean range of motion (relative to the contralateral wrist) was 83% for palmar flexion, 91% for extension, 94% for radial deviation, 92% for ulnar deviation, and 98%/94% for pronation/supination angles. Grip strength was 90% of the mean uninjured side. The average radiographic measurements were 23.6° for radial inclination angle, 6.1° for palmar (volar) tilt angle, and 0 mm for ulnar variance. The proportion of fractures for which the Gartland and Werley score was categorized as either good or excellent was 89%. Minor complications occurred in 14 patients, although none of these events were considered to be directly related to the implant.

Conclusion.—After a 2-year follow-up period, the use of an angle stable implant for unstable distal radius fractures provides adequate fixation with minimal loss of reduction. This device is associated with good functional and radiologic outcome for the patient and is indicated for distal radius fractures classified as Orthopaedic Trauma Association (OTA) Type 23-A2/A3, OTA Type 23-B2/B3, and OTA Type 23-C.

▶ Injuries to the triangular fibrocartilage complex (TFCC) concomitant with distal radius fractures often affect the postoperative outcomes of patients. The authors mentioned in the methodology that ulnar fractures were involved in 37% of fractures of the radius, with most involving distal radioulnar joint dislocations. They did not refer to the treatment of ulnar fractures[1] or to the evaluation and treatment of the associated TFCC injuries[2,3] in this study. TFCC injuries are found in 40% to 50% of intra-articular fractures of the distal radius.[2] It is true that many of the concomitant TFCC injuries can heal spontaneously only by cast immobilization after reduction of the fractures of the distal radius. However, in this study the postoperative immobilization period of the wrist was only 10 to 14 days, which might be too short to allow the TFCC injuries to repair spontaneously. Rigid fixation and anatomical reduction of the distal radius using locking screws cause surgeons to decrease the postoperative immobilization period. Evaluation of concomitant TFCC injuries is necessary during surgery or just after immobilization of the wrist. If TFCC injuries are suspected, their treatment should be considered.

R. Kakinoki, MD, PhD

References

1. Protopsaltis TS, Ruch DS. Triangular fibrocartilage complex tears associated with symptomatic ulnar styloid nonunions. *J Hand Surg Am.* 2010;35:1251-1255.
2. Fujitani R, Omokawa S, Akahane M, et al. Predictors of distal radioulnar joint instability in distal radius fractures. *J Hand Surg Am.* 2011;36:1919-1925.
3. Ruch DS, Yang CC, Smith BP. Results of acute arthroscopically repaired triangular fibrocartilage complex injuries associated with intra-articular distal radius fractures. *Arthroscopy.* 2003;19:511-516.

Ulnar Variance: Correlation of Plain Radiographs, Computed Tomography, and Magnetic Resonance Imaging With Anatomic Dissection

Laino DK, Petchprapa CN, Lee SK (NYU Hosp for Joint Diseases)
J Hand Surg 37A:90-97, 2012

Purpose.—Several techniques used to measure ulnar variance on a posteroanterior wrist radiograph have been described. It remains unclear whether they accurately represent the true ulnar variance of the patient.

The purpose of this study was to correlate ulnar variance measurements on plain radiographs, computed tomography (CT), magnetic resonance imaging (MRI), and anatomic dissection.

Methods.—Posteroanterior (PA) radiographs, coronal and sagittal CT scans, and coronal MRI scans were obtained on 8 fresh-frozen cadaver wrists. The ulnar variance was measured by 5 reviewers. The specimens were then dissected, exposing the wrist joint. The ulnar variance was measured directly on each specimen using digital calipers. The inter-rater reliability was calculated for each imaging modality. The bias for each imaging modality was calculated using the digital caliper measurements as the true ulnar variance.

Results.—Intraclass correlation coefficients demonstrated excellent inter-rater reliability for each imaging modality. The average bias from the true variance was the following: PA radiograph, 0.77 mm; coronal CT, 0.96 mm; sagittal CT, 0.96 mm; MRI with articular cartilage, 0.73 mm; MRI excluding cartilage, 0.49 mm. The variance measured on all imaging modalities tended to underestimate the magnitude of the true variance.

Conclusions.—Ulnar variance measured on coronal MRI best reflected the true ulnar variance as measured directly using calipers. The CT scans demonstrated the greatest deviation from the true variance. However, differences were small and might not be clinically meaningful. All imaging modalities demonstrated excellent inter-rater reliability, with MRI being highest. All imaging modalities tended to underestimate the magnitude of the true variance.

Clinical Relevance.—The imaged underestimation of true ulnar variance should be taken into account when performing surgical procedures that alter the relative lengths of the radius and ulna.

▶ Accurate measurement of ulnar variance is important when assessing patients with ulnar-sided wrist pain. Numerous methods have been described and their accuracy determined.[1-3] These have traditionally been performed using plain posteroanterior (PA) radiographs. The authors have conducted a cadaveric study to examine the accuracy of ulnar variance measurements using 3 imaging modalities—plain radiographs, CT, and MRI—and compared this to anatomic dissection. Of the 3 radiological techniques studied, measurements taken from the coronal MRI were found to be the most accurate; yet all underestimated the true variance when compared to cadaveric analysis.

With increasing use of advanced imaging in the management of patients with ulnar-sided wrist pain, I commend the authors on their attempts to determine which modality most accurately quantifies true ulnar variance. There are a few methodological concerns, however, with the study. First, the magnet used was a 1.5 T. Since 1 measurement used coronal MRI sequences, accounting for the cartilage thickness, this would have been more accurately measured using a stronger (3.0 T) magnet. Second, all imaging was performed with the wrists in neutral rotation. As ulnar variance increases with forearm pronation,[4] performing the study with the wrists in this position may have resulted in a more clinically relevant simulation. The authors acknowledge the difficulties involved in measuring ulnar variance on CT and MRI scans and describe their technique. They provide the interrater reliability for each imaging modality but do not comment on its validity. A further weakness of the study, which the authors acknowledge, is being underpowered with only 8 cadavers used. The authors noted that with coronal MRI sequences, the articular cartilage could be visualized. An area of interest would have been if the authors had noted any differences in triangular fibrocartilage thickness because of varying degrees of ulnar variance.

Not withstanding these limitations, I believe the authors should be congratulated on their attempts to determine the accuracy of the use of CT and MRI to quantify ulnar variance. Although coronal MRI scans best reflected true ulnar variance, the authors acknowledge that the differences were small and may not be clinically relevant. They noted all imaging techniques underestimated the true ulnar variance, a finding that should be considered by the treating surgeon.

S. Kakar, MD, MRCS

References

1. Palmer AK, Glisson RR, Werner FW. Ulnar variance determination. *J Hand Surg Am.* 1982;7:376-379.
2. Kristensen SS, Thomassen E, Christensen F. Ulnar variance determination. *J Hand Surg.* 1986;11B:255-257.
3. Steyers CM, Blair WF. Measuring ulnar variance: a comparison of techniques. *J Hand Surg.* 1988;14A:607-612.
4. Tomaino MM. The importance of the pronated grip x-ray view in evaluating ulnar variance. *J Hand Surg.* 2000;25A:352-357.

Subluxation of the Distal Radioulnar Joint as a Predictor of Foveal Triangular Fibrocartilage Complex Tears
Ehman EC, Hayes ML, Berger RA, et al (Mayo Clinic, Rochester, MN)
J Hand Surg 36A:1780-1784, 2011

Purpose.—The triangular fibrocartilage complex (TFCC) with its ulnar foveal attachment is the primary stabilizer of the distal radioulnar joint (DRUJ). The purpose of this study was to describe a technique for measuring the degree of subluxation of the DRUJ in wrist magnetic resonance imaging (MRI) examinations to predict tears involving the foveal attachment of the TFCC.

Methods.—We measured DRUJ geometry in wrist MRI examinations of 34 patients who were found to have foveal TFCC tears at surgery. We compared the results with DRUJ geometry in 11 asymptomatic controls. Subluxation of the ulnar head was assessed using transaxial MRI images obtained at the level of the DRUJ with the wrist in pronation. We quantified subluxation with a line spanning the sigmoid notch of the radius and a perpendicular line through the center of curvature of the articulating surface of the ulna. We calculated the ratio of the lengths of the dorsal and volar segments and normalized it to the center of the sigmoid notch.

Results.—A total of 34 patients with intraoperatively confirmed tears of the foveal attachment of the TFCC had a mean dorsal ulnar subluxation measurement of 16% ± 4%, whereas the 11 controls had a mean subluxation measurement of 5% ± 4%.

Conclusions.—The results confirm the hypothesis that subluxation of the ulnar head relative to the sigmoid notch of the radius, as assessed by MRI with the wrist in pronation, is a predictor of tears of the foveal attachment of the TFCC.

Type of Study/Level of Evidence.—Diagnostic II.

▶ This article is significant because the amount of dorsal subluxation of the ulnar head relative to the sigmoid notch of the radius can be used as a predictor for diagnosing foveal tears of the triangular fibrocartilage complex (TFCC).

Strengths of the study are the strict inclusion and exclusion criteria used and the simple and reproducible formula used for measuring the amount of dorsal subluxation. Weaknesses of the study, as also stated by the authors, are possible inclusion bias in the group receiving surgery and the fact that only one type of destabilizing wrist pathology was examined.

The importance of this study's findings lies in its confirmation that foveal tears of the TFCC are commonly associated with dorsal subluxation of the ulna on the sigmoid notch. The study demonstrates a useful and simple way of predicting the presence of a foveal TFCC tear based on a preoperative MRI (specifically axial images of the wrist in pronation where the radius and ulna demonstrate the greatest cross-sectional profile at the distal radioulnar joint [DRUJ]).

In my experience, it is usually not difficult to visualize and palpate whether dorsal subluxation of the ulna on the radius and possibly DRUJ instability exist in comparison with the opposite, unaffected wrist. Therefore, the clinical utility of the findings in this study is questionable. If a patient presents with ulnar-sided wrist pain with or without DRUJ instability and has failed nonoperative treatments, the clinician will likely end up evaluating the wrist arthroscopically and at that time determine with his or her own eyes if a foveal TFCC tear or other pathology is present. This would occur regardless of whether a preoperative MRI was performed and also regardless of the findings of that study. As stated in the article and confirmed in the literature, the sensitivity, specificity, and accuracy of MRIs for the diagnosis of foveal TFCC tears vary widely. I have ordered preoperative MRIs less and less over the years because I have not found them to be critical to the treatment of the patient. One can argue that ordering a preoperative MRI is mostly for the patient's sake, to possibly confirm for the patient that there is an objective reason to put scalpel to skin. I strongly believe that arthroscopic visualization is still the gold standard for the diagnosis of intra-articular wrist pathology, including TFCC tears. I do not see myself measuring the exact amount of percentage dorsal subluxation of the ulna on the sigmoid notch to determine whether or not a foveal tear might be present; however, this article does add to our knowledge base of this relatively common condition.

S. S. Shin, MD, MMSc

12 Flexor Tendon

Flexor Tendon Repair With a Knotless Barbed Suture: A Comparative Biomechanical Study

Marrero-Amadeo IC, Chauhan A, Warden SJ, et al (Indiana Univ Schools of Medicine, Indianapolis)
J Hand Surg 36A:1204-1208, 2011

Purpose.—To test the hypothesis that a flexor tendon repair with only a knotless barbed suture technique provides a repair with a greater maximal load to failure and 2-mm gapping resistance than a traditional technique using a 4-strand core plus a running-locking epitendinous suture.

Methods.—We assigned 41 fresh-frozen cadaveric flexor digitorum profundus tendons for repair by either a traditional technique using a 4-strand core (Tajima and horizontal mattress) plus a running-locking epitendinous suture (n = 20) or a bidirectional barbed suture technique using a knotless, 4-strand core secured with 3 transverse passes (n = 21). A biomechanical study was performed on each tendon-suture construct and the tendons were linearly distracted to failure at 100 mm/min. The maximal tensile load to failure, 2-mm gapping tensile load, and mode of failure were determined and statistically compared.

Results.—The average maximal load to failure was not significantly different between the traditional repair (48 ± 12 N) and the barbed suture repair (50 ± 14 N). The average 2-mm gapping load was also insignificantly different between the traditional repair (42 ± 12 N) and the barbed suture repair (32 ± 9 N). The traditional repair failed by knot unraveling and suture rupture 35% and 65% of the time, respectively. The barbed suture repair failed by suture pull-out and rupture 67% and 33% of the time, respectively. The average load to failure by suture rupture was insignificantly different between the traditional repair (51 ± 13 N) and the barbed suture repair (63 ± 16 N). The average load to failure by knot unraveling using the traditional repair was 43 ± 11 N, whereas the average load to failure by suture pull-out using the barbed suture repair was 43 ± 8 N.

Conclusions.—The barbed suture repair did not demonstrate a significant difference in maximal load to failure and 2-mm gapping resistance compared with the traditional method of repair.

Clinical Relevance.—This study examines the biomechanical differences between 2 types of flexor-tendon repair, which can help guide the surgical management for these injuries.

▶ Barbed tendon repair was proposed decades ago and has elicited both positive and negative comments. Some surgeons have shown both clinical and experimental findings to support the use of this method, but others do not consider it superior to other methods. The current report is in the latter group. The findings of this report and previous studies indicate that the barbed suture has strength similar to any of the current 4-strand repairs, and the barbed suture is less resistant to gapping.

My understanding of these seemingly conflicting findings is that the barbed suture has advantages over most 2-strand repairs; thus, even in the late 20th century, this method did appear more beneficial than most of the then-popular methods. However, 4- or 6-strand repairs are now known to double or triple the strength of 2-strand repairs, and the strength of these multistrand repairs is no lower than the barbed suture—and many are in fact stronger. The barbed suture approximates the strength of a typical 4-strand repair. In other words, the barbed suture is not superior to the most currently used methods. Considering the availability of special sutures with barbs and lack of superior repair strength, it is not necessary to change our practice to use this method. Nevertheless, for surgeons who have been familiar with this technique, it could be a wonderful option to repair the tendon. It will be valuable to have English-language reports based on a large patient series and analysis of the clinical outcomes of barbed suture tendon repair; I am aware that such reports currently exist in non-English European publications.

I currently use a 6- or 4-strand repair method and 4-0 conventional sutures to make core repairs in the flexor tendons and do not intend to change to barbed sutures.

J. B. Tang, MD

Gliding Resistance and Triggering After Venting or A2 Pulley Enlargement: A Study of Intact and Repaired Flexor Tendons in a Cadaveric Model

Bunata RE, Simmons S, Roso M, et al (Univ of North Texas Health Science Ctr, Fort Worth; John Peter Smith Hosp (Tarrant County Hosp District), Fort Worth, TX)
J Hand Surg 36A:1316-1322, 2011

Purpose.—This study compared the effect of 2 techniques of pulley management—venting and pulley enlargement (complete A2 incision with pulley repair and sheath closure using a retinacular graft)—on gliding resistance and on the incidence of triggering following zone 2 flexor tendon repairs in human cadaver specimens.

Methods.—*In vitro* gliding resistance and the incidence of triggering were determined in 10 human cadaver specimens under 5 progressive conditions:

(1) intact, (2) tendon repair (both tendons cut and repaired with the sheath intact), (3) condition 2 plus 50% venting of the distal A2 pulley, (4) condition 2 with venting extended to 66% of distal A2, and (5) condition 4 plus pulley enlargement. Triggering was determined in the same specimens by 2 computational algorithms that detected force changes in the load cells used to measure gliding resistance.

Results.—Tendon repair increased gliding resistance from the intact condition by an average of 229%. Gliding resistance was reduced in conditions 3, 4, and 5 from the repair condition by 15%, 25%, and 22%, respectively. Triggering commenced with tendon repair in some specimens, and its incidence increased with 50% venting. Further venting reduced triggering, but not as effectively as pulley enlargement did.

Conclusions.—In this cadaveric study, venting and pulley enlargement reduce gliding resistance by equivalent amounts. Triggering persisted despite venting. The surgeon should carefully examine tendon repairs for free gliding. Pulley enlargement might be more effective than venting in reducing the incidence of triggering.

Clinical Relevance.—This basic science, biomechanical study is intended to improve understanding of zone 2 tendon repair behavior, including gliding resistance and triggering, thereby improving flexor tendon repair results.

▶ The authors examined 2 currently controversial methods: venting or enlargement plasty of the flexor pulley. Using a cadaveric model, both methods decreased gliding resistance and "freed" tendon motion. This is the most current of a series of studies conducted by the authors investigating pulley enlargement using cadaveric models. The results largely corroborate the studies in my group and support venting or enlargement pulley plasty. However, it is difficult to obtain a clear conclusion regarding which of the 2 methods is preferable from the current report. The results of this study appear to favor the enlargement pulley plasty because it causes less triggering.

I began to perform sheath enlargement plasty in 1990. I was not particularly concerned about how much of the pulley was included in the sheath plasty at that time; I wrote "sheath enlargement plasty" in 1993, but it is possible that a part of the A2 pulley was actually included.[1] I obtained good outcomes without tendon rupture over a 2-year period; I continued to use sheath enlargement plasty until I found that simple partial venting is a valid option and does not lead to tendon bowstringing. Currently, I perform only venting, without reconstruction of the incised sheath/pulley. I believe both methods lead to essentially the same clinical outcomes, but enlargement plasty may be unnecessary because it does not further improve the results. I should point out that I have no experience with incising the entire A2 pulley and performing an interposition graft to enlarge the sheath and prevent bowstringing. I doubt whether such a complete cut (even with graft reconstruction) would be necessary and would avoid the danger of tendon bowstringing; thus I suggest that neither venting nor enlargement plasty extend over the entire A2 pulley.

J. B. Tang, MD

Reference

1. Tang JB, Zhang QG, Ishii S. Autogenous free sheath grafts in reconstruction of injured digital flexor tendon sheath at the delayed primary stage. *J Hand Surg Br.* 1993;18:31-32.

Surgical Repair of Multiple Pulley Injuries—Evaluation of a New Combined Pulley Repair

Schöffl V, Küpper T, Hartmann J, et al (Friedrich Alexander Univ Erlangen-Nuremberg, Germany; Aachen Technical Univ, Germany; Dept of Pediatrics, Klinikum Bamberg, Germany)
J Hand Surg 37A:224-230, 2012

Purpose.—We report on a combined repair of multiple annular pulley tears using 1 continuous palmaris longus tendon graft to restore strength and function.

Methods.—We treated 6 rock climbers with grade 4 pulley injuries (multiple pulley injuries) using the combined repair technique and re-evaluated them after a mean of 28 months.

Results.—All patients had excellent Buck-Gramcko scores; the functional outcome was good in 4, satisfactory in 1, and fair in 1. The sport-specific outcome was excellent in 5 and satisfactory in 1. Proximal interphalangeal joint flexion deficit slightly increased in 1 patient and remained the same in the other 5. Climbing level after the injury was the same as before in 4 and decreased slightly in 2 climbers.

Conclusions.—The technique is effective with good results and has since become our standard treatment. Nevertheless, it is limited in patients with flexion contracture of the proximal interphalangeal joint.

Type of Study/Level of Evidence.—Therapeutic III.

▶ The authors describe a unique technique to reconstruct injuries to multiple annular and cruciate pulleys. While this is a small case series with the limitations of such a study due to the relatively rare incidence of the injury, this type of study may be the best there is to offer. The article does a good job of reviewing the available literature, and their results seem reasonable and honest. They recognize that proximal interphalangeal joint contractures are difficult to deal with, and because they are unevenly distributed among studies, it is difficult to make comparisons. The biomechanics behind their reconstruction seem sound, and I would consider using their technique in these injuries. My recommendations for future research would be a biomechanics study evaluating different reconstruction techniques to see which reconstruction would be the best. They reference a study (*J Biomech* 2006) that was a mathematical model that helped them determine where the placement of the pulley would be ideal with respect to the PIP joint but did not compare different reconstruction techniques. My personal bias is a cadaver model over mathematical models with the understanding that cadaver models do not take into account healing and evaluate only at time zero. However, these models (cadaver or mathematical) along with case series will most likely be the best science given the rarity of the injury, which would make prospective, randomized trials difficult to accomplish.

P. Tang, MD, MPH

Flexor carpi ulnaris tenotomy alone does not eliminate its contribution to wrist torque
de Bruin M, Smeulders MJC, Kreulen M (Academic Med Ctr, Amsterdam, The Netherlands)
Clin Biomech 26:725-728, 2011

Background.—Flexor carpi ulnaris muscle tenotomy and transfer to the extensor side of the wrist are common procedures used to improve wrist position and dexterity in patients with cerebral palsy. Our aim was to determine whether this muscle still influences wrist torque even after tenotomy of its distal tendon.

Methods.—Intra-operatively, we determined in vivo maximal wrist torque in hemiplegic cerebral palsy patients (n = 15, mean age 17 years) in three conditions: 1) with the arm and the muscle intact; 2) after tenotomy of the flexor carpi ulnaris just proximal to the pisiform bone, with complete release from its insertion; and 3) after careful dissection of the belly of the muscle from its fascial surroundings up until approximately halfway its length.

Findings.—After tenotomy of the flexor carpi ulnaris muscle, the maximal wrist torque decreased 18% whereas dissection of the muscle resulted in an additional decrease of 18%.

Interpretation.—We conclude that despite the tenotomy of its distal tendon, the flexor carpi ulnaris still contributes to the flexion torque at the wrist through myofascial force transmission. Quantification of this phenomenon will help in the study of the effects of fascial dissection on the functional results of tendon transfer surgery.

▶ The authors demonstrated that tenotomy of the flexor carpi ulnaris (FCU) reduced only 18% of the total torque of wrist flexion because the fascia over the FCU still served in wrist flexion. Tenotomy and proximal muscle belly dissection for quite a long distance are necessary to reduce the wrist flexion torque caused by transection of the FCU. While treating patients with radial nerve palsy, the flexor carpi radialis (FCR) or FCU is often transferred to the extensor digitorum communis (EDC) to reconstruct finger extension. The results of this study indicate that both finger extension and wrist flexion occur simultaneously after FCU transfer to the EDC extensor when dissection of the FCU muscle belly is inadequate. To deteriorate the simultaneous finger extension and wrist flexion, it is reasonable to transfer the FCU to the EDC passing over the ulna laterally, because the FCU must be dissected proximally for quite a long distance to join the EDC after passing over the ulna. In some muscles, it is known that the fascia over the muscles can help retain the original function of the muscle following tenotomy. Considering the function of the fascia of such muscles, the tendons of these muscles should be transferred to those muscles producing motions that are synchronous with those of the transferred tendons.

R. Kakinoki, MD, PhD

Repair of Flexor Digitorum Profundus to Distal Phalanx: A Biomechanical Evaluation of Four Techniques
Lee SK, Fajardo M, Kardashian G, et al (Hosp for Special Surgery, NY)
J Hand Surg 36A:1604-1609, 2011

Purpose.—Many techniques for repair of the flexor digitorum profundus to the distal phalanx show excessive gapping with variable clinical results. The purpose of this study was to test the biomechanical characteristics of an anchor-button (AB) technique, as compared to 3 other techniques.

Methods.—Twenty-four fresh-frozen human cadaveric fingers were randomized to 4 groups, 6 in each: group 1, 2-strand Bunnell suture button pullout technique; group 2, modified Kessler suture and 2 retrograde anchors; group 3: locking Krakow suture with 2 retrograde anchors; group 4, AB technique incorporating a 2-part repair, consisting of a locking dorsal Krakow suture with 2 retrograde anchors and a locking palmar Krakow suture fixed with a button. Tendon-to-bone gapping was measured after cyclical loading. Ultimate load to failure was measured at the end of 500 cycles.

Results.—The AB technique resulted in significantly less gapping when compared to the other techniques. It also resulted in a significantly stronger repair compared to all the other groups with an average load to failure comparable to the native tendon-to-bone interface.

Conclusions.—The AB repair might allow for early active postoperative motion after repair of flexor digitorum profundus avulsion injuries and tendon reconstruction procedures; however, the soft tissue effects of this multistrand technique are unknown in clinical repairs.

▶ This article compares 4 techniques of flexor digitorum profundus (FDP) tendon repair, including a new technique, the "anchor button" technique. In this technique, 2 anchors and a suture button are used to repair the FDP tendon, whereas in the other techniques in this study, only one of these constructs is used. As one might predict, the anchor button technique yielded the strongest load to failure and least gapping and even approximated that of the native tendon–bone interface. Therefore, this technique may be the strongest of any FDP tendon repair yet described in the literature.

Strengths of the study are the study protocol itself and the number of specimens used (dictated by the authors' power analysis of the literature). Weaknesses of the study are the variability in suture materials and sizes used for the groups and investigator bias.

The authors have found, at least biomechanically, a technique for FDP tendon repair that appears to be very strong and likely amenable to early active motion postoperatively. Obviously, clinical studies comparing these techniques would be very useful as well as studies that would compare different flexor tendon rehabilitation protocols for the anchor-button technique. However, one begs the following question: does this new technique make a difference clinically? That is, is 115 N of failure strength really needed for good clinical results, or is 30 N all that is needed? Kudos to the authors, however, for coming up with an innovative technique that seems to be the strongest yet.

My technique of choice for repairs of FDP tendon ruptures is using 2 modified Kessler sutures with 2 retrograde Mitek Microfix anchors, the Group 2 repair. My personal opinion, however, is that less than ideal results are common with this surgery, even with the best of repairs, no matter which technique is used. I believe that postoperative scar tissue formation and swelling are the main reasons why the amount of active range of motion ultimately gained may be poor, no matter how happy I am intraoperatively with the repair.

S. S. Shin, MD, MMSc

13 Elbow

Validity of Goniometric Elbow Measurements: Comparative Study with a Radiographic Method
Chapleau J, Canet F, Petit Y, et al (Université de Montreal, Canada; Hôpital du Sacré-Coeur de Montréal, Canada)
Clin Orthop Relat Res 469:3134-3140, 2011

Background.—A universal goniometer is commonly used to measure the elbow's ROM and carrying angle; however, some authors question its poor intertester reliability.

Questions/Purposes.—We (1) assessed the validity of goniometric measurements as compared with radiographic measurements in the evaluation of ROM of the elbow and (2) determined the reliability of both.

Methods.—The ROM and carrying angle of 51 healthy subjects (102 elbows) were measured using two methods: with a universal goniometer by one observer three times and on radiographs by two independent examiners. Paired t-test and Pearson's correlation were used to compare and detect the relationship between mean ROM. The maximal error was calculated according to the Bland and Altman method.

Results.—The intraclass correlation coefficients (ICC) ranged from 0.945 to 0.973 for the goniometric measurements and from 0.980 to 0.991 for the radiographic measurements. The two methods correlated when measuring the total ROM in flexion and extension. The maximal errors of the goniometric measurement were 10.3° for extension, 7.0° for flexion, and 6.5° for carrying angle 95% of the time. We observed differences for maximum flexion, maximal extension, and carrying angle between the methods.

Conclusion.—Both measurement methods differ but they correlate. When measured with a goniometer, the elbow ROM shows a maximal error of approximately 10°.

Clinical Relevance.—The goniometer is a reasonable and simple clinical tool, but for research protocols, we suggest using the radiographic method because of the higher level of precision required.

▶ This article highlights the pitfalls of accurately measuring elbow range of motion. To identify whether patients have shown improvement (or loss) of motion we need to be able to accurately measure it.

Because most patients being treated for a stiff elbow do not require serial radiographs in their course of treatment, this study helps to define the correlation between the gold standard measurement of elbow range of motion from radiographs and clinical measurement with a goniometer.

121

This article reminds us that no matter how precise we think we are with our measurements, there is always error, in this case up to 12°. Because there is inherent error in any x-ray technique, the error of measurement is actually greater than what the authors report. In addition, the patient population we are most interested in, patients with elbow stiffness, often have bony landmarks that are difficult to palpate, abnormal anatomy from prior trauma, and other physical characteristics that make measurement error invariably higher than healthy, thin volunteers.

So, how does this help us as clinicians? First of all, it reminds us to be careful with our measurements. Knowing that in a perfect testing environment the error is up to 12°, we need to use a goniometer with long limbs, accurately place the center of the goniometer on the lateral epicondyle, and make sure that the limbs are in line with the humerus and radius. Second, remind patients to use internal landmarks as their goal for recovery of motion. I have found that patients frequently perseverate on the numbers marked on their continuous passive motion machines that are often meaningless. Redirecting the patient's attention to functional milestones, reaching hand to mouth or hand to ear, are much more reliable and functionally relevant to the patient than reaching the magic mark of 130° of flexion. Lastly, it is important to remember that although we measure an actual number, having a goniometer and measuring within a degree or 2 is misleading. Having an accurate measuring device does not increase clinical accuracy of the measurement.

A. Daluiski, MD

Contralateral Elbow Radiographs Can Reliably Diagnose Radial Head Implant Overlengthening
Athwal GS, Rouleau DM, MacDermid JC, et al (Univ of Western Ontario, London, Ontario, Canada)
J Bone Joint Surg Am 93:1339-1346, 2011

Background.—Excessive lengthening of the radius with use of a radial head implant, a common cause of capitellar wear and clinical failure, is difficult to identify on radiographs of the injured elbow. The purpose of this study was to determine if a novel measurement technique based on radiographs of the contralateral elbow could be used to accurately estimate the magnitude of overlengthening due to the radial head implant. In part I of this study, we examined the side-to-side consistency of radiographic landmarks used in the measurement technique. In part II, the technique was validated in a cadaveric model with simulated radial head implant overlengthening.

Methods.—In part I of the study, a side-to-side comparison of elbow joint dimensions was performed with use of 100 radiographs from fifty patients. In part II, radial head prostheses of varying lengths (leading to 0, 2, 4, 6, and 8 mm of overlengthening) were implanted in four pairs of cadaveric specimens (eight elbows). Radiographic measurements were performed by two examiners blinded to the implant size to determine if radiographs of the contralateral elbow could be used to diagnose, and provide a valid estimate of the magnitude of, implant overlengthening. Intrarater and interrater reliability ratios, absolute measurement errors, and diagnostic accuracy were determined.

Results.—No significant side-to-side differences (p > 0.2) in radiographic measurements were identified between paired elbows. In the cadaveric model, the measurement technique involving use of radiographs of the contralateral elbow was successful in predicting the implant size (± 1 mm) in 104 (87%) of the 120 scenarios tested. The sensitivity of the technique— i.e., the ability of the test to correctly identify overlengthening (within ± 1 mm) when it was present—was 98%, with a positive likelihood ratio of 49 and a negative likelihood ratio of 0.02. The reliability of the radiographic measurements, based on repeated measurements performed by a single blinded orthopaedic surgeon on two separate occasions or based on separate measurements performed by two different orthopaedic surgeons, was excellent (intraclass correlation coefficient > 0.95).

Conclusions.—A measurement technique based on radiographs of the contralateral elbow can be used to diagnose and calculate the magnitude of radial overlengthening due to the use of an incorrectly sized radial head implant.

▶ This is a very interesting study evaluating a new measurement technique to identify whether a radial head prosthesis is long compared with the native side. This is a cumbersome set of measurements requiring a 6-step process that identifies how many millimeters longer the prosthesis is compared with the native radius. It requires the elbow be flexed to 45° for the radiographs, something that is often problematic for the patient with limited or no motion of the elbow.

The true benefit of this article is that it continues to increase the awareness of the detrimental effects of implanting a radial head prosthesis that is too long. It reminds us to exercise care when measuring and replacing the radial head. Although the authors reference a biomechanics study evaluating the effect of a radial head that is too short, I am unaware of any publications showing clinical deficits in patients with radial head replacements that are shorter than the native side. In contrast, a large number of the patients that I treat with a surgical release for their stiff elbow have radial heads that are longer than they should be. In these patients, knowing whether the prosthesis is 1 versus 3 mm too long is not material. In addition, this method does not offer guidance to the surgeon requiring help intraoperatively, although the authors have written several other articles that are useful in this regard. Although this measurement is not required to treat most patients that have stiffness or lateral-sided elbow pain after a radial head replacement, using this tool will add an interesting additional data point from which to make our decision. I will be again using this in my clinical practice.

A. Daluiski, MD

A Randomized Study Comparing Corticosteroid Injection to Corticosteroid Iontophoresis for Lateral Epicondylitis

Stefanou A, Marshall N, Holdan W, et al (Henry Ford Hosp, Detroit, MI; Wayne State Univ, Detroit, MI)
J Hand Surg 37A:104-109, 2012

Purpose.—We designed a prospective, randomized study to evaluate the effects of iontophoresis delivery of dexamethasone versus corticosteroid injection therapy on patient outcomes.

Methods.—We randomized 82 patients to 10 mg dexamethasone via iontophoresis using a self-contained patch with a 24-hour battery; 10 mg dexamethasone injection; or 10 mg triamcinolone injection. All patients received the same hand therapy protocol. Primary outcomes tracked were change in grip strength (flexion vs extension), pain, and function scores on a validated questionnaire. The secondary outcome was return-to-work status. Patients were evaluated at baseline, completion of physical therapy, and 6-month follow-up.

Results.—The iontophoresis patients had statistically significant improvement in grip strength at the conclusion of hand therapy compared with baseline. They were also more likely to get back to work without restriction. By 6-month follow-up, all groups had equivalent results for all measured outcomes.

Conclusions.—Dexamethasone via iontophoresis produced short-term benefits because for this group grip strength and unrestricted return to work were significantly better. This study suggests that this iontophoresis technique for delivery of corticosteroid may be considered a treatment option for patients with lateral epicondylitis.

▶ This is an interesting study examining the efficacy of small, self-contained iontophoresis patches that deliver dexamethasone for the treatment of lateral epicondylitis. As with many treatments for lateral epicondylitis, by 6 months, all study groups showed similar improvement using several outcomes measures. Clinically, patients complain of pain. Because a simple visual analogue scale pain score was not reported as an independent variable in this study, it is still unclear as to how therapeutically useful this modality is in reducing pain. Using composite scores comprised of multiple questions and work status confuses the matter and adds to the uncertainty as to how much of the modest improvement can be attributed to each specific treatment.

Clinically, I have not found iontophoresis administered by a hand therapist to be a particularly effective treatment for this common condition. If the stand-alone iontophoresis units that reside in therapy offices show questionable efficacy, it is difficult to be convinced that a single-use, disposable unit would be better. The study does, however, bring up several interesting points that may merit further investigation. The portability and sustained therapeutic exposure to an active drug make this modality something I will consider for patients refractory to other conservative measures I use even though the exact efficacy for tennis elbow or other conditions has yet to be conclusively shown.

A. Daluiski, MD

Effectiveness of Different Methods of Resistance Exercises in Lateral Epicondylosis—A Systematic Review
Raman J, MacDermid JC, Grewal R (Univ of Western Ontario, London, Ontario, Canada; St Joseph's Health Centre, London, Ontario, Canada)
J Hand Ther 25:5-26, 2012

Study Design.—Systematic Review.

Introduction.—Lateral epicondylosis (LE) is relatively common with an annual incidence in the general population of 1% to 3%. Systematic reviews have identified exercise is effective, but have not established specific exercise parameters.

Purpose.—The purpose of this systematic review was to synthesize the quality and content of clinical research addressing type and dosage of resistance exercises in lateral epicondylosis.

Methods.—Computerized bibliographic databases (1990—2010) were searched using relevant keywords; bibliographies of included papers were hand searched. Of 594 screened abstracts, 11 articles (12 studies) met inclusion criteria. Articles were randomly allocated to pairs of reviewers who independently verified data extraction and appraised the full text, using a structured critical appraisal tool with 24 items. Data extraction was limited by a lack of consistent reporting of elements of exercise dosage.

Results.—The mean quality rating of the studies was 72%, with 2 papers exceeding 75% quality. Of the 12 studies, 9 addressed the effects of isotonic (eccentric/concentric) exercises, 2 studied the effect of isometric and one studied isokinetic exercises. The exercise programs ranged over a period of 4 to 52 weeks. Exercises were prescribed 1 to 6 times per day, with an average duration of 15 minutes per session, and average of 15 repetitions (range: 3 to 50), with 1 to 4 sets per session.

Conclusion.—All the studies reported that resistance exercise resulted in substantial improvement in pain and grip strength; eccentric exercise was most studied. Strengthening using resistance exercises is effective in reducing pain and improving function for lateral epicondylosis but optimal dosing is not defined.

Level of Evidence.—2a.

▶ This systematic review attempts to synthesize evidence extracted from a series of studies investigating the benefits of resistive exercises in subjects with lateral epicondylosis in an effort to qualify optimal exercise type, dosage, and frequency. As is the case with many systematic reviews, few studies meet the inclusionary criteria, and fewer meet the high-quality criteria for randomized controlled trials. Additionally, because of variations in interventions and outcome measures between studies, the data cannot be statistically analyzed, and the effect of resistance exercise is difficult to isolate. What remains is a narrative review that compares different exercise types with pointed references to study weaknesses, such as a lack of detailed descriptions of exercise parameters. The article fails to provide an overarching conclusion or suggestion and at best provides a general statement supporting a protocol of eccentric exercises as having the best, albeit weak, evidence. Of greatest value is the recommendation that future studies include better reporting methods, detailed exercise regimen, and a description for how specific load is calculated for individuals in an exercise routine. In my own practice, I have seen the greatest improvement in patients who received a progressive exercise regime (isometric to eccentric, followed by concentric) of wrist extension exercises in conjunction with stretching, proximal strengthening, and attention to posture.

A. Wolff, OTR/L, CHT

Contralateral Elbow Radiographs Can Reliably Diagnose Radial Head Implant Overlengthening
Athwal GS, Rouleau DM, MacDermid JC, et al (Univ of Western Ontario, London, Canada)
J Bone Joint Surg Am 93:1339-1346, 2011

Background.—Excessive lengthening of the radius with use of a radial head implant, a common cause of capitellar wear and clinical failure, is difficult to identify on radiographs of the injured elbow. The purpose of this study was to determine if a novel measurement technique based on radiographs of the contralateral elbow could be used to accurately estimate the magnitude of overlengthening due to the radial head implant. In part I of this study, we examined the side-to-side consistency of radiographic landmarks used in the measurement technique. In part II, the technique was validated in a cadaveric model with simulated radial head implant overlengthening.

Methods.—In part I of the study, a side-to-side comparison of elbow joint dimensions was performed with use of 100 radiographs from fifty patients. In part II, radial head prostheses of varying lengths (leading to 0, 2, 4, 6, and 8 mm of overlengthening) were implanted in four pairs of cadaveric specimens (eight elbows). Radiographic measurements were performed by two examiners blinded to the implant size to determine if radiographs of the contralateral elbow could be used to diagnose, and provide a valid estimate of the magnitude of, implant overlengthening. Intrarater and interrater reliability ratios, absolute measurement errors, and diagnostic accuracy were determined.

Results.—No significant side-to-side differences ($p > 0.2$) in radiographic measurements were identified between paired elbows. In the cadaveric model, the measurement technique involving use of radiographs of the contralateral elbow was successful in predicting the implant size (± 1 mm) in 104 (87%) of the 120 scenarios tested. The sensitivity of the technique— i.e., the ability of the test to correctly identify overlengthening (within

± 1 mm) when it was present—was 98%, with a positive likelihood ratio of 49 and a negative likelihood ratio of 0.02. The reliability of the radiographic measurements, based on repeated measurements performed by a single blinded orthopaedic surgeon on two separate occasions or based on separate measurements performed by two different orthopaedic surgeons, was excellent (intraclass correlation coefficient >0.95).

Conclusions.—A measurement technique based on radiographs of the contralateral elbow can be used to diagnose and calculate the magnitude of radial overlengthening due to the use of an incorrectly sized radial head implant.

▶ The goal of this study was to identify a method for diagnosing and estimating the magnitude of radial head implant overlengthening postoperatively. The authors defined and validated a measurement technique based on radiographs of the contralateral elbow that is accurate for diagnosing and calculating the magnitude of radial head implant overlengthening. The technique requires bilateral anteroposterior elbow radiographs, with the elbow flexed 45°, the forearm in neutral rotation and made orthogonal to the forearm, and a commercially available image viewing program with a calibrated length tool. The joint measurements were made at 4 locations: (1) the lateral side of the lateral ulnohumeral facet, (2) the medial side of the lateral ulnohumeral facet, (3) the lateral side of the medial ulnohumeral facet, and (4) the medial side of the medial ulnohumeral facet. The lateral joint measurements demonstrated better correlations than did the medial joint measurements. The described measurement technique, based on radiographs of the contralateral normal elbow, was found to be accurate in predicting radial head implant length. The authors point out that although this method was effective for diagnosing implant overlengthening in the postoperative situation, the focus should remain on preventing this problem by inserting an implant of correct length at the time of the primary surgery.

E. Cheung, MD

Restoration of Elbow Flexion with Functioning Free Muscle Transfer in Arthrogryposis: A Report of Two Cases
Doi K, Arakawa Y, Hattori Y, et al (Ogori Daiichi General Hosp, Yamaguchi Prefecture, Japan)
J Bone Joint Surg Am 93:e105, 2011

Background.—The characteristics of arthrogryposis include nonprogressive, multiple joint contractures present at birth because of neurogenic, myopathic (amyoplasia), or connective tissue disorders. Upper extremity amyloplasia is most seriously expressed as an inability to flex the elbow because of extension contracture of the elbow. Children must be able to flex one elbow to become functionally independent, including self-feeding and performing self-care of the face and hair. Extension of both elbows is needed for independent toileting. Surgical intervention in amyloplasia is designed to achieve active elbow flexion, and many procedures are used. The long-term results with free muscle transfer using the gracilis muscle for restoration of elbow flexion were noted in two patients with arthrogryposis.

Case Reports.—Case 1: Boy, 3 months, had amyoplasia of both upper extremities without lower limb involvement. The pectoralis major and latissimus dorsi muscles were hypoplastic and unavailable for transfer. Preoperative physiotherapy improved passive elbow flexion to 90 degrees on the right side and 100 degrees on the left. At age 1 year 8 months, free gracilis muscle transfer was done. The contralateral gracilis muscle and skin paddle were harvested and placed in the subcutaneous plane on the anterior part of the deltoid muscle in the upper arm. The distal tendinous part was passed through the subcutaneous tunnel in the arm's distal part and fixed to the radial tuberosity via an incision over the cubital fossa. The motor nerve of the gracilis muscle was tunneled under the clavicle and sutured to the middle and distal branches of the accessory nerve in the supraclavicular area. Nutrient vessels of the muscle transplant and the thoracromial artery and cephalic vein in the infraclavicular region were linked via microvascular anastomoses. The muscle's proximal origin was fixed to the clavicle's lateral half using anchoring sutures under maximal traction with shoulder flexion at 30 degrees and abduction at 30 degrees and elbow flexion at 100 degrees. Both transferred muscles survived without vascular compromise. Three months after surgery the muscles were reinnervated; 1 month later muscle contraction was visible. Electromyographic biofeedback exercises strengthened the transferred muscles. Eleven years postoperatively, the patient's active range of elbow flexion was 50 to 130 degrees on the right and 50 to 130 degrees on the left. His elbow flexion was about 30% of normal in adults, but he could perform all school and daily activities without difficulty or assistance.

Case 2: Girl, 17 months, had amyoplasia of both upper arms, with hypoplastic pectoralis major and latissimus dorsi muscles but no lower limb involvement. Physiotherapy achieved about 70 degrees of passive elbow flexion before free gracilis muscle transfer was done at age 2 years 4 months on the right and 2 years 8 months on the left. Both muscle transfers survived without vascular complications. Twenty-one months after the second transfer the patient had elbow contractures that limited her ability to flex the elbows to 70 degrees. Posterior capsulotomy of the elbow with triceps lengthening was done. Three years after her second free muscle transfer, her active elbow flexion was 40 to 100 degrees on the left and 40 to 105 degrees on the right. She still had shoulder contracture, but could lift light objects and feed herself.

Conclusions.—Free muscle transfer achieved optimal function when suitable donor muscles for pedicle transfer were unavailable. For best results, this approach involves a demanding surgical technique and requires both passive elbow flexion of at least 90 degrees preoperatively and closely supervised postoperative management.

▶ The authors begin their article with an interesting discussion of the most commonly performed surgical procedures for restoration of elbow flexion in patients with arthrogryposis. They discuss the advantages and disadvantages of 3 different tendon transfers using the triceps, pectoralis major, and latissimus dorsi, and the Steindler flexorplasty, in which the origin of the flexor-pronator muscle group is shifted proximally. They then discuss the advantages of free gracilis muscle transfers.

The major strength of the article is that it provides a comprehensive description of the technical aspects of free gracilis muscle transfers, including proper tensioning of the muscle. There are 2 weaknesses of the article. The first is that it is somewhat disorganized and does not follow logical sequence. For example, prerequisites for the procedure are discussed at the end of the article rather than at the beginning. The second weakness is that the authors discuss the importance in patients with bilateral disease of restoring flexion in 1 elbow for self-feeding and self-care of the hair and face and maintaining extension in the other elbow for independent toilet care. Yet, in the 2 cases they present, they performed bilateral gracilis muscle transfers but provide no explanation for their rationale in doing so. Regardless, the article should be in the file of every hand surgeon who treats children with arthrogryposis.

M. A. Posner, MD

A Randomized Study Comparing Corticosteroid Injection to Corticosteroid Iontophoresis for Lateral Epicondylitis

Stefanou A, Marshall N, Holdan W, et al (Henry Ford Hosp, Detroit, MI; Wayne State Univ, Detroit, MI)
J Hand Surg 37A:104-109, 2012

Purpose.—We designed a prospective, randomized study to evaluate the effects of iontophoresis delivery of dexamethasone versus corticosteroid injection therapy on patient outcomes.

Methods.—We randomized 82 patients to 10 mg dexamethasone via iontophoresis using a self-contained patch with a 24-hour battery; 10 mg dexamethasone injection; or 10 mg triamcinolone injection. All patients received the same hand therapy protocol. Primary outcomes tracked were change in grip strength (flexion vs extension), pain, and function scores on a validated questionnaire. The secondary outcome was return-to-work status. Patients were evaluated at baseline, completion of physical therapy, and 6-month follow-up.

Results.—The iontophoresis patients had statistically significant improvement in grip strength at the conclusion of hand therapy compared with baseline. They were also more likely to get back to work without restriction. By 6-month follow-up, all groups had equivalent results for all measured outcomes.

Conclusion.—Dexamethasone via iontophoresis produced short-term benefits because for this group grip strength and unrestricted return to work were significantly better. This study suggests that this iontophoresis technique for delivery of corticosteroid may be considered a treatment option for patients with lateral epicondylitis.

Type of Study/Level of Evidence.—Therapeutic II.

▶ Overall, the title, abstract, methodology, and discussion in this article are concise and easy to follow. Primary outcome is evident with differential grip strength improvement in the iontophoresis group, both at the end of treatment and at the end of the study compared with the injection treatment group,which only showed improvement at the end of the study (Table 2 in the original article).

This means of measuring differential grip strength can be diagnostic to lateral epicondylitis and support the study outcome that the use of the iontophoresis technique for delivery of corticosteroid may be the better treatment option.

Functional or secondary outcomes, such as return to work or normal activities of daily living, was determined based on baseline, completion of physical therapy, and the 6-month follow-up. This was again acheived and presented in a clear and concise manner.

One concern is with the statement, "Recent studies suggest that lateral epicondylitis might not be a inflammatory process." No study or author was specifically listed for this. Referring back to the references does not provide clear study or research.

Another concern is in the statement, "This device can potentially deliver higher levels of medication over 24 hours than in a traditional therapy session." The dosage for iontophoresis stays the same whether delivered in the home-going integrated battery system or in the clinical setting of traditional iontophoresis. The dosage is just introduced over a longer period of time in the intergrated electrodes. The integrated battery electrodes are in 40 mA or 80 mA, and the potential for dosage in clinical settings is variable. The authors provided a good discussion in reference to an iontophoresis group that is patient-managed without formal therapy, which may produce similar results. Also, stating that the population that underwent surgery within each group was too small for comprehensive comparison was a useful inclusion.

Regarding the final statement that "the integrated battery offers technical and lifestyle advantages over traditional iontophoresis," I agree with the lifestyle aspect, but not with the technical. Not enough evidence is provided to support that allowing the corticocosteroid to be in place for 24 hours potentially delivers higher levels of medication. The dosage delivered stays the same. Traditional therapy does make use of treatment time while iontophoresis is in use, for education, instruction, and therapy.

S. Kranz, CHT

Clinical and Ultrasonographic Results of Ultrasonographically Guided Percutaneous Radiofrequency Lesioning in the Treatment of Recalcitrant Lateral Epicondylitis

Lin C-L, Lee J-S, Su W-R, et al (Natl Cheng Kung Univ Hosp, Tainan, Taiwan)
Am J Sports Med 39:2429-2435, 2011

Background.—In patients with lateral epicondylitis recalcitrant to nonsurgical treatments, surgical intervention is considered. Despite the numerous therapies reported, the current trend of treatment places particular emphasis on minimally invasive techniques.

Purpose.—The authors present a newly developed minimally invasive procedure, ultrasonographically guided percutaneous radiofrequency thermal lesioning (RTL), and its clinical efficacy in treating recalcitrant lateral epicondylitis.

Study Design.—Case series: Level of evidence, 4.

Methods.—Thirty-four patients (35 elbows), with a mean age of 52.1 years (range, 35-65 years), suffered from symptomatic lateral epicondylitis for more than 6 months and had exhausted nonoperative therapies. They were treated with ultrasonographically guided RTL. Patients were followed up at least 6 months by physical examination and 12 months by interview. The intensity of pain was recorded with a visual analog scale (VAS) score. The functional outcome was evaluated using grip strength, the upper limb Disability of Arm, Shoulder and Hand (Quick-DASH) outcome measure, and the Modified Mayo Clinic Performance Index (MMCPI) for the elbow. The ultrasonographic findings regarding the extensor tendon origin were recorded, as were the complications.

Results.—At the time of the 6-month follow-up, the average VAS score in resting (from 4.9 to 0.9), palpation (from 7.6 to 2.5), and grip (from 8.2 to 2.9) had improved significantly compared with the preoperative condition ($P < .01$). The grip strength (from 20.6 to 27.0 kg) and QuickDASH score (from 54.3 to 21.0) had also improved significantly ($P < .01$). The MMCPI score improved from "poor" to "excellent." The ultrasonographic finding revealed that the thickness of the common extensor tendon origin did not change significantly. At the final follow-up (mean, 14.3 months; range, 12-21 months), the patients reported a 78% reduction in pain compared with the preoperative status. No major complications were noted in any patient.

Conclusion.—Ultrasonographically guided RTL for recalcitrant lateral epicondylitis was found to be a minimally invasive treatment with satisfactory results in this pilot investigation. This innovative method can be considered as an alternative treatment of recalcitrant lateral epicondylitis before further surgical intervention.

▶ This level 4 study describes the utility of ultrasound-guided percutaneous radio-frequency lesioning (RTL) in the treatment of recalcitrant lateral epicondylitis. This technique requires specialized equipment as well as operators who are skilled in both ultrasonography and percutaneous techniques. The general theory behind RTL is that heat dissipation from an active electrode will denature the target tissue, inducing healing and regeneration. In addition, RTL is theorized to denervate peripheral nerve endings, hence resolving pain in the affected area. The nature of this study is retrospective and the subjects were those who had failed at least 6 months of other forms of nonoperative care. Results were favorable overall, with an improvement in visual analog pain scores, grip strength, the Disability of Arm, Shoulder and Hand measure, and Modified Mayo Clinic Performance Index. Only 5 of 34 patients required a second round of RTL, and 4 of those 5 ultimately experienced satisfactory results. In sum, the authors present another nonoperative treatment option for what is universally regarded as a pathologic quandary. Lateral epicondylitis is incompletely understood with regard to etiology as well as optimal treatment. This study typifies some of the weaknesses inherent in studies that evaluate a particular therapeutic intervention without a matched cohort. Further, RTL was initiated at least 6 months after initial presentation. Other modalities had been utilized prior to RTL in this study, and it is therefore unclear as to whether there was a carryover effect or whether the natural tendency of the disease process to wane over time manifested itself. Nonetheless, for those who have access and are skilled enough to perform this technique, there are data to support the use of RTL in the treatment of lateral epicondylitis. Of course, prospective randomized studies are lacking and would contribute valuable information to the ever-expanding literature on lateral epicondylitis.

S. M. Jacoby, MD

A Randomized Study Comparing Corticosteroid Injection to Corticosteroid Iontophoresis for Lateral Epicondylitis
Stefanou A, Marshall N, Holdan W, et al (Henry Ford Hosp, Detroit, MI; Wayne State Univ, Detroit, MI)
J Hand Surg 37A:104-109, 2012

Purpose.—We designed a prospective, randomized study to evaluate the effects of iontophoresis delivery of dexamethasone versus corticosteroid injection therapy on patient outcomes.

Methods.—We randomized 82 patients to 10 mg dexamethasone via iontophoresis using a self-contained patch with a 24-hour battery; 10 mg dexamethasone injection; or 10 mg triamcinolone injection. All patients received the same hand therapy protocol. Primary outcomes tracked were change in grip strength (flexion vs extension), pain, and function scores on a validated questionnaire. The secondary outcome was return-to-work status. Patients were evaluated at baseline, completion of physical therapy, and 6-month follow-up.

Results.—The iontophoresis patients had statistically significant improvement in grip strength at the conclusion of hand therapy compared with baseline. They were also more likely to get back to work without restriction. By 6-month follow-up, all groups had equivalent results for all measured outcomes.

Conclusion.—Dexamethasone via iontophoresis produced short-term benefits because for this group grip strength and unrestricted return to work were significantly better. This study suggests that this iontophoresis technique for delivery of corticosteroid may be considered a treatment option for patients with lateral epicondylitis.

Types of Study/Level of Evidence.—Therapeutic II.

▶ This therapeutic level II study aims to compare the effects of corticosteroid iontophoresis (dexamethasone) via a self-contained patch delivered over a 24-hour period with injection of either of 2 long-acting corticosteroids: triamcinolone and dexamethasone.

Primary outcome measures include grip strength; PRTEE (patient-rated tennis elbow evaluation), which includes pain and function; as well as secondary outcomes, including return to work status. This study is unique in that iontophoresis was powered by an electrode with an integrated battery that allowed for delivery over a 24-hour period, thereby potentially delivering higher levels of medication than during a traditional iontophoresis session. The authors correctly point out that lateral epicondyle enthesopathy is oftentimes a self-limited process that requires appropriate rest, behavioral and/or activity modification, as well as patient education to receive an unacceptable result. Multiple prior studies have shown the effectiveness of numerous interventions for the treatment of this disabling condition. The strength of this study is that it is well designed and includes 3 treatment limbs to compare effectiveness based on mode of delivery: a novel form of iontophoresis versus steroid injection. Since the 2 injection limbs had similar outcomes, this fact confirms the authors' hypothesis that this novel mode of delivery may be more important than the specific medication administered. An added benefit is that the application of this patch is straightforward and can save time, allowing the therapist to focus on education, instruction, and therapy. This study adds yet another viable intervention to treat a condition that most often responds to a tincture of time, therapeutic modalities, and patient education.

S. M. Jacoby, MD

Effect of Lateral Epicondylosis on Grip Force Development
Chourasia AO, Buhr KA, Rabago DP, et al (Univ of Wisconsin, Madison)
J Hand Ther 25:27-37, 2012

Study Design.—Case-Control.

Introduction.—Although it is well known that grip strength is adversely affected by lateral epicondylosis (LE), the effect of LE on rapid grip force generation is unclear.

Purpose of the Study.—To evaluate the effect of LE on the ability to rapidly generate grip force.

Methods.—Twenty-eight participants with LE (13 unilateral and 15 bilateral LE) and 13 healthy controls participated in this study. A multiaxis profile dynamometer was used to evaluate grip strength and rapid grip force generation. The ability to rapidly produce force is composed of the electro-mechanical delay and rate of force development. Electromechanical delay is defined as the time between the onset of electrical activity and the onset of muscle force production. The Patient-rated Tennis Elbow Evaluation (PRTEE) questionnaire was used to assess pain and functional disability. Magnetic resonance imaging was used to evaluate tendon degeneration.

Results.—LE-injured upper extremities had lower rate of force develop-ment (50 lb/sec, confidence interval [CI]: 17, 84) and less grip strength (7.8 lb, CI: 3.3, 12.4) than noninjured extremities. Participants in the LE group had a longer electromechanical delay (-59%, CI: 29, 97) than controls. Peak rate of force development had a higher correlation ($r = 0.56$; $p<0.05$) with PRTEE function than grip strength ($r = 0.47$; $p<0.05$) and electromechanical delay ($r = 0.30$; $p>0.05$) for participants with LE. In addition to a reduction in grip strength, those with LE had a reduction in rate of force development and an increase in electromechanical delay.

Conclusions.—Collectively, these changes may contribute to an increase in reaction time, which may affect risk for recurrent symptoms. These find-ings suggest that therapists may need to address both strength and rapid force development deficits in patients with LE.

Level of Evidence.—3B.

▶ The purpose of this article was to evaluate the effect of lateral epicondylitis (LE) on sensorimotor ability to rapidly generate force. The design was a case-controlled study that compared 28 persons with LE (+ LE) with 13 healthy persons without LE (−LE). Data included strength assessment with the pain-free grip test in the elbow-extended position using a novel rate-of-force—generated multiaxis profile (MAP) dynamometer, a hydraulic dynamometer, MRI, pain visual analog scale (VAS), and the Patient-Rated Tennis Elbow Evaluation (PRTEE). Besides measuring grip strength and rate of force, the MAP dynamometer also measured electromechanical delay of grip strength.

The results of the study were (1) reduced grip strength in the + LE group regard-less of the dynamometer used; (2) the dominant extremity generating more force; (3) significantly less rate of peak force, regardless of dominance, in the injured extremity; (4) less submaximal rate of force generation in the injured extremities; (5) a grouped effect of electromechanical delay with all + LE compared with all −LE; and (6) increased MRI signal intensity for all + LE persons.

The following correlations were noted: high correlations between MAP grip strength and PRTEE function ($r = -0.56$) and peak rate of force with PRTEE func-tion ($r = -0.47$) and significant correlations between grip strength, rate of force development, and self-reported pain with PRTEE function but not with VAS pain.

Strength of the study is that it showcases a novel approach to studying force generation in the elbow, such as what is occurring in the literature for other joints. A priori power calculation was performed before the study; however, because of the dropout rate, they failed to meet the 50 subjects expected. Limitations of the study are small sample, only chronic LE persons, and lack of blinding of assessors other than the radiologist. Clinical recommendations include the plausible consideration of the use of plyometrics in rehabilitation versus focusing on resistive exercises only, if this fits the patient profile.

V. O'Brien, OTD, OTR/L, CHT

Effectiveness of Different Methods of Resistance Exercises in Lateral Epicondylosis—A Systematic Review
Raman J, MacDermid JC, Grewal R (Univ of Western Ontario, London, Ontario, Canada; St Joseph's Health Centre, London, Ontario, Canada)
J Hand Ther 25:5-26, 2012

Study Design.—Systematic Review.

Introduction.—Lateral epicondylosis (LE) is relatively common with an annual incidence in the general population of 1% to 3%. Systematic reviews have identified exercise is effective, but have not established specific exercise parameters.

Purpose.—The purpose of this systematic review was to synthesize the quality and content of clinical research addressing type and dosage of resistance exercises in lateral epicondylosis.

Methods.—Computerized bibliographic databases (1990–2010) were searched using relevant keywords; bibliographies of included papers were hand searched. Of 594 screened abstracts, 11 articles (12 studies) met inclusion criteria. Articles were randomly allocated to pairs of reviewers who independently verified data extraction and appraised the full text, using a structured critical appraisal tool with 24 items. Data extraction was limited by a lack of consistent reporting of elements of exercise dosage.

Results.—The mean quality rating of the studies was 72%, with 2 papers exceeding 75% quality. Of the 12 studies, 9 addressed the effects of isotonic (eccentric/concentric) exercises, 2 studied the effect of isometric and one studied isokinetic exercises. The exercise programs ranged over a period of 4 to 52 weeks. Exercises were prescribed 1 to 6 times per day, with an average duration of 15 minutes per session, and average of 15 repetitions (range: 3 to 50), with 1 to 4 sets per session.

Conclusion.—All the studies reported that resistance exercise resulted in substantial improvement in pain and grip strength; eccentric exercise was most studied. Strengthening using resistance exercises is effective in reducing pain and improving function for lateral epicondylosis but optimal dosing is not defined.

Level of Evidence.—2a.

▶ Lateral epicondylosis (LE) has been reported on frequently in surgical and therapeutic literature. This systematic review aimed to investigate the current evidence specific to resistance exercises, to find exercise modalities details, and hopefully establish the evidence for therapeutic dosage parameters. The systematic review was completed using MacDermid's critical appraisal form (CAF), a quality scale to evaluate the study designs and outcomes.[1,2] The CAF has been used in previous systematic reviews of therapeutic interventions.[3,4] This is a 24-item form with a maximum score of 48 that is expressed in percentages to denote quality of evidence: high quality, more than 75%; moderate quality, 51% to 75%; low quality, less than 50%.

Databases were searched from January 1990 to December 2010, revealing 12 studies that fit their criteria: these included 7 randomized controlled trials (RCT), 4 nonrandomized clinical trials, and 1 cohort study. Of these studies, 2 reported on the effect of isometric exercise, 1 reported on the effect of isokinetic eccentric exercise, 7 reported on isotonic eccentric exercises, and 2 reported on the effect of isotonic concentric and eccentric exercise. Ten of the studies were of moderate quality and 2 were of high quality. All studies compared resistive exercises with conventional therapy modalities or procedures. Because of the variability of all therapies reported, data were not pooled; therefore, a meta-analysis was not possible. Seven reported a positive effect with resistance exercises when compared with conventional interventions, and 4 studies showed a positive effect with resistive exercises over time, but not when compared with the control or alternative group. One study reported that wrist manipulation, when compared with conventional interventions, was more effective.

In the synthesis of the studies, resistance exercises were found to reduce pain and increase strength and function for those with LE. However, this result must be cautiously accepted, as is noted in this systematic review. The many limitations of this group of studies are well documented in this systematic review. One of the major limitations was the small number of quality studies on which to base recommendations. Although eccentric exercise was found to have moderate evidence for LE, this was because that was the most studied. The recommendations continue with weak evidence for isotonic or isokinetic exercises. The limitations of the studies include: lack of report of patient exercise compliance, widely ranged follow-up periods from 1 week to 1 year, and the range of types of resistive exercises, which was not well documented as to resistance, repetitions, duration, and how or whether the exercises were upgraded.

Outcome measures between the studies were multiple and were not always those validated specifically for this population, thus making it difficult to determine the outcome goal of each study or to make a generalized statement of functional improvement. The measures included the Disabilities of the Arm, Shoulder, and Hand survey, the modified Nirschl/Pettrone score, the Mayo elbow performance score, the visual analog scale for pain and function or the patient-rated forearm evaluation questionnaire, Short Form-36, and the global measure of improvement, as well as impairment outcomes of range of motion and pain-free grip strength. Of note, return to work status was not identified as part of the studies.

The systematic review concludes with a list of recommendations for future studies, including: improved quality of studies using the Consolidated Standards of Reporting Trials criteria, studies with control and wait-and-see groups, clear reporting of resistive exercises, clear reporting of frequency and duration of repetitions with exercise upgrades, inclusion of patient adherence to exercises, and use of outcome measures that are validated for this population, which include ratings of pain, function, and return to work status.

V. O'Brien, OTD, OTR/L, CIIT

References

1. MacDermid JC. An introduction to evidence-based practice for hand therapists. *J Hand Ther.* 2004;17:105-117.
2. MacDermid JC. Critical appraisal of study quality for psychometric articles. Evaluationform. In: Law M, MacDermid J, eds. *Evidence-Based Rehabilitation.* Thorofare, MN: Slack Inc; 2008:387-388.
3. Valdes K, Marik T. A systematic review of conservative interventions for osteoarthritis of the hand. *J Hand Ther.* 2010;23:334-350.
4. Michlovitz SL, Harris BA, Watkins MP. Therapy interventions for improving joint range of motion: a systematic review. *J Hand Ther.* 2004;17:118-131.

Modular Prosthetic Reconstruction of Major Bone Defects of the Distal End of the Humerus
Funovics PT, Schuh R, Adams SB Jr, et al (Med Univ of Vienna, Austria)
J Bone Joint Surg Am 93:1064-1074, 2011

Background.—Bone defects of the distal end of the humerus require complex reconstructions, for which standard prostheses may be insufficient. We investigated the outcomes of distal humeral reconstruction with use of a modular prosthesis.

Methods.—Fifty-three elbows in fifty-two patients underwent reconstruction with a modular prosthesis (twelve total humeral replacements and forty-one distal humeral replacements) after tumor resection (thirty-eight elbows) or because of massive joint degeneration (fifteen elbows). In the tumor group, twenty-three patients (twenty-four elbows) had metastatic disease and fourteen had a primary tumor. Degenerative defects of the distal end of the humerus were caused by pseudarthrosis (six elbows), prosthetic failure (five), trauma (two), osteomyelitis (one), and supracondylar fracture (one). The mean duration of follow-up for all patients was twenty-eight months (median, thirteen months; range, one to 219 months).

Results.—The mean Inglis-Pellicci score in the tumor group was 84 points, and the mean Musculoskeletal Tumor Society score was 78%. Patients with total humeral reconstruction had worse scores than those with distal humeral reconstruction. Twenty-four patients died of disease at a mean of thirteen months after surgery. Local tumor control was achieved in all patients. In the revision group, the mean Inglis-Pellicci score was 76 points. The Inglis-Pellicci score was significantly better for patients in the tumor group. Eight patients (15%) had a deep periprosthetic infection, requiring amputation in one patient (2%) and prosthetic removal in two patients (4%). Four patients (8%) had the implants revised for aseptic loosening.

Conclusions.—Modular prostheses of the distal end of the humerus provide a stable reconstruction of the elbow with satisfactory function and disease control in patients with a tumor, but careful patient selection is required when the prostheses are used for revision surgery in patients without a tumor.

▶ Modular elbow prostheses can be used as a salvage surgery for reconstruction of bone defects of the distal end of the humerus after tumor resection or for massive bone defects after failed reconstructive surgery. Elbows in which the modular implant was used following failed elbow surgery for massive defects had worse outcomes, suggesting that previous surgery, extensive scarring, a history of infection, and poor bone stock can adversely affect results. Also, radiation therapy must be factored into the increased infection rate in oncology patients. The high rate of patients with metastatic disease emphasizes the role of a surgical procedure with fast recovery and successful tumor control. The most severe complication in this series, similar to other studies reporting on complex elbow reconstruction using allograft prosthetic composites, was infection. The overall infection rate was 15% (8 of 53 elbows), resulting in removal of the prosthesis in 2 patients and amputation in another patient. The authors note that they have thus altered their antibiotic regimen to prolonged prophylaxis over 5 days. Also, they mention that silver-coated modular prostheses of the femur and tibia have been shown to reduce infection rates and could provide improvements for humeral reconstructions. This operation should perhaps be avoided in patients with a history of infection or osteoporotic bone. The study is limited by its relatively small numbers and its retrospective nature. Also, the tumor group differed from the nontumor group in overall patient demographics, and a high number of the patients with tumor eventually succumbed to their disease.

E. Cheung, MD

Anterior subcutaneous transposition of ulnar nerve with fascial flap and complete excision of medial intermuscular septum in cubital tunnel syndrome: A prospective patient cohort
Hamidreza A, Saeid A, Mohammadreza D, et al (Shahid Beheshti Univ of Med Sciences, Iran; Bushehr Univ of Med Sciences, Iran; et al)
Clin Neurol Neurosurg 113:631-634, 2011

Objective.—Regarding the frequency of cubital tunnel syndrome, varieties of treatment modalities, and ambiguity of anterior subcutaneous transposition of ulnar nerve method, we aimed to evaluate the efficacy of this procedure in patients with cubital tunnel syndrome referred to Taleghani hospital between 2006 and 2009.

Methods.—This study was a case series including all referred patients with definite diagnosis of cubital tunnel syndrome, treated by anterior subcutaneous transposition. Treatment results were measured according to modified Bishop rating system, and were ranked into excellent, good, fair, and poor. Variables such as gender, age (less/more than 45 years), causation, and initial severity, determined by Dellon criteria preoperatively, were analyzed by Fisher's exact test.

Results.—This study was performed on 26 eligible cases including 29 elbows, 38% males and 62.1% females, with mean age of 44.5 years (ranging 23–72 years). In a 12 months follow-up post-operatively, 62% showed excellent, 20.7% good, and 17.3% fair, with no poor result. In a 1–12 months follow-up post-operatively, results showed improvement, and initial severity and old age were demonstrated to significantly affect treatment results ($P < 0.07$).

Conclusion.—Though considered standard of care, the present study suggests that criteria for surgical techniques of ulnar nerve decompression, e.g. simple decompression vs. more extensive repair as in the present cohort, should be revised by controlled prospective studies.

▶ The authors present their experience with anterior subcutaneous transposition of the ulnar nerve for the management of cubital tunnel syndrome. Strengths of the study include its prospective design and choice of outcome measurements. Limitations of the study include its small sample size (26 patients), length of follow-up, and lack of novelty.

The study looked at the modified Bishop rating scale results at 3, 6, and 12 months. At each interval, the percentages of good/excellent results versus fair/poor results were continuing to change, with an increasing number of good/excellent results over time, drawing into question whether 1-year follow-up is adequate. Gender and etiology (trauma vs idiopathic) were not associated with outcome, while increasing patient age and presurgical severity were predictors of worse outcomes (also shown by numerous previous studies).

There have been numerous previous studies demonstrating the efficacy of anterior subcutaneous transposition of the ulnar nerve for cubital tunnel syndrome, so there is nothing particularly new demonstrated by this series. Furthermore, there are many studies demonstrating the efficacy of in situ decompression, medial epicondylectomy, and submuscular transposition in the management of cubital tunnel syndrome.

Although this series offers support for those surgeons who prefer this technique over other surgical options, it does not address the more pertinent question of which technique, if any, is superior. When is in situ release alone, whether open or endoscopic, adequate? Does nerve subluxation always require transposition? Do severe cases need submuscular transposition?

In short, this small prospective series supports previous studies showing that anterior subcutaneous transposition is an acceptable treatment for cubital tunnel syndrome.

G. Gaston, MD

Predictors of Functional Outcome Change 18 Months After Anterior Ulnar Nerve Transposition

Shi Q, MacDermid J, Grewal R, et al (McMaster Univ, Hamilton, Ontario, Canada; St Joseph's Health Centre, London, Ontario, Canada)
Arch Phys Med Rehabil 93:307-312, 2012

Objective.—To determine which variables derived from the electrodiagnostic examination were predictive of patient self-reported symptoms and disability at 18 months after anterior ulnar nerve transposition.

Design.—Retrospective cohort study.

Setting.—Electrodiagnostic laboratories affiliated with a tertiary care center.

Participants.—Patients (N = 73) with cubital tunnel syndrome (CuTS).

Interventions.—Patients were randomly assigned to one of the anterior transpositions of the ulnar nerve (subcutaneous or submuscular).

Main Outcome Measures.—Outcome was a patient-rated ulnar elbow evaluation (PRUNE). Predictors were all variables derived from the electrodiagnostic examination and characteristics of participants, as well as the preoperative clinical status. A stepwise multivariable linear regression analysis was used to determine the relative importance of the selected variables on the change in PRUNE scores.

Results.—Above-elbow compound muscle action potentials amplitude and proportional compound muscle action potentials amplitude decreasing from above elbow to below elbow were predictors of change score of the PRUNE at 18 months after operation ($R^2 = 16\%$). Sex and preoperative PRUNE also showed predictive information ($R^2 = 14\%$ and 15%, respectively).

Conclusions.—CuTS is predominantly a clinical diagnosis. Electrophysiologic studies are important supplemental examinations for the diagnosis of CuTS because they not only contribute to diagnosis, but are also important prognostic features. Females may have more improvement with regard to functional outcomes than males when undergoing surgical intervention.

▶ This article provides interesting data on patients with cubital tunnel syndrome undergoing anterior transposition. Seventy-three patients with cubital tunnel syndrome underwent anterior (subcutaneous vs submuscular) transposition. Patients were evaluated using preoperative and postoperative electrodiagnostic testing as well as the Patient-Rated Ulnar Elbow Evaluation (PRUNE) preoperatively and postoperatively. This series evaluated factors predictive of outcome. Gender appears to make a difference in outcomes. Women have a larger improvement following ulnar nerve transposition, even after controlling for a reported higher symptom and disability level preoperatively.

Preoperative electrodiagnostic testing was predictive of outcome: less-compromised electrical studies suggest larger improvement in patient-reported symptoms postoperatively. Patients with axonal loss as demonstrated by EDS (more severe motor findings) do more poorly. However, more importantly, more than 20% of patients classified as McGowan stage III did not meet the electrodiagnostic testing criteria for diagnosis of cubital tunnel syndrome. Interestingly, improvement in electrodiagnostic testing postoperatively was noted (100%), although half of the arms had persistent abnormalities postoperatively.

The authors conclude that electrodiagnostic testing is helpful not so much for diagnosis of cubital tunnel syndrome but much more as predictive of outcomes following surgery.

J. Adams, MD

A Tailored Approach to the Surgical Treatment of Cubital Tunnel Syndrome
Keith J, Wollstein R (Univ of Pittsburgh Med Ctr, PA; Veterans Administration of Pittsburgh, PA)
Ann Plast Surg 66:637-639, 2011

Multiple studies have compared the outcome of surgery for cubital tunnel syndrome (CUTS), yet there remains no clear guidelines for treatment. We describe an approach to CUTS that includes tailoring the procedure to the pathology found at surgery. Patients treated surgically were retrospectively reviewed. Following in situ neurolysis, nerve stability within the cubital tunnel was assessed, and the nerve was left in situ, or transposed accordingly. We evaluated demographic information, presenting features, intraoperative and postoperative findings. Statistics included paired t test and logistic regression analysis. A total of 63 patients (standard deviation = 10.3 years) were reviewed. Fourteen nerves were transposed (22.5%). Postoperatively, sensation (71%), static 2-point discrimination, and motor strength improved. Grip strength compared with the uninvolved side was 94.8% postoperatively. Overall, 90% of the patients reported improvement in function. Our results compare favorably with other studies. Since CUTS originates from numerous causes, basing the operative plan on intraoperative findings produces excellent results.

▶ The implication of this article is that the choice between a simple decompression, a transposition, or a medial epicondylectomy is determined by intraoperative findings. Essentially, however, the authors' main point can be summed up as: perform an in situ release, but if the nerve subluxes, then convert to an anterior transposition, although they also note that a prominent medial head of the triceps should be excised as well. This is not a novel algorithm as Palmer and Hughes[1] previously suggested: "after in situ decompression, the nerve (should be) assessed for signs of persistent compression or nerve subluxation. The elbow is placed through a full range of motion, and if the nerve is found to subluxate, then transposition is necessary." Additionally, Kevin Chung[2] noted that subluxation is a known (though potentially acceptable) complication associated with in situ release. None of these articles, however, demonstrate that a subluxating nerve was definitely detrimental. Intuitively, a nerve rubbing across the medial epicondyle seems to be a potential problem, and the benefits of transposing the nerve in this scenario would seem to outweigh the theoretical risks of more extensive dissection and transposition, including post-surgical fibrosis, iatrogenic kinking, or failed transposition.

J. Frankenhoff, MD

References

1. Palmer BA, Hughes TB. Cubital tunnel syndrome. *J Hand Surg Am.* 2010;35:
153-163.
2. Chung KC. Treatment of ulnar nerve compression at the elbow. *J Hand Surg Am.*
2008;33:1625-1627.

Subcutaneous Anterior Transposition Versus Decompression and Medial Epicondylectomy for the Treatment of Cubital Tunnel Syndrome
Capo JT, Jacob G, Maurer RJ, et al (Univ of Medicine and Dentistry of New Jersey, Newark; Orthopedic Surgeons of Central Pennsylvania, Mechanicsburg)
Orthopedics 34:e713-e717, 2011

A review of the literature often fails to uncover the best procedure for the treatment of cubital tunnel syndrome. This article compares 2 frequently used methods (subcutaneous anterior transposition vs decompression and medial epicondylectomy) for their effectiveness in relieving both subjective and objective symptoms of cubital tunnel syndrome. Between August 1991 and October 1993, nineteen patients underwent surgical decompression by a single surgeon for ulnar neuropathy at the elbow. Factors evaluated included upper extremity range of motion, elbow valgus stress, grip strength, pinch, 2-point discrimination, and pre- and postoperative nerve conduction. A standardized questionnaire was administered to assess subjective relief of symptoms.

In the transposition group, grip strength averaged 71.2% of normal and pinch strength 86.6% of normal, and 2-point discrimination averaged 8.0 mm. The derived subjective assessment score was 23.2 of a possible 40. The average ulnar motor conduction velocity across the elbow was 50.1 m/sec preoperatively and 56.3 m/sec postoperatively. In the medial epicondylectomy group, grip strength averaged 79.5% of normal and pinch strength 81.7% of normal, and 2-point discrimination averaged 8.0 mm. The average ulnar motor conduction velocity across the elbow was 45.7 m/sec preoperatively and 55.7 m/sec postoperatively. No statistically significant difference existed between the 2 groups for the aforementioned indexes. These results do not indicate a difference between the outcomes of the patients undergoing either of the procedures. Because epicondylectomy is less technically demanding, with less soft tissue dissection of the nerve, it may be preferred over ulnar transposition.

▶ This small, nonrandomized, retrospective case series comparing 2 historically common treatments for cubital tunnel syndrome adds extremely little to the literature on this subject. It is unclear why the authors were inclined to publish 20-year-old data on fewer than 20 patients with less than 2-year follow-up, in light of the vast information available from meta-analyses published within just the past few years.[1,2] The current relevant debates in cubital tunnel syndrome are whether more complicated procedures are superior to a simple in situ decompression, as well as the emergence of minimally invasive endoscopic methods. The authors discuss their bias toward medial epicondylectomy, claiming less invasiveness and trauma as compared to transposition and a reduction in ulnar nerve strain with elbow flexion as compared to in situ decompression alone. Although these advantages may have theoretical merit, this study falls short in design, power, and impact to prove these points.

J. Isaacs, MD

References

1. Zlowodzki M, Chan S, Bhandari M, Kalliainen L, Schubert W. Anterior transposition compared with simple decompression for treatment of cubital tunnel syndrome. A meta-analysis of randomized, controlled trials. *J Bone Joint Surg Am.* 2007;89:2591-2598.
2. Macadam SA, Gandhi R, Bezuhly M, Lefaivre KA. Simple decompression versus anterior subcutaneous and submuscular transposition of the ulnar nerve for cubital tunnel syndrome: a meta-analysis. *J Hand Surg Am.* 2008;33:1314.e1-1314.e12.

14 Elbow: Trauma

The Epidemiology of Radial Head and Neck Fractures
Duckworth AD, Clement ND, Jenkins PJ, et al (Royal Infirmary of Edinburgh, Scotland, UK)
J Hand Surg 37A:112-119, 2012

Purpose.—The aim of this study was to define the epidemiological characteristics of proximal radial fractures.

Methods.—Using a prospective trauma database of 6,872 patients, we identified all patients who sustained a fracture of the radial head or neck over a 1-year period. Age, sex, socioeconomic status, mechanism of injury, fracture classification, and associated injuries were recorded and analyzed.

Results.—We identified 285 radial head (n = 199) and neck (n = 86) fractures, with a patient median age of 43 years (range, 13–94 y). The mean age of male patients was younger when compared to female patients for radial head and neck fractures, with no gender predominance seen. Gender did influence the mechanism of injury, with female patients commonly sustaining their fracture following a low-energy fall. Radial head fractures were associated more commonly with complex injuries according to the Mason classification, while associated injuries were related to age, the mechanism of injury, and increasing fracture complexity.

Conclusions.—Radial head and neck fractures have distinct epidemiological characteristics, and consideration for osteoporosis in a subset of patients is recommended.

Type of Study/Level of Evidence.—Prognostic IV.

▶ The main strength of this study is that it documents prospectively collected data on a large series of patients with radiologically confirmed radial head or neck fractures and is also from a well-demarcated population. A weakness of the study is the intraobserver and interobserver error associated with the interpretation of the elbow radiographs. Larger numbers might have demonstrated statistically significant correlations with deprivation, particularly those correlations that approached significance, such as incidence. The overall incidence of radial head and neck fractures was 55.4 per 100 000 population (95% confidence interval, 49–62). Ninety-nine percent of radial neck fractures were Mason type I or type II injuries. These findings suggest that proximal radial fractures, particularly radial neck fractures, are frequently low-energy fragility fractures associated with osteoporosis. Appropriate investigation with dual-energy x-ray absorptiometry scanning should potentially be considered in these patients, particularly in postmenopausal women who present with these injuries.

E. Cheung, MD

Interobserver Reliability of Radial Head Fracture Classification: Two-Dimensional Compared with Three-Dimensional CT
Guitton TG, on behalf of the Science of Variation Group (Massachusetts General Hosp, Boston)
J Bone Joint Surg Am 93:2015-2021, 2011

Background.—The Broberg and Morrey modification of the Mason classification of radial head fractures has substantial interobserver variation. This study used a large web-based collaborative of experienced orthopaedic surgeons to test the hypothesis that three-dimensional reconstructions of computed tomography (CT) scans improve the interobserver reliability of the classification of radial head fractures according to the Broberg and Morrey modification of the Mason classification.

Methods.—Eighty-five orthopaedic surgeons evaluated twelve radial head fractures. They were randomly assigned to review either radiographs and two-dimensional CT scans or radiographs and three-dimensional CT images to determine the fracture classification, fracture characteristics, and treatment recommendations. The kappa multirater measure (κ) was calculated to estimate agreement between observers.

Results.—Three-dimensional CT had moderate agreement and two-dimensional CT had fair agreement among observers for the Broberg and Morrey modification of the Mason classification, a difference that was significant. Observers assessed seven fracture characteristics, including fracture line, comminution, articular surface involvement, articular step or gap of ≥2 mm, central impaction, recognition of more than three fracture fragments, and fracture fragments too small to repair. There was a significant difference in kappa values between three-dimensional CT and two-dimensional CT for fracture fragments too small to repair, recognition of three fracture fragments, and central impaction. The difference between the other four fracture characteristics was not significant. Among treatment recommendations, there was fair agreement for both three-dimensional CT and two-dimensional CT.

Conclusions.—Although three-dimensional CT led to some small but significant decreases in interobserver variation, there is still considerable disagreement regarding classification and characterization of radial head fractures. Three-dimensional CT may be insufficient to optimize interobserver agreement.

▶ With the widespread use and availability of axial imaging studies and 3D reconstructions of CT scans, our understanding of fractures is changing. Our existing classifications for most fractures are based on plain film radiographs, which may not be adequate to describe 3D anatomy. The use of CT scanning, particularly with 2D and 3D reconstructions, may be helpful to improve interobserver and intraobserver reliability of fracture classification schemes. It will be interesting to see how fracture classification systems may change over time (or remain the same) with more reliance on CT scans. In this series, the authors used a web-based collaboration with a large number of observers and evaluated interobserver reliability of fracture classification and assessment of fracture characteristics using plain radiographs and 2D and 3D CT scans. Although there was some improved reliability with the use of CT scans, there still remained substantial differences in the ability of different observers to characterize radial head fractures even with axial imaging studies.

J. Adams, MD

The epidemiology of fractures of the proximal ulna
Duckworth AD, Clement ND, Aitken SA, et al (Royal Infirmary of Edinburgh, UK)
Injury 43:343-346, 2012

Introduction.—The aim of our study was to report the epidemiological characteristics of fractures of the proximal ulna.

Methods.—From our prospective trauma database of 6872 fractures, we identified all acute fractures of the proximal ulna from a 1-year period between July 2007 and June 2008. Age, gender, mode of injury, fracture classifications, associated injuries and treatment were the factors documented and analysed.

Results.—There were 78 fractures of the proximal ulna with a mean age of 57 years (15−97). Males ($n = 35$) sustained their fracture at a significantly younger age than females ($p = 0.041$), with no gender predominance seen ($p = 0.365$). The overall fracture distribution was a unimodal older male and unimodal older female type-F curve. The most common mode of injury was a simple fall from standing height ($n = 52$, 67%), with younger patients more likely to sustain their injuries following a high-energy mechanism such as sports or a motor vehicle collision ($p < 0.001$). Seventeen (22%) patients sustained associated injuries to the ipsilateral limb, with an associated proximal radial fracture most frequent ($n = 13$, 17%). Open fractures were seen in five (6.4%) patients. A total of 64 patients had a fracture of the olecranon, with the Mayo 2A most frequently seen ($n = 47$, 60%).

Conclusions.—Fractures of the proximal ulna are fragility fractures that predominantly occur in elderly patients. Given the number of elderly patients sustaining these injuries, research is needed to determine the role of non-operative treatment for these fractures, particularly in patients with multiple co-morbidities and low functional demands (Fig 1).

▶ This epidemiologic study sought to establish the incidence of fractures of the proximal ulna. The study center is an established trauma center in Scotland (the Royal Infirmary of Edinburgh), which serves a large catchment area without any

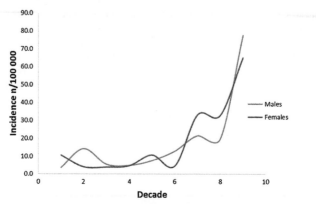

FIGURE 1.—The incidence of proximal ulna fractures, categorised by age and gender. (Reprinted from Duckworth AD, Clement ND, Aitken SA, et al. The epidemiology of fractures of the proximal ulna. *Injury.* 2012;43:343-346, Copyright 2012, with permission from Elsevier.)

other trauma center caring for these patients. Patients were identified through an established prospective fracture database over a 1-year period.

Fig 1 delineates fracture incidence by age and gender. There was a peak with advanced age past the 7th decade in both groups. Olecranon fractures occurred at an incidence of 12 per 100 000 individuals and were the most common fracture type of the proximal ulna. They occurred typically in a low-energy setting, commonly a fall from standing height. Notably, there was an almost 25% incidence of concomitant injury to the same limb, most commonly a proximal radius fracture, highlighting the importance of careful evaluation to exclude more complex injuries.

Most importantly, the series suggests that these are typically fragility fractures, and there may be a role for evaluation and treatment of coexisting osteopenia or osteoporosis or a potential preventative role. Lastly, the authors suggest that in some patients of advanced age or low demand, perhaps the risks and benefits of surgery should be carefully weighed, as some selected patients and fractures may be most amenable to nonoperative treatment.

J. Adams, MD

Staged Versus Acute Definitive Management of Open Distal Humerus Fractures

Min W, Ding BC, Tejwani NC (Univ of California, Sacramento; Baylor Univ Med Ctr, Dallas, TX; NYU Hosp for Joint Diseases)
J Trauma 71:944-947, 2011

Background.—Open distal humerus fractures are associated with soft tissue and bony injury. This study compares the results of a staged protocol using initial joint spanning external fixation and delayed definitive fixation to acute definitive fixation.

Methods.—Treated open distal humerus fractures were retrospectively reviewed, with patients examined at 2 weeks, 6 weeks, 12 weeks, 26 weeks, and 52 weeks after definitive surgery. Outcomes were determined radiographically by union rate and clinically by range of motion, Short Musculoskeletal Function Assessment, Short Form-36, and Mayo Elbow Performance Index.

Results.—Fourteen treated patients with open AO/OTA type 13-C3 distal humerus fractures, with average patient age 52.7 years and average follow-up 98.6 weeks, were identified. All fractures were treated with initial irrigation and debridement emergently and either spanning external fixation in eight patients or primary definitive internal fixation in six patients. All fractures healed, with average time to osseous healing, in 25.7 weeks versus 23.4 weeks ($p = 0.7$) in staged versus primary definitive treatment, respectively. Elbow range of motion on final follow-up was 73.75° versus 94.17° ($p = 0.22$). Complications included nonunions, heterotopic ossification, infection, and persistent ulnar nerve deficit. Average functional outcomes scores for staged management versus primary internal fixation were Short Form-36, 50.2 versus 68.2 ($p = 0.065$); Short Musculoskeletal Function Assessment, 33.5 versus 12.5 ($p = 0.078$); and Mayo Elbow Performance Index, 55.6 versus 84.2 ($p = 0.011$), respectively.

Conclusions.—Open distal humerus fractures had poor outcomes relative to normative functional scores; however, this is possibly due to more severe soft tissue injuries that were felt better managed with staged management at the time of presentation.

▶ This retrospective study evaluated 14 patients with type C3 open distal humerus fracture treated with either a staged protocol of external fixation and delayed open reduction, internal fixation (ORIF; 8 cases) versus ORIF on the day of presentation (6 cases). The decision to perform either approach was made intraoperatively based on associated soft tissue injuries and surgeons' discretion. This study demonstrated that, although not statistically significant, the arc of motion on the final follow-up was higher in the acute fixation group (94 degrees vs 74 degrees). Complications were surprisingly higher in the staged group. This included bridging heterotopic ossification (2 of 8 vs 0 of 6) and persistent ulnar nerve deficit requiring neurolysis (6 of 8 vs 1 of 6). Unfortunately, no significance calculations were reported on these complications. Functional outcome was assessed using the SF-36 (Medical Outcomes Trust, Boston), Short Musculoskeletal Functional Assessment, and Mayo Elbow Performance Index (MEPI) scores. All showed an improved score with the primary fixation group, with the MEPI score showing a significant difference. The authors attribute the differences in outcome to the possibility of worse injuries being relegated to the staged group. It would have been helpful to look at the patients' injury patterns and associated injuries to prove that they were "matched," thus eliminating this bias. I believe this study is important because it demonstrates, in even this small number of patients, that primary treatment of this difficult injury is acceptable and even has improved outcomes and a reduced complication rate compared to a staged protocol.

J. Capo, MD

Comparison of Olecranon Plate Fixation in Osteoporotic Bone: Do Current Technologies and Designs Make a Difference?

Edwards SG, Martin BD, Fu RH, et al (Georgetown Univ School of Medicine, Washington, DC; et al)
J Orthop Trauma 25:306-311, 2011

Objectives.—The purpose of this study is to determine if recent innovations in olecranon plates have any advantages in stabilizing osteoporotic olecranon fractures.

Methods.—Five olecranon plates (Acumed, Synthes-SS, Synthes-Ti, US Implants/ITS, and Zimmer) were implanted to stabilize a simulated comminuted fracture pattern in 30 osteoporotic cadaveric elbows. Specimens were randomized by bone mineral density per dual-energy x-ray absorptiometry scan. Three-dimensional displacement analysis was conducted to assess fragment motion through physiological cyclic arcs of motion and failure loading, which was statistically compared using one-way analysis of variance and Tukey honestly significant difference post hoc comparisons with a critical significance level of $\alpha = 0.05$.

Results.—Bone mineral density ranged from 0.546 g/cm² to 0.878 g/cm² with an average of 0.666 g/cm². All implants limited displacement of the fragments to less than 3 mm until sudden, catastrophic failure as the bone of the proximal fragment pulled away from the implant. The maximum load sustained by all osteoporotic specimens ranged from 1.6 kg to 6.6 kg with an average of 4.4 kg. There was no statistical difference between the groups in terms of cycles survived and maximum loads sustained.

Conclusions.—Cyclic physiological loading of osteoporotic olecranon fracture fixation resulted in sudden, catastrophic failure of the bone—implant interface rather than in gradual implant loosening. Recent plate innovations such as locking plates and different screw designs and positions appear to offer no advantages in stabilizing osteoporotic olecranon fractures. Surgeons may be reassured that the current olecranon plates will probably adequately stabilize osteoporotic fractures for early motion in the early postoperative period, but not for heavy activities such as those that involve over 4 kg of resistance.

▶ This is a biomechanical study evaluating the effectiveness of 5 different olecranon plates in treating osteoporotic olecranon fractures in a cadaver model. A 5-mm osteotomy was created, cyclic load was applied, and displacement at the osteotomy site was detected using an optical tracking system (Fig 3 in the original article). The outcomes reported were number of cycles and load applied at failure. Using these parameters, no statistical differences were appreciated. This article does not give us any new or useful data. The purpose was to tell if locking plates are more effective than nonlocking plates, but unfortunately only one of the 5 plates used was nonlocking. A final load to failure of each construct may have given the readers some useful comparative data. I am also concerned about the accuracy of the model because the motion sensors were applied to the bone with tissue adhesive and not rigidly fixed with pins.

J. Capo, MD

Radial Head and Neck Fractures: Functional Results and Predictors of Outcome
Duckworth AD, Watson BS, Will EM, et al (Royal Infirmary of Edinburgh, UK; et al)
J Trauma 71:643-648, 2011

Background.—The purpose of this study was to determine the functional outcomes and predictive factors of radial head and neck fractures.

Methods.—Over an 18-month period, we performed a prospective study of 237 consecutive patients with a radiographically confirmed proximal radial fracture (156 radial head and 81 radial neck). Follow-up was carried out over a 1-year period using clinical and radiologic assessment, including the Mayo Elbow Score (MES). Multivariate regression analysis was used to determine significant predictors of outcome according to the MES.

Results.—Of the 237 patients enrolled in the study, 201 (84.8%) attended for review, with a mean age of 44 years (range, 16—83 years; standard deviation, 17.3). One hundred eighty-seven (93%) patients achieved excellent or good MESs. The mean MES for Mason type-I (n = 103) and type-II (n = 82) fractures was excellent, with only two patients undergoing surgical intervention. For Mason type-III (n = 11) and type-IV (n = 5) fractures, the flexion arc, forearm rotation arc, and MES in the nonoperatively treated patients were not significantly different (all $p \geq 0.05$) from those managed operatively. Regression analysis revealed that increasing age, increasing fracture complexity according to the AO-OTA classification, increasing radiographic comminution, and operative treatment choice were independently significant predictors of a poorer outcome (all $p < 0.05$).

Conclusions.—A majority of radial head and neck fractures can be treated nonoperatively, achieving excellent or good results. Age, fracture classification, radiographic comminution, and treatment choice are important factors that determine recovery.

▶ The purpose of this study was to prospectively analyze consecutive patients with uncomplicated radial head and neck fractures to determine factors that directly influence patient outcomes.

The strengths of the study include its prospective design, its use of an independent assessor for clinical evaluation, its substantial sample size (n = 237), and its high follow-up rate (84%). This study would have been strengthened through the use of a validated patient-rated outcome measure and longer-term follow-up. Another limitation is the heterogeneity of the study cohort, which makes interpretation of the results difficult. By combining simple nondisplaced fractures with complex articular injuries in the same analysis, it is difficult to draw a conclusion other than that more complicated fracture patterns tend to have worse outcomes. Increasing age and operative management are potential indicators of increased fracture complexity rather than independent factors influencing patient outcome. The subanalysis of Mason type III and IV fractures with respect to operative versus nonoperative management is likely underpowered, and, because of a lack of randomization, it is limited by selection bias, with both factors acknowledged by the authors.

The article adds to the literature that supports nonoperative management of uncomplicated type I and II radial head and neck fractures. Despite its widespread use, the Mason classification system has been shown to have poor to moderate intrauser and interuser reliability,[1,2] and this study suggests that it is also a poor predictor of functional outcome. The article suggests that further work is required to create better treatment algorithms for radial head and neck fractures, as well as a more useful classification system, and it does further confirm that the majority of radial head and neck fractures (Mason I and II) can achieve good to excellent results with nonoperative treatment.

R. Demcoe, MD

R. Grewal, MD

References

1. Morgan SJ, Groshen SL, Itamura JM, Shankwiler J, Brien WW, Kuschner SH. Reliability evaluation of classifying radial head fractures by the system of Mason. *Bull Hosp Jt Dis.* 1997;56:95-98.
2. Guitton TG, Ring D. Interobserver reliability of radial head fracture classification: two-dimensional compared with three-dimensional ct. *J Bone Joint Surg Am.* 2011;93:2015-2021.

A Fragment-Specific Approach to Type IID Monteggia Elbow Fracture–Dislocations

Beingessner DM, Nork SE, Agel J, et al (Harborview Med Ctr, Seattle, WA; et al)
J Orthop Trauma 25:414-419, 2011

Objectives.—To describe the pattern of injury, surgical technique, and outcomes of Monteggia Type IID fracture dislocations.

Design.—Retrospective review of prospectively collected clinical and radiographic patient data in an orthopaedic trauma database.

Setting.—Level I university-based trauma center.

Patients/Participants.—All patients with Monteggia Type IID fracture–dislocations admitted from January 2000 to July 2005.

Intervention.—Review of patient demographics, fracture pattern, method of fixation, complications, additional surgical procedures, and clinical and radiographic outcome measures. Main Outcome Measurements: Clinical outcomes: elbow range of motion, complications. Radiographic outcomes: characteristic fracture fragments, quality of fracture reduction, healing time, degenerative changes, and heterotopic ossification.

Results.—Sixteen patients were included in the study. All fractures united. There were six complications in six patients, including three contractures with associated heterotopic ossification, one pronator syndrome and late radial nerve palsy, one radial head collapse, and one with prominent hardware.

Conclusions.—Monteggia IID fracture–dislocations are complex injuries with typical specific fracture fragments. Anatomic fixation of all injury components and avoidance of complications where possible can lead to a good outcome in these challenging injuries.

▶ The purposes of the article are to describe the typical injury pattern associated with Jupiter Type IID Monteggia elbow fracture-dislocations and to outline a surgical technique based on the specific fragments most commonly involved. The article is a retrospective review of 16 patients with Jupiter Type IID Monteggia elbow fracture-dislocations treated at a single institution by the technique presented in the article.

The strength of the study lies in its systematic and well-thought-out operative plan. The authors break down this injury into its primary components and classify them using widely utilized systems (Hotchkiss; Regan-Morrey). The operative technique described is logical and addresses all components of the injury complex, including the ligamentous component. The primary limitation of this study is its retrospective design. The radial head and coronoid fragments are well characterized as noted earlier; however, the remainder of the fragments are not addressed. There is repeated mention of an anterior oblique fragment and the osseous insertions of the medial collateral ligament and lateral ulnar collateral ligament; however, there is no indication of how frequently these occur. One of the primary goals of the article was to describe the injury pattern in Monteggia IID fracture-dislocations, and the article would have been strengthened had these fragments been characterized in more detail.

The article adds to the orthopedic literature by better characterizing the constellation of injuries associated with Jupiter IID Monteggia fracture-dislocation and proposes a systematic surgical technique for its treatment. Additionally, it provides relevant clinical information regarding the average postoperative range of motion, complications, and time to union, which is beneficial for perioperative discussions with patients sustaining this complex injury.

In general, this is a well-done retrospective review, which will aid surgeons treating this rare and challenging injury.

R. Demcoe, MD
R. Grewal, MD

Operative Fixation of Medial Humeral Epicondyle Fracture Nonunion in Children
Smith JT, McFeely ED, Bae DS, et al (Children's Hosp Boston, MA)
J Pediatr Orthop 30:644-648, 2010

Background.—There is little information regarding the clinical presentation and/or surgical treatment of symptomatic medial humeral epicondyle nonunions. The purpose of this investigation was to describe the presenting symptoms and evaluate the results of surgical fixation of medial epicondyle nonunions.

Methods.—Eight patients with symptomatic medial humeral epicondyle nonunions were evaluated after open reduction and internal fixation of the medial epicondyle. Average age at the time of initial injury was 11.3 years (range: 9.2 to 13.9 y). Outcome was assessed with radiographs and a questionnaire that included 3 self-reported functional outcome tools at a mean of 4.7 years (range: 1.5 to 7.5 y) after the surgery.

Results.—Common presenting symptoms and signs included medial elbow pain and prominence, pain with lifting weights or throwing, limited range of motion, valgus instability, and ulnar nerve compression. After open reduction and internal fixation, patients reported improved pain score from a mean of 6.2 to 0.5. All patients returned to athletics. Mean postoperative QuickDASH (Disability of Arm, Shoulder, and Hand) score (and SD) was 6.8 ± 11.7; mean Mayo Elbow Performance Score was 85.8 ± 14.6; and mean Timmerman-Andrews Elbow Score was 87.5 ± 10.4. Radiographic union was achieved in all but one patient postoperatively and there were no operative complications.

Conclusions.—Open reduction and internal fixation of symptomatic medial humeral epicondyle nonunion results in improved pain and good elbow function.

Level of Evidence.—Retrospective Case Series. Therapeutic Level IV.

▶ There is controversy regarding the treatment of displaced medial epicondylar fractures. Some authors present compelling long-term data on nonoperative treatment, yet most elbow surgeons have seen the occasional symptomatic nonunion.

This retrospective review does not attempt to resolve the controversy; rather, it examines the surgical treatment of those nonunions that are symptomatic.

Over a 7-year span, 137 patients were treated for medial epicondylar fracture, and 9 (21%) went on to symptomatic nonunion. Eight patients formed the basis of this study. The surgery was done 7 months to 8 years (average, 12 months) after the injury. All 8 patients had pain with lifting or throwing, as well as pain over the epicondyle. Four had valgus instability, and 5 ulnar nerve symptoms.

Surgery consisted of 1- or 2-headed screws to repair the nonunion. Concomitant ulnar nerve decompression was done in 5, transposition in 3, and contracture release in 4.

One patient had to return for repeat contracture release, and 5 of the 8 had the screws removed. Seven of the 8 went on to union. No patient had a decrease in range of motion. Pain levels went down, all patients returned to sports, and range of motion increased in patients undergoing capsulectomies.

Although the study group is small, the authors provide insight into the post-injury patient with a symptomatic medial epicondylar nonunion. Open reduction and internal fixation was safe and effective in the reported group. All 8 patients had their ulnar nerve treated with decompression or transposition, suggesting that this should be part of any attempt to gain union of the medial epicondyle. Five of 8 patients had symptoms from the prominent hardware; this should cause a treating surgeon to give consideration to utilizing a headless screw, so long as it gains adequate fixation.

R. F. Papandrea, MD

Closed Reduction and Early Mobilization in Fractures of the Humeral Capitellum
Puloski S, Kemp K, Sheps D, et al (Univ of Calgary, Alberta, Canada; Univ of Alberta, Edmonton, Canada)
J Orthop Trauma 26:62-65, 2012

Seven consecutive patients with an isolated fracture of the humeral capitellum were treated by a single surgeon at a Level II care facility according to a simple treatment algorithm. Closed reduction was attempted in all cases using a standard technique. After reduction, the arm was splinted at 90° of flexion and mobilized at 14 days. All patients completed a clinical and radiographic follow-up consisting of a radiographic evaluation of reduction, elbow range of motion, Disabilities of the Arm, Shoulder and Hand Questionnaire, and a subjective rating of patient satisfaction. None of the patients required conversion to open reduction internal fixation or excision. Disabilities of the Arm, Shoulder and Hand Questionnaire scores ranged from 6 to 13 points (out of 100; mean, 9). The mean flexion/extension arc of motion obtained was 126° with minimal loss of rotation. Patient satisfaction was rated as excellent in five patients and good in two. All fractures appeared united at the most recent clinical and radiographic review. Closed reduction and early mobilization appears to be a safe and effective method of treating displaced fractures of the humeral capitellum with clinical results comparable to that of open reduction internal fixation.

▶ This retrospective review offers a relatively simple closed reduction technique for the treatment of type 1 displaced capitellar fractures. The study describes both a technical trick as well as data on 7 consecutive patients treated with this particular technique. Type 1 capitellar fractures, also called Hahn-Steinthal fragments, represent shear fractures that typically are the result of a direct load applied to the elbow in a fully extended posture. The authors note that when the fracture is comminuted and not amenable to either closed reduction or open reduction internal fixation (ORIF), primary excision is indicated. This article describes a technique in which the patient is fully sedated for muscle relaxation. The elbow is brought into full extension with the forearm fully supine. The elbow is then flexed with gentle traction and varus tension, ensuring that the radial head "locks" the fragment at roughly 40° of flexion. A posterior splint is applied, and active range of motion was initiated 14 days following reduction. All 7 fractures appeared united at final follow-up, and the Disabilities of the Arm, Shoulder and Hand scores were favorable. None of the patients required subsequent ORIF, while only 1 patient exhibited a serious flexion contracture of 45°, a finding later attributed to posterior comminution. In light of the complications associated with ORIF, the authors make a strong argument to attempt closed reduction for capitellar shear fractures. However, caution must be exercised with comminuted fragments, intra-articular extension, or patients with osteopenic bone. In addition, the benefit of early range of motion following stable internal fixation should be considered in the context of prolonged elbow immobilization required after a closed reduction. Although the authors report that there were no cases of significant decreased range of motion, other than the 1 fracture with posterior comminution, one must consider the limited sample size in this study. In sum, displaced capitellar shear fractures may be amenable to closed reduction and immobilization, but one should also consider the possibility of loss of fixation and immobilization-induced stiffness.

S. M. Jacoby, MD

15 Brachial Plexus

Fascicular Topography of the Suprascapular Nerve in the C5 Root and Upper Trunk of the Brachial Plexus: A Microanatomic Study From a Nerve Surgeon's Perspective
Siqueira MG, Foroni LHL, Martins RS, et al (Univ of São Paulo Med School, Brazil; et al)
Neurosurgery 67:ons402-ons406, 2010

Background.—In patients with supraclavicular injuries of the brachial plexus, the suprascapular nerve (SSN) is frequently reconstructed with a sural nerve graft coapted to C5. As the C5 cross-sectional diameter exceeds the graft diameter, inadequate positioning of the graft is possible.

Objective.—To identify a specific area within the C5 proximal stump that contains the SSN axons and to determine how this area could be localized by the nerve surgeon, we conducted a microanatomic study of the intraplexal topography of the SSN.

Methods.—The right-sided C5 and C6 roots, the upper trunk with its divisions, and the SSN of 20 adult nonfixed cadavers were removed and fixed. The position and area occupied by the SSN fibers inside C5 were assessed and registered under magnification.

Results.—The SSN was monofascicular in all specimens and derived its fibers mainly from C5. Small contributions from C6 were found in 12 specimens (60%). The mean transverse area of C5 occupied by SSN fibers was 28.23%. In 16 specimens (80%), the SSN fibers were localized in the ventral (mainly the rostroventral) quadrants of C5, a cross-sectional area between 9 o'clock and 3 o'clock from the surgeon's intraoperative perspective.

Conclusion.—In reconstruction of the SSN with a sural nerve graft, coaptation should be performed in the rostroventral quadrant of C5 cross-sectional area (between 9 and 12 o'clock from the nerve surgeon's point of view in a right-sided brachial plexus exploration). This will minimize axonal misrouting and may improve outcome (Fig 2).

▶ This is an anatomic cadaver study to assess the intrafascicular anatomy of the suprascapular nerve (SSN) within the brachial plexus. The goal of the study was to provide nerve surgeons with more information on the anatomy of the SSN so that they could have a clearer plan on surgical reconstruction. The authors found that the majority of the axons to the SSN come from the C5 nerve root and that the most frequent position of these fibers within the C5 root was in the rostral ventral position (Fig 2).

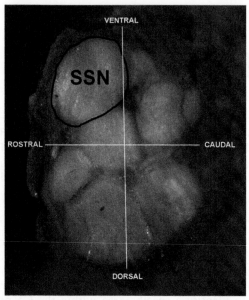

FIGURE 2.—C5 root with fascicles completely individualized, including the fascicle formed by the fibers of the suprascapular nerve (SSN) divided in quadrants. The area occupied by SSN fibers is outlined. (Reprinted from Siqueira MG, Foroni LHL, Martins RS, et al, Fascicular topography of the suprascapular nerve in the C5 root and upper trunk of the brachial plexus: a microanatomic study from a nerve surgeon's perspective. *Neurosurgery.* 2010;67:ons402-ons406, with permission from the Congress of Neurological Surgeons.)

This study adds to the available literature because the dissection and results were designed from the surgeon's perspective. This information should direct surgeons in their placement of sural nerve cable grafts when performing an intraplexal SSN reconstruction. They should change from current practice, in which grafts are put at random to a guided placement of the graft to the C5 root in the rostroventral position.

There continues to be several ways to reconstruct the SSN with direct cable graft reconstruction versus more distal nerve transfers. The information from this study may improve intraplexal reconstruction outcomes. However, at this point, the superior technique remains unclear, and further clinical studies of functional outcomes are needed.

C. Curtin, MD

Contralateral spinal accessory nerve for ipsilateral neurotization of branches of the brachial plexus: a cadaveric feasibility study

Tubbs RS, Mortazavi MM, Shoja MM, et al (Children's Hosp, Birmingham, AL; Indiana Univ, Indianapolis; et al)
J Neurosurg 114:1538-1540, 2011

Object.—Additional nerve transfer options are important to the peripheral nerve surgeon to maximize patient outcomes following nerve injuries.

Potential regional donors may also be injured or involved in the primary disease. Therefore, potential contralateral donor nerves would be desirable. To the authors' knowledge, use of the contralateral spinal accessory nerve (SAN) has not been explored for ipsilateral neurotization procedures. In the current study, therefore, the authors aimed to evaluate the SAN as a potential donor nerve for contralateral nerve injuries by using a novel technique.

Methods.—In 10 cadavers, the SAN was harvested using a posterior approach, and tunneled subcutaneously to the contralateral side for neurotization to various branches of the brachial plexus. Measurements were made of the SAN available for transfer and of its diameter.

Results.—The authors found an SAN length of approximately 20 cm (from transition of upper and middle fibers of the trapezius muscle to approximately 2—4 cm superior to the insertion of the trapezius muscle onto the spinous process of T-12) available for nerve transposition. The average diameter was 2.5 mm.

Conclusions.—Based on these findings, the contralateral SAN may be considered for ipsilateral neurotization to the suprascapular and axillary nerves.

▶ This is a cadaver study looking at the feasibility of harvesting the spinal accessory nerve (SAN) and using it as a donor for a contralateral nerve injury. The authors found that using the posterior approach, they could harvest 20 cm of SAN length. This was enough to reach the contralateral axillary and suprascapular nerves.

Nerve surgeons are always looking for new donor nerves for nerve transfers. The patient with a total plexus palsy has limited resources, and each additional donor nerve can greatly improve the function of the arm. This is an interesting feasibility study, especially because the posterior approach to the spinal accessory and suprascapular nerve is familiar to many nerve surgeons.

The major concern with this study is whether there are enough axons remaining in the terminal portion of the spinal accessory nerve to restore function. Vathana et al[1] found that there were 863 axons in the distal SAN, and it is unclear what kind of functional recovery this number of axons would yield. Unfortunately, with too few axons, the outcome may be only an "academic" success.

This study pursues an innovative idea and shows that this nerve transfer is feasible. However, work is needed to assess clinical applicability. This type of research is critical to expanding our reconstructive options for these devastating injuries.

C. Curtin, MD

Reference

1. Vathana T, Larsen M, de Ruiter GC, Bishop AT, Spinner RJ, Shin AY. An anatomic study of the spinal accessory nerve: extended harvest permits direct nerve transfer to distal plexus targets. *Clin Anat.* 2007;20:899-904.

Reinnervation of thenar muscle after repair of total brachial plexus avulsion injury with contralateral C7 root transfer: report of five cases

Wang L, Zhao X, Gao K, et al (Fudan Univ, Shanghai, People's Republic of China)
Microsurgery 31:323-326, 2011

Objective.—In this report, we present the findings of reinnervation of the thenar muscle in five patients who underwent the contralateral C7 nerve root transfers for repair of total brachial plexus root avulsions.

Patients and Methods.—Five (2 children and 3 adults) of 32 patients who received two-staged procedures of the contralateral C7 nerve root transfers to the median nerves showed reinnervation of thenar muscle were evaluated. The patients also received other procedures including the intercostal nerve transfer to the musculocutaneous nerve, the spinal accessory nerve to the suprascapular nerve, and the ipsilateral phrenic nerve to the musculocutaneous nerve before the contralateral C7 nerve root transfers. The patients were followed up from 24 to 118 months after surgery.

Results.—Varied degrees of functional restorations were achieved after different procedures. The strength of abductor pollicis brevis (APB) muscle with Grade M2 was found in four patients. The incomplete interference pattern in the APB muscle was detected by electromyogram (EMG) in two patients, and the minority motor unit potential (MUP) was detected in other two patients. The strength of APB muscle was found with Grade M1 in one patient with EMG showing MUP.

Conclusion.—The findings from our series show reinnervation of thenar muscles after repair of the median nerve with the contralateral C7 nerve root transfer, which provides evidence for further investigation of reconstruction of the brachial plexus root avulsion injury with this procedure.

▶ Contralateral C7 root transfers are rarely performed and only in cases in which viable axons from the ipsilateral limb are insufficient to optimize motor recovery after a brachial plexus injury. This study focused on 5 patients out of 32 with global avulsion injuries that recovered thenar muscle tone after C7 transfers to the median nerve via a 2-stage vascularized ulnar nerve graft. It is unclear what happened to the remaining 27 patients. Nonetheless, with more than adequate follow-up, none of the 5 patients recovered meaningful thenar function. The authors had better success with intercostal to biceps nerve transfers, as is consistent with available literature. They were also able to achieve at least S3 sensation via the C7 transfer, which is commendable. It is unfortunate that the study did not report on more proximal median nerve function, which may also have recovered, nor on the incidence of complications from the C7 loss on the contralateral side. I agree with the authors that although this study demonstrates that the contralateral C7 nerve transfer has the potential to recover some median nerve function, additional work to optimize this transfer is required before it can be more widely adopted.

D. A. Zlotolow, MD

Minimum 4-Year Follow-Up on Contralateral C7 Nerve Transfers for Brachial Plexus Injuries

Chuang DC-C, Hernon C (Chang Gung Univ, Taoyuan, Taiwan)
J Hand Surg 37A:270-276, 2012

Purpose.—Contralateral C7 (CC7) transfer for brachial plexus injuries (BPI) can benefit finger sensation but remains controversial regarding restoration of motor function. We report our 20-year experience using CC7 transfer for BPI, all of which had at least 4 years of follow-up.

Methods.—A total of 137 adult BPI patients underwent CC7 transfer from 1989 to 2006. Of these patients, 101 fulfilled the inclusion criteria for this study. A single surgeon performed all surgeries. A vascularized ulnar nerve graft, either pedicled or free, was used for CC7 elongation. The vascularized ulnar nerve graft was transferred to the median nerve (group 1, 1 target) in 55 patients, and to the median and musculocutaneous nerves (group 2, 2 targets) in 23 patients. In another 23 patients (group 3, 2 targets, 2 stages), the CC7 was transferred to the median nerve (17 patients) or to the median and musculocutaneous nerve (6 patients) during the first stage, followed by functioning free muscle transplantation for finger flexion.

Results.—We considered finger flexion strength greater or equal to M3 to be a successful functional result. Success rates of CC7 transfer were 55%, 39%, and 74% for groups 1, 2, and 3, respectively. In addition, the success rate for recovery of elbow flexion (strength M3 or better) in group 2 was 83%.

Conclusions.—In reconstruction of total brachial plexus root avulsion, the best option may be to adopt the technique of using CC7 transfer to the musculocutaneous and median nerve, followed by FFMT in the early stage (18 mo or less) for finger flexion. Such a technique can potentially improve motor recovery of elbow and finger flexion in a shorter rehabilitation period (3 to 4 y) and, more importantly, provide finger sensation to the completely paralytic limb.

Type of Study/Level of Evidence.—Therapeutic II.

▶ This article is important in the evolution of thought for the treatment of patients with total arm brachial plexus injury. Unfortunately, total arm palsy is the most common type in adults, and treatment strategies are highly varied among brachial plexus centers. The results are relatively unsatisfactory, especially when all nerve roots are avulsed. One of the most difficult problems is crossing the elbow to regain useful motor function. The authors propose their strategy and describe the history of how they evolved to this point. They describe their use of the contralateral C7 (CC7) nerve transfer, which they admit is controversial in the world of brachial plexus surgery. They offer a novel modification, where in a second stage, they capture the regenerating axons in the median nerve and use this as the donor nerve for a free functioning muscle transfer. Doing this, they achieve 74% success with M3 finger flexion, a relatively high percentage for this devastating injury. The authors also describe and compare the routes of the nerve graft—cross-chest, cross-neck subcutaneous, cross-neck prevertebral—and give their justification for cross-neck subcutaneous as their preferred technique. A major worrisome feature of CC7 transfer is the possibility of donor site morbidity. The Mayo group recently reported on permanent major donor site morbidity, which contributed to them abandoning the use of CC7 transfer in their practice. Nevertheless, this current study is valuable to take note of the possibility of the modified CC7 with secondary functioning free muscle transplantation as a strategy for reconstruction of the brachial plexus total arm palsy, especially in cases of 5-root avulsion.

A. Chong, MD

Clinimetric Evaluation of Questionnaires Used to Assess Activity After Traumatic Brachial Plexus Injury in Adults: A Systematic Review
Hill BE, Williams G, Bialocerkowski AE (Epworth HealthCare, Melbourne, Australia; Univ of Western Sydney, Sydney, Australia)
Arch Phys Med Rehabil 92:2082-2089, 2011

Objectives.—To identify upper limb questionnaires used in the brachial plexus injury (BPI) literature to assess activities and to evaluate their clinimetric properties.

Data Sources; Study Selection; Data Extraction.—This systematic review was undertaken in 2 stages. In stage 1, 10 electronic databases and 1 Internet journal were searched for quantitative studies (ie, randomized controlled trials, comparative studies, case series, and case studies) that evaluated outcome after BPI, irrespective of language or date of publication, from date of database inception to September 2010. All outcome instruments used were extracted and classified using the *International Classification of Functioning, Disability and Health framework*. Questionnaires were identified that apportioned >50% of the total score to the assessment of upper limb activity. In stage 2, 4 electronic databases were searched for papers that evaluated the clinimetric properties of all identified activity questionnaires with respect to peripheral nerve injuries of the upper limb. Two independent reviewers assessed the clinimetric properties of identified questionnaires according to standardized criteria.

Data Synthesis.—Stage 1 identified 4324 papers, of which 265 met the inclusion criteria. One hundred and three outcome measures were identified, the majority of which assess body function or body structure. Twenty-nine questionnaires assessed upper limb activity. Two questionnaires, the ABILHAND and Disability of the Arm, Shoulder and Hand (DASH), attributed >50% of the overall score to activity of the upper limb. The DASH had some published evidence of clinimetric properties in individuals with peripheral nerve injuries. Neither had been clinimetrically evaluated for BPI, nor met all quality criteria.

Conclusions.—Day-to-day activities of the upper limb are infrequently evaluated after BPI. While attempts have been made to measure activity, there is a paucity of clinimetric evidence on activity questionnaires for individuals with BPI. We recommend that a core set of items be developed which evaluate activity, as well a body structure, body function, and participation.

▶ The outcomes reported in the brachial plexus literature are highly variable and mostly revolve around motor strength. Some other parameters measured are range of motion, function, sensibility, and pain. These other 4 parameters are infrequently reported, making it difficult to compare studies with any data other than motor strength. The more important data of whether a patient can function better after treatment is generally not reported, making the outcomes reporting for brachial plexus injury deficient in information that is most important to know. The authors recognize this problem, and they look into brachial plexus literature and recommend that a core set of items be developed that evaluate activity as well as body structure, body function, and participation. They report that the functional questionnaires of the Disability of the Arm, Shoulder and Hand and the ABILHAND attribute less than 50% of the score to upper limb function as opposed to other scores in the literature, which they exclude and give reasons for. The overall message of the article is a valuable one: the brachial plexus community needs to report on more than just motor strength. What a patient can actually do before and after treatment is what we should really be interested in.

J. Yao, MD

Combined nerve transfers for repair of the upper brachial plexus injuries through a posterior approach

Lu J, Xu J, Xu W, et al (Fudan Univ, Shanghai, China)
Microsurgery 32:111-117, 2012

The upper brachial plexus injury leads to paralysis of muscles innervated by C5 and C6 nerve roots. In this report, we present our experience on the use of the combined nerve transfers for reconstruction of the upper brachial plexus injury. Nine male patients with the upper brachial plexus injury were treated with combined nerve transfers. The time interval between injury and surgery ranged from 3 to 11 months (average, 7 months). The combined nerve transfers include fascicles of the ulnar nerve and/or the median nerve transfer to the biceps and/or the brachialis motor branch, and the spinal accessory nerve (SAN) to the suprascapular nerve (SSN) and triceps branches to the axillary nerve through a posterior approach. At an average of 33 months of follow-up, all patients recovered the full range of the elbow flexion. Six out of nine patients were able to perform the normal range of shoulder abduction with the strength degraded to M3 or M4. These results showed that the technique of the combined nerve transfers, specifically the SAN to the SSN and triceps branches to the axillary nerve through a posterior approach, may be a valuable alternative in the repair of the upper brachial plexus injury. Further evaluations of this technique are necessary.

▶ This study details the management via nerve transfers of late-presenting upper trunk/C5/C6 injuries to the brachial plexus. It is relatively small in number, and patients with vascular injury or previous clavicle fracture were not excluded.

The authors advocate the use of combined nerve transfers as a means of providing emergent re-innervation to muscle. In itself there is nothing new in this approach, as the transfers of Oberlin and its modification and that of Somsak are routine tools in the armory of the peripheral nerve surgeon.

The authors comment that the use of nerve transfers may be helpful where supraclavicular exploration is not feasible. In countries with large distances between specialist centers it is inevitable that some patients will present late, and the approach used is, of course, very reasonable.

Interestingly, the authors clearly comment on the desirability of urgent brachial plexus exploration and repair via the supraclavicular approach as being their procedure of choice. In that sense, this article bucks a relatively recent trend toward using nerve transfers as a universal panacea for treatment of brachial plexus injuries. The risk inherent in adopting this strategy is of course that surgeons deskill in exploring the supraclavicular plexus and managing the acute repair. Overall, a very balanced analysis is presented here with good results from combined transfers.

In our unit, serving a large population in a relatively small land mass and with long-established referral patterns, we are in a fortunate position to receive and treat very early supraclavicular brachial plexus lesions. In patients with significant concomitant injury, surgery is inevitably delayed, and we adopt a similar strategy to that described. In my experience, the Somsak transfer is technically significantly easier in a slim patient. With a larger Western type patient, I prefer the beach-chair position to the semiprone position described in this article, with an incision at the superior margin of the delto-tricepital interval, allowing triceps and subcutaneous fat to fall away under gravity. A distal spinal accessory to suprascapular or branch to supraspinatus transfer is still possible, and this obviates the need to reposition the patient for an Oberlin transfer.

M. Fox, MD

Hemi-Contralateral C7 Transfer in Traumatic Brachial Plexus Injuries: Outcomes and Complications

Sammer DM, Kircher MF, Bishop AT, et al (Mayo Clinic, Rochester, MN)
J Bone Joint Surg Am 94:131-137, 2012

Background.—In brachial plexus injuries with nerve root avulsions, the options for nerve reconstruction are limited. In select situations, half or all of the contralateral C7 (CC7) nerve root can be transferred to the injured side for brachial plexus reconstruction. Although encouraging results have been reported, CC7 transfer has not gained universal popularity. The purpose of this study was to critically evaluate hemi-CC7 transfer for restoration of shoulder function or median nerve function in patients with severe brachial plexus injury.

Methods.—A retrospective review of all patients with traumatic brachial plexus injury who had undergone hemi-CC7 transfer at a single institution during an eight-year period was performed. Complications were evaluated in all patients regardless of the duration of follow-up. The results of electro-diagnostic studies and modified British Medical Research Council (BMRC) motor grading were reviewed in all patients with more than twenty-seven months of follow-up.

Results.—Fifty-five patients with traumatic brachial plexus injury underwent hemi-CC7 transfer performed between 2001 and 2008 for restoration of shoulder function or median nerve function. Thirteen patients who underwent hemi-CC7 transfer to the shoulder and fifteen patients who underwent hemi-CC7 transfer to the median nerve had more than twenty-seven months of follow-up. Twelve of the thirteen patients in the shoulder group demonstrated electromyographic evidence of reinnervation, but only three patients achieved M3 or greater shoulder abduction motor function. Three of the fifteen patients in the median nerve group demonstrated electromyographic evidence of reinnervation, but none developed M3 or greater composite grip. All patients experienced donor-side sensory or motor changes; these were typically mild and transient, but one patient sustained severe, permanent donor-side motor and sensory losses.

Conclusions.—The outcomes of hemi-CC7 transfer for restoration of shoulder motor function or median nerve function following posttraumatic brachial plexus injury do not justify the risk of donor-site morbidity, which includes possible permanent motor and sensory losses.

▶ This study is essential reading for any surgeon contemplating a contralateral C7 nerve transfer. It contains sufficient numbers to make a real comment and comes from a highly respected unit with real experience in the Mayo Clinic.

While it is retrospective in nature, the follow-up was sufficient, and clearly the postoperative data collection was good, with follow-up of motor and sensory recovery clinically augmented with electromyography data.

It is important that a unit with a well-established brachial plexus surgical pedigree does not recommend the procedure of hemicontralateral C7 transfer, deeming the risk of donor site morbidity to be unjustifiable. This will, of course, inform opinion on the complete contralateral C7 transfer in addition.

Our unit has learned from the experience of others in this regard, and we do not routinely perform reconstructive procedures using the contralateral C7 nerve root. We are in the fortunate position of being able to reimplant some avulsions that are referred early but would not contemplate contralateral C7 use even in the late referral. We believe jeopardizing the function of the normal arm is not justifiable and hampers rehabilitation, which is almost more important than the technical surgery in this patient group.

M. Fox, MD

16 Arm and Humerus

Radial nerve palsy associated with humeral shaft fracture. Is the energy of trauma a prognostic factor?
Venouziou AI, Dailiana ZH, Varitimidis SE, et al (Univ of Thessalia, Biopolis, Larissa, Greece)
Injury 42:1289-1293, 2011

Background.—Radial nerve palsy associated with humeral shaft fractures is the most common nerve lesion complicating fractures of long bones. The purpose of the study was to review the outcome of surgical management in patients with low energy and high energy radial nerve palsy after humeral shaft fractures.

Methods.—Eighteen patients were treated operatively for a humeral shaft fracture with radial nerve palsy. The mean age was 32.2 years and the mean follow up time was 66.1 months (range: 30–104). The surgical management included fracture fixation with early nerve exploration and repair if needed. The patients were divided in two groups based on the energy of trauma (low vs. high trauma energy). The prevalence of injured and unrecovered nerves and time to nerve recovery were analysed.

Results.—Five patients sustained low and 13 high energy trauma. All patients with low energy trauma had an intact (4) or entrapped (1) radial nerve and recovered completely. Full nerve recovery was also achieved in five of 13 patients with high energy trauma where the nerve was found intact or entrapped. Signs of initial recovery were present in a mean of 3.2 weeks (range: 1–8) for the low energy group and 12 weeks (range: 3–23) for the high energy group ($p = 0.036$). In these patients, the average time to full recovery was 14 and 26 weeks for the low and high energy trauma group respectively. Eight patients with high energy trauma had severely damaged nerves and failed to recover, although microsurgical nerve reconstruction was performed in 4 cases. Patients with high energy trauma had a prolonged fracture healing time (18.7 weeks on average) compared to those with low energy fractures (10.4 weeks), ($p = 0.003$).

Conclusions.—The outcome of the radial nerve palsy following humeral fractures is associated to the initial trauma. Palsies that are part of a low energy fracture uniformly recover and therefore primary surgical exploration seems unnecessary. In high energy fractures, neurotmesis or severe contusion must be expected. In this case nerve recovery is unfavourable and the patients should be informed of the poor prognosis and the need of tendon transfers.

▶ The authors present a retrospective review of patients with humeral shaft fractures and concomitant radial nerve palsy treated operatively, with the goal of determining whether nerve recovery would be the same in high-energy injuries and low-energy injuries. Surgery was indicated based on each patient's fracture, not the status of the radial nerve, with 48 patients included. In the 18 patients with radial nerve palsy, all 5 in the low-severity group and 5 of 13 in the high-severity group had an intact nerve and full recovery, with a nonsignificant slower recovery in high-energy injury patients. There were 4 lacerated and 4 irreparable nerves in the high-energy injury group, which showed no recovery, despite primary repair in 3 cases and nerve grafting in 1 case. This article reinforces previous literature that guides us to observe patients with humerus fracture and radial nerve palsy in which the nerve is intact. When there is a high-energy injury with open fracture or significant crush, there are 2 main take-home points. First, nerve exploration is indicated due to the higher incidence of laceration, incarceration, or avulsion. Second, even in nerves with laceration suitable to repair, recovery may be poor. The authors go so far as to advise against repairing lacerated nerves, recommending tendon transfer instead. However, they provide no clarity as to what other factors, other than the energy level of the injury, may impact recovery following nerve repair, such as patient age or comorbidities, which are known to impact recovery. Because of the small numbers in this and similar studies, the question as to what to do with a lacerated radial nerve in a high-energy injury remains unanswered. Further research is necessary to garner sufficient numbers of patients with radial nerve repair following fracture, with analysis based on injury, age, comorbidities, and repair type, before it can be stated that nerve repair is not indicated.

F. T. D. Kaplan, MD

Radial Nerve Disruption Following Application of a Hinged Elbow External Fixator: A Report of Three Cases
Baumann G, Nagy L, Jost B (Univ Hosp Balgrist, Zurich, Switzerland)
J Bone Joint Surg Am 93:e51.1-e51.4, 2011

Background.—The use of a hinged or articulated elbow external fixator can be helpful for patients with elbow instability, after extensive capsular release of elbow contractures, after ligamentous reconstruction, for distraction interposition arthroplasty, and to manage complex elbow fracture-dislocations. These devised maintain elbow stability but allow the patient to mobilize the elbow soon after surgery. Transient, but not permanent, radial nerve palsy has been reported after a hinged external fixator has been applied. Three cases were reported of radial nerve palsy caused by complete nerve disruption after a hinged external fixator was used to manage complex elbow injuries.

Case Reports.—Case 1: Man, 47, fell on his right, dominant arm but did not fracture or dislocate it. After 7 years, ulnar nerve decompression with a medial epicondylectomy was performed to manage posttraumatic ulnar nerve irritation, but symptoms persisted. Marked medial and lateral elbow instability prompted reconstruction with semitendininosus tendon autografts, anterior-ward ulnar nerve transposition, and elbow stabilization using a hinged external fixator, with pins placed percutaneously. Complete radial nerve palsy was noted immediately, and the external fixator was removed 4 weeks later. Injury level was at the division of the sensory and posterior interosseous nerves in the area of the distal humerus pin. No sensory radial nerve action potentials were discernible after 12 months, and the extensor carpi radialis, extensor digitorum communis, and abductor pollicis longus muscles exhibited high spontaneous activity but no voluntary activity. A complete lesion of the common radial artery was suspected, but the patient refused further treatment.

Case 2: Man, 74, fell on his left, nondominant arm, suffering a simple posterior elbow dislocation that was treated with closed reduction. The elbow remained unstable even after open repair of the radial and ulnar collateral ligaments, so a hinged external fixator was applied. The humeral half-pins were hand-drilled and placed percutaneously through a small incision, tunneling until contacting bone. Complete radial nerve palsy was noted postoperatively, with surgical exploration 1 day postoperatively showing complete disruption of the radial nerve and loss of substance of over 4 cm at the level of the distal humeral pin. The external fixator was removed 4 weeks later. The elbow demonstrated complex medial-lateral instability with anterior radial head dislocations in flexion and pronation. Autologous toe extensor tendon grafts were used to reconstruct the anular ligament and medial and lateral collateral ligaments. After 5 weeks the patient had satisfactory stability and elbow mobility, so tendon transfers to the wrist, finger, and thumb extensions were done. After 3 months the patient had free, stable elbow motion, 145° of flexion, 10° loss of extension, and 30° of active wrist extension.

Case 3: Woman, 55, fell while skiing and completely dislocated her right, dominant elbow with a comminuted radial head fracture. Closed reduction was performed and a long arm cast applied. Redislocation of the elbow in the cast was observed immediately and persisted despite two further attempts at closed reduction and cast immobilization. After 6 weeks open reduction was done through a posterior approach. Medial and lateral collateral ligaments were reattached, with insertion of a radial head prosthesis. A hinged external fixator was applied, with pins placed percutaneously.

Complete radial nerve palsy was seen immediately after surgery. Electrodiagnostic testing 4 weeks later suggested severe nerve injury. A week later, the radial nerve was explored when the external fixator was removed, showing complete disruption of the nerve at the level of the distal humeral pin. Secondary reconstruction was done 3 months later. After another 3 months, the elbow was stable with 100° arc of elbow motion and almost full forearm rotation. Radial nerve reconstruction was performed along with a pronator teres tendon transfer for wrist extension. After 3 months active wrist extension was 40° and grip strength was 10 kg. However, the patient had no active thumb or finger extension.

Conclusions.—Three patients experienced elbow instability that was managed using a hinged external fixator and suffered complete loss of radial nerve function at the site of the distal humeral pin. All experienced complete radial nerve paralysis, and two of the three had segmental nerve defects. Applying the hinged external fixator is a challenging procedure. It is highly likely that this procedure is complicated by major nerve injury related to percutaneous placement of the humeral pins more often than has been reported. The best approach appears to be placing these pins through an open approach spreading bluntly down to bone and inserting them under direct visualization.

▶ This case series highlights an underreported, important, and preventable complication, namely, iatrogenic injury to the radial nerve. The authors describe 3 patients in whom an articulated external fixator was applied for indications of elbow trauma or reconstruction, with percutaneous placement of the pins. These cases were complicated by complete palsy and documented transection in the 2 patients who underwent further surgery.

Although previous reports have suggested that percutaneous application of an external fixator about the elbow may be performed safely, this study highlights the complex anatomy about this region. The safest approach for application of an external fixator in this region is via an open incision for placement of the pins to identify and protect the radial nerve.

J. Adams, MD

Predictors of Functional Outcome Change 18 Months After Anterior Ulnar Nerve Transposition
Shi Q, MacDermid J, Grewal R, et al (McMaster Univ, Hamilton, Ontario, Canada; St Joseph's Health Centre, London, Ontario, Canada)
Arch Phys Med Rehabil 93:307-312, 2012

Objective.—To determine which variables derived from the electrodiagnostic examination were predictive of patient self-reported symptoms and disability at 18 months after anterior ulnar nerve transposition.

Design.—Retrospective cohort study.

Setting.—Electrodiagnostic laboratories affiliated with a tertiary care center.

Participants.—Patients (N = 73) with cubital tunnel syndrome (CuTS).

Interventions.—Patients were randomly assigned to one of the anterior transpositions of the ulnar nerve (subcutaneous or submuscular).

Main Outcome Measures.—Outcome was a patient-rated ulnar elbow evaluation (PRUNE). Predictors were all variables derived from the electrodiagnostic examination and characteristics of participants, as well as the preoperative clinical status. A stepwise multivariable linear regression analysis was used to determine the relative importance of the selected variables on the change in PRUNE scores.

Results.—Above-elbow compound muscle action potentials amplitude and proportional compound muscle action potentials amplitude decreasing from above elbow to below elbow were predictors of change score of the PRUNE at 18 months after operation ($R^2 = 16\%$). Sex and preoperative PRUNE also showed predictive information ($R^2 = 14\%$ and 15%, respectively).

Conclusions.—CuTS is predominantly a clinical diagnosis. Electrophysiologic studies are important supplemental examinations for the diagnosis of CuTS because they not only contribute to diagnosis, but are also important prognostic features. Females may have more improvement with regard to functional outcomes than males when undergoing surgical intervention.

▶ The authors' stated objective was to determine those electrodiagnostic findings that correlated best with the patient-related ulnar elbow evaluation following ulnar nerve transposition at the elbow for cubital tunnel syndrome. Although this term is commonly used when referring to any ulnar nerve compression at the elbow, it should refer only to ulnar nerve compression in the cubital tunnel, the anatomical site where the nerve passes between the 2 heads of the flexor carpi ulnaris under Osborne's ligament, which is also called the arcuate ligament. When the ulnar nerve is compressed at other sites at the elbow, such as the epicondylar groove and proximal to the groove, the diagnosis should be ulnar nerve compression at the elbow.

The article is probably of greater interest to physicians who perform electrodiagnostic studies than to surgeons who determine when surgery is necessary and then decompress and transpose the nerve, either in a subcutaneous or submuscular fashion, which were the operative procedures performed on the patients in this study. The authors' disappointment in the McGowan grading system to evaluate effectively the postoperative results should have been anticipated. The McGowan grading system was originally described as a preoperative system that rated only intrinsic muscle function, and the most severe stage III complete paralysis of the interossei muscles is uncommon.

The authors acknowledge that the diagnosis of ulnar nerve compression at the elbow is essentially a clinical diagnosis, and that electrodiagnostic studies are complementary and supplemental. Their conclusion that patients with severe preoperative electrodiagnostic findings usually have poor postoperative clinical results was not surprising.

M. A. Posner, MD

17 Shoulder: Anatomy and Instability

Injury of the Suprascapular Nerve During Latarjet Procedure: An Anatomic Study
Lädermann A, Denard PJ, Burkhart SS (Geneva Univ Hosps, Switzerland; The San Antonio Orthopaedic Group, TX)
Arthroscopy 28:316-321, 2012

Purpose.—The purpose of this study was to evaluate the relation between the specific exit point of the screws securing the coracoid graft and the suprascapular nerve during the Latarjet procedure.

Methods.—Ten fresh-frozen shoulder specimens were dissected after having undergone an open Latarjet procedure.

Results.—The mean distance from the posterior exit site of the superior screw to the suprascapular nerve at the base of the scapular spine was only 4 mm. Two of the superior screws were directly in contact with the major branch of the suprascapular nerve, and 2 screws were also in contact with minor branches of the suprascapular nerve. As for the inferior screw, there was contact with the major branch in 1 case and with minor branches of the suprascapular nerve in 6 cases. In the axial plane, the screws were not in contact with the suprascapular nerve if the angle relative to the glenoid was less than or equal to 10°.

Conclusions.—The proximity of the suprascapular nerve to the posterior glenoid rim puts this nerve at risk during insertion of the screws used for the Latarjet procedure. Placement of screws within 10° of the face of the glenoid in the axial plane is safe and will avoid the potential for suprascapular nerve injury (Figs 1B and 4A, B).

▶ This anatomic study provides a useful guideline for the placement of screws during the fixation of the coracoid in the Latarjet procedure. Through their cadaveric study, the authors identified the relation of the exit point of the screws to the suprascapular nerve (Fig 1B). This article suggests that the "safe zone" extends to within 10° of the face of the glenoid. Importantly, the authors point out that their model did not create a glenoid bone defect. In cases with bone loss, the screws exit the posterior cortex more laterally and farther from the suprascapular nerve. The authors point out that their model produces the most narrow safe zone (Fig 4A, B).

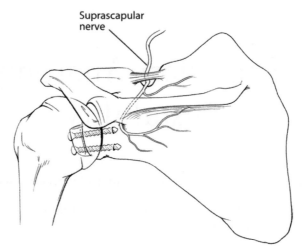

Suprascapular
nerve

FIGURE 1.—(B) The infraspinatus branches of the suprascapular nerve are at risk during screw placement for Latarjet reconstruction. (Reprinted from Lädermann A, Denard PJ, Burkhart SS. Injury of the suprascapular nerve during latarjet procedure: an anatomic study. *Arthroscopy.* 2012;28:316-321, Copyright 2012, with permission from the Arthroscopy Association of North America.)

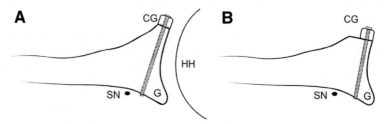

FIGURE 4.—Relation between screw placement (A) without glenoid bone loss and (B) with glenoid bone loss. A screw inserted at the same angle will exit the posterior cortex medially as the point of origin is moved farther anteriorly to a greater distance from the posterior glenoid. Therefore, in the absence of glenoid bone loss, a screw inserted for a Latarjet procedure at a given angle will exit the posterior glenoid closer to the suprascapular nerve. In addition, in the setting of glenoid bone loss, the angle of screw placement actually changes slightly. To achieve a congruent arc, the graft must be placed flush with the glenoid. With bone loss, the graft is flush with a portion of the glenoid that is more parallel to the posterior glenoid. In the absence of bone loss, a graft is placed flush farther out on the arc of the glenoid, which is oriented at a more medial angle. (Reprinted from Lädermann A, Denard PJ, Burkhart SS. Injury of the suprascapular nerve during latarjet procedure: an anatomic study. *Arthroscopy.* 2012;28:316-321, Copyright 2012, with permission from the Arthroscopy Association of North America.)

It is important to note that case reports of iatrogenic suprascapular nerve injury with the Latarjet procedure are quite rare. However, the authors also correctly note that such an injury may go unnoticed in the postoperative period or be compensated for by other motor branches.

This article provides useful information for fixation of the coracoid in a Latarjet procedure as well as during fixation of additional glenoid bone grafting procedures.

A. K. Harrison, MD

Analysis of Risk Factors for Glenoid Bone Defect in Anterior Shoulder Instability

Milano G, Grasso A, Russo A, et al (Catholic Univ, Rome, Italy; Villa Valeria Clinic, Rome, Italy; Villa Ulivella Clinic, Florence, Italy; et al)
Am J Sports Med 39:1870-1876, 2011

Background.—Glenoid bone defect is frequently associated with anterior shoulder instability and is considered one of the major causes of recurrence of instability after shoulder stabilization.

Hypothesis.—Some risk factors are significantly associated with the presence, size, and type of glenoid bone defect.

Study Design.—Cohort study (prognosis); Level of evidence, 2.

Methods.—One hundred sixty-one patients affected by anterior shoulder instability underwent morphologic evaluation of the glenoid by computed tomography scans to assess the presence, size, and type of glenoid bone defect (erosion or bony Bankart lesion). Bone loss greater than 20% of the area of the inferior glenoid was considered "critical" bone defect (at risk of recurrence). Outcomes were correlated with the following predictors: age, gender, arm dominance, frequency of dislocation, age at first dislocation, timing from first dislocation, number of dislocations, cause of first dislocation, generalized ligamentous laxity, type of sport, and manual work.

Results.—Glenoid bone defect was observed in 72% of the cases. Presence of the defect was significantly associated with recurrence of dislocation compared with a single episode of dislocation, increasing number of dislocations, male gender, and type of sport. Size of the defect was significantly associated with recurrent dislocation, increasing number of dislocations, timing from first dislocation, and manual work. Presence of a critical defect was significantly associated with number of dislocations and age at first dislocation. Bony Bankart lesion was significantly associated with male gender and age at first dislocation.

Conclusion.—The number of dislocations and age at first dislocation are the most significant predictors of glenoid bone loss in anterior shoulder instability.

▶ Recently, emphasis has been placed on preoperative identification of patients with anterior shoulder instability due to bony deficiency. Failure to recognize these patients can place them at risk for continued instability following a soft tissue reconstruction that fails to address the bony deficiency. However, which patients are at highest risk for glenoid bone defects have not been fully elucidated. Milano et al sought to identify risk factors for glenoid bone defects in anterior shoulder instability. They analyzed the association between glenoid bone defects detected by CT scan and associated risk factors with shoulder instability in a cohort of patients. Following a pre hoc power analysis, 161 consecutive patients with unilateral anterior shoulder instability with at least 1 episode of dislocation and an unaffected contralateral shoulder were evaluated with bilateral CT scans. Glenoid en face views were then evaluated with the described "Pico" method for the presence of a glenoid bone defect, percentage size of the glenoid bone defect, presence of a critical bone defect (defined as 20% or greater glenoid bone loss), and type of bone defect, either erosion or fracture/bony Bankart.

Glenoid bone defects were detected in 72%, with erosion in 49% and bony Bankart in 23%. The average size of defect was 7% (range, 0%-33%), and a critical bone defect was present in 7.5%. The strongest predictors for both presence and increasing size of a glenoid bone defect were recurrence of dislocation and increasing number of dislocations. Male gender also had a significant association with presence of a bone defect. Patients with recurrent dislocation had on average 5% greater glenoid bone defects than patients with an acute dislocation. Manual laborers had 2.5% greater bone defects than sedentary workers. Presence of a critical defect (> 20%) was associated with increased number of dislocations, while increased age at first dislocation had a protective effect. Presence of a bony Bankart lesion was associated with male gender.

Overall, the work of Milano et al was a well-executed, appropriately powered radiologic evaluation of a single cohort of patients identified with anterior shoulder instability. Their work further validates the theory that recurrent instability leads to progressive glenoid bone erosion. Clinically, their study highlights the importance of obtaining an advanced imaging study to evaluate patients with strong risk factors for severe bone loss, specifically recurrent dislocators, and those with an increasing number of dislocations. Their work identifies 2 groups at risk for progressive osseous erosion: the recurrently unstable young man and the manual laborer. For these groups, early surgical treatment may be advisable to halt progression of the osseous erosion cascade. Future research should report results of surgical treatment of patients with critical bone defects.

J. M. Wiater, MD

18 Shoulder: Arthroplasty

Shoulder arthroplasty in patients aged fifty-five years or younger with osteoarthritis

Bartelt R, Sperling JW, Schleck CD, et al (Mayo Clinic, Rochester, MN)
J Shoulder Elbow Surg 20:123-130, 2011

Background.—The younger patient with glenohumeral arthritis presents a challenge because of concerns about activity and frequency of failure. The purpose of this study was to define the results, complications, and frequency of revision surgery in this group.

Materials and Methods.—Between 1986 and 2005, 46 total shoulder arthroplasties and 20 hemiarthroplasties were performed in 63 patients who were aged 55 years or younger and had chronic shoulder pain due to glenohumeral osteoarthritis. All 63 patients had complete preoperative evaluation, operative records, and minimum 2-year follow-up (mean, 7.0 years) or follow-up until revision.

Results.—Nine shoulders underwent a revision operation. The implant survival rate was 92% (95% confidence interval, 77%-100%) at 10 years for total shoulder arthroplasty and 72% (95% confidence interval, 54%-97%) for hemiarthroplasty (Kaplan-Meier result). Patients who underwent total shoulder arthroplasty had less pain ($P = .01$), greater active elevation ($P = .05$), and higher satisfaction ($P = .05$) at final follow-up compared with those who underwent hemiarthroplasty. Complete radiographs were available for 47 arthroplasties with a minimum 2-year follow-up or follow-up until revision (mean, 6.6 years). More than minor glenoid periprosthetic lucency or a shift in component position was present in 10 of 34 total shoulder arthroplasties. Moderate to severe glenoid erosion was present in 6 of 13 hemiarthroplasties.

Conclusions.—This study indicates that there is intermediate- to long-term pain relief and improvement in motion with shoulder arthroplasty in young patients with osteoarthritis. These results favor total shoulder arthroplasty in terms of pain relief, motion, and implant survival.

▶ Determining the best surgery for younger patients with glenohumeral osteoarthritis is challenging. Because of the frequently higher activity level and increased longevity in this population, concern for implant loosening has led many to recommend hemi-arthroplasty in younger patients. This is despite the evidence that pain control is better in patients who undergo total shoulder arthroplasty compared to hemi-arthroplasty.[1,2] In an attempt to shed light on this dilemma, the authors retrospectively reviewed all shoulder arthroplasties at their institution over a 20-year period, finding 5% performed in patients aged 55 or younger.

In patients with at least 2 years of follow-up, 46 underwent total shoulder arthroplasty and 20 had a hemi-arthroplasty. With an average follow-up of 6 years in the total shoulder arthroplasty group and 9.3 years in the hemi-arthroplasty group, the total shoulder group had an estimated 5-year revision-free survival of 100% and a 10-year rate of 92%, compared to the hemi-arthroplasty rates of 85% at 5 years and 72% at 10 years. There were three total shoulder patients who underwent revision: 1 for loosening and 2 for infection. In the hemi-arthroplasty group, there were 6 revisions: 5 for painful glenoid arthritis and 1 for infection. In the radiologic evaluation in the hemi-arthroplasty group, half of the patients had glenohumeral subluxation and all had glenoid erosion. For the total shoulder patients, half of the patients had subluxation, 25% had humeral lucency, and 62% had glenoid lucency.

Based on their findings, the authors conclude that total shoulder arthroplasty is preferred in patients aged 55 or younger. Although these midterm results are favorable, it is important to remember that the average follow-up was 6 years in the total shoulder group and that the majority had developed lucency about the glenoid at final follow-up. This is concerning, because progressive lucency is likely to occur, portending the need for revision. In contrast, there is a high percentage of patients in the hemi-arthroplasty group with joint subluxation and glenoid erosion, which was the main indication for revision surgery in this group. The authors show us that total shoulder arthroplasty patients have better midterm outcomes; however, concerns for prosthetic loosening remain.

F. T. D. Kaplan, MD

References

1. Bryant D, Litchfield R, Sandow M, Gartsman GM, Guyatt G, Kirkley A. A comparison of pain, strength, range of motion, and functional outcomes after hemiarthroplasty and total shoulder arthroplasty in patients with osteoarthritis of the shoulder. A systematic review and meta-analysis. *J Bone Joint Surg Am.* 2005;87:1947-1956.
2. Radnay CS, Setter KJ, Chambers L, Levine WN, Bigliani LU, Ahmad CS. Total shoulder replacement compared with humeral head replacement for the treatment of primary glenohumeral osteoarthritis: a systematic review. *J Shoulder Elbow Surg.* 2007;16:396-402.

Prevalence of Neurologic Lesions After Total Shoulder Arthroplasty
Lädermann A, Lübbeke A, Mélis B, et al (Geneva Univ Hosps, Switzerland; Centre Orthopédique Santy, Lyon, France)
J Bone Joint Surg Am 93:1288-1293, 2011

Background.—Clinically evident neurologic injury of the involved limb after total shoulder arthroplasty is not uncommon, but the subclinical prevalence is unknown. The purposes of this prospective study were to determine the subclinical prevalence of neurologic lesions after reverse shoulder arthroplasty and anatomic shoulder arthroplasty, and to evaluate the correlation of neurologic injury to postoperative lengthening of the arm.

Methods.—All patients undergoing either a reverse or an anatomic shoulder arthroplasty were included during the period studied. This study focused on the clinical, radiographic, and preoperative and postoperative electromyographic evaluation, with measurement of arm lengthening in patients who had reverse shoulder arthroplasty according to a previously validated protocol.

Results.—Between November 2007 and February 2009, forty-one patients (forty-two shoulders) underwent reverse shoulder arthroplasty (nineteen shoulders) or anatomic primary shoulder arthroplasty (twenty-three shoulders). The two groups were similar with respect to sex distribution, preoperative neurologic lesions, and Constant score. Electromyography performed at a mean of 3.6 weeks postoperatively in the reverse shoulder arthroplasty group showed subclinical electromyographic changes in nine shoulders, involving mainly the axillary nerve; eight resolved in less than six months. In the anatomic shoulder arthroplasty group, a brachial plexus lesion was evident in one shoulder. The prevalence of acute postoperative nerve injury was significantly more frequent in the reverse shoulder arthroplasty group (p = 0.002), with a 10.9 times higher risk (95% confidence interval, 1.5 to 78.5). Mean lengthening (and standard deviation) of the arm after reverse shoulder arthroplasty was 2.7 ± 1.8 cm (range, 0 to 5.9 cm) compared with the normal, contralateral side.

Conclusions.—The occurrence of peripheral neurologic lesions following reverse shoulder arthroplasty is relatively common, but usually transient. Arm lengthening with a reverse shoulder arthroplasty may be responsible for these nerve injuries.

▶ Certainly, neurologic injury is a documented complication with both anatomic and reverse shoulder arthroplasty. A previous report (Van Hoof et al) documented the strain on variable segments of the brachial plexus after reverse shoulder arthroplasty. However, this study by Lädermann et al is the first prospective evaluation of neurologic lesions in both anatomic and reverse shoulder arthroplasty. The authors found acute postoperative nerve injury was significantly more common in reverse shoulder arthroplasty compared with anatomic shoulder arthroplasty. Nine patients had subclinical electromyogram changes after reverse shoulder arthroplasty, and the axillary nerve was most commonly involved. The study also examined arm lengthening in reverse shoulder arthroplasty and was hypothesized as a cause for nerve injury. However, the smaller study size limited the authors' ability to determine the degree to which arm lengthening is responsible for neurologic injuries.

This study serves to educate the shoulder arthroplasty surgeon regarding the prevalence of neurologic lesions after shoulder arthroplasty and, in particular, provides more specific information about the frequency with which these injuries are seen in reverse shoulder arthroplasty. This information not only informs the surgeon but should also be used to councel the patient preoperatively.

This study did exclude patients with comorbidities that may cause neuropathies such as diabetes mellitus. However, this patient population may be at greater risk for exacerbation of neurologic function and would be important for further study. Additionally, further study with larger sample sizes may allow determination of the role arm lengthening may have in neurologic lesions after reverse shoulder arthroplasty.

A. K. Harrison, MD

Early Results of Reverse Shoulder Arthroplasty in Patients with Rheumatoid Arthritis
Young AA, Smith MM, Bacle G, et al (Centre Orthopédique Santy, Lyon, France)
J Bone Joint Surg Am 93:1915-1923, 2011

Background.—Rheumatoid arthritis affecting the shoulder is typically associated with rotator cuff compromise and can also result in severe glenoid erosion. Since reverse shoulder arthroplasty is capable of addressing both rotator cuff disorders and glenoid bone deficiencies, our aim was to evaluate the outcome of reverse shoulder arthroplasty in patients with rheumatoid arthritis and either or both of these associated conditions.

Methods.—We performed eighteen primary reverse total shoulder arthroplasties in sixteen patients with rheumatoid arthritis involving the shoulder as well as associated rotator cuff compromise and/or severe erosion of the glenoid bone between 2002 and 2007. Patients were assessed with use of the Constant score, patient satisfaction score, subjective shoulder value, range of shoulder motion, and imaging studies.

Results.—The mean Constant score improved from 22.5 to 64.9 points at a mean of 3.8 years (range, 2.1 to 7.0 years) postoperatively. The patients were either very satisfied or satisfied with the outcome of the surgery in seventeen of the eighteen shoulders. The mean subjective shoulder value was 68.6% postoperatively. Active forward elevation improved from 77.5° to 138.6°, and external rotation with the arm in 90° of abduction improved from 16.9° to 46.1°. The mean Constant score improved from 28.0 points to 74.3 points in shoulders in which the teres minor muscle was normal before the surgery, and it improved from 20.8 to 54.6 points in shoulders with an atrophic teres minor muscle. Scapular notching was observed in ten of the eighteen shoulders. A fracture involving the acromion, acromial spine, coracoid, or greater tuberosity was observed either intraoperatively or postoperatively in four of the eighteen shoulders. One case of transient axillary nerve injury was noted. There were no cases of dislocation, infection, or component loosening. None of the patients required revision surgery for any reason.

Conclusions.—Comparatively good outcomes were observed in the short to intermediate term after reverse shoulder arthroplasty in patients with rheumatoid arthritis. However, surgeons should be aware of the risk of intraoperative and postoperative fractures in this patient group.

▶ This study provides an important current report on the results of reverse total shoulder arthroplasty in a very select but important patient population: patients with rheumatoid arthritis. Although recent studies of reverse shoulder arthroplasty in this patient population have suggested improved functional outcomes, the first study of this population by Rittmeister and Kerschbaumer documented a high complication rate. This led many to recommend against reverse total shoulder arthroplasty for patients with rheumatoid arthritis. However, the report by Rittmeister and Kerschbaumer included cases done through a transacromial approach, which led to complications unique to this approach. This study, as well as most recent reports, includes cases done through a deltopectoral approach.

This study outlines the complications unique to reverse total shoulder arthroplasty, such as acromial or coracoid fractures. The authors correctly advise caution for reverse shoulder arthroplasty in patients with rheumatoid arthritis as we continue to gain experience and knowledge of this implant. This study provides evidence of improved objective outcomes using current techniques and experience, suggesting that this procedure is not only safe but can be effective in providing improved pain relief and function for this patient population.

A. K. Harrison, MD

Preoperative Patient Expectations of Total Shoulder Arthroplasty
Henn RF III, Ghomrawi H, Rutledge JR, et al (Hosp for Special Surgery, NY)
J Bone Joint Surg Am 93:2110-2115, 2011

Background.—Very little data exist regarding patients' preoperative expectations of the outcome of total shoulder arthroplasty. We hypothesized that younger patients and patients with worse function and worse general health would have greater expectations of total shoulder arthroplasty.

Methods.—Ninety-eight patients who underwent unilateral primary total shoulder arthroplasty at one institution were studied prospectively. The preoperative evaluation included the American Shoulder and Elbow Surgeons (ASES) score, Shoulder Activity Scale, Short Form-36 (SF-36), and visual analog scale scores for shoulder pain, fatigue, and general health. Expectations were evaluated with use of the Hospital for Special Surgery's Shoulder Surgery Expectations Survey.

Results.—Relief of daytime pain, relief of nighttime pain, and improvement of shoulder range of motion were very important to 86%, 82%, and 84% of the patients, respectively. Expectations were not associated with education, history of previous joint replacement, or comorbidities. Greater expectations were associated with younger age, worse general health on the visual analog scale, and worse ASES scores ($p < 0.05$ for all), with correlation coefficients ranging from 0.25 to 0.28. Multivariate analysis showed that younger age was the only independent predictor of greater expectations ($p < 0.05$).

Conclusions.—Younger patients had greater expectations of total shoulder arthroplasty, which may have implications for outcome and implant longevity.

▶ The authors have completed a very well-organized study on patient expectations of total shoulder arthroplasty. Previously, there was minimal information on this important topic. This prospective study carefully examined those outcome measurements that were most important to patients. A variety of factors were analyzed including patient comorbidities, history of prior joint arthroplasty, and educational level. Interestingly, the data from this study clearly indicate that younger patients had greater expectations about total shoulder arthroplasty. This information is very valuable when discussing the expected outcome of total shoulder arthroplasty with patients.

J. Sperling, MD

Total Shoulder Arthroplasty with an All-Polyethylene Pegged Bone-Ingrowth Glenoid Component: A Clinical and Radiographic Outcome Study
Wirth MA, Loredo R, Garcia G, et al (Univ of Texas Health Science Ctr at San Antonio; et al)
J Bone Joint Surg Am 94:260-267, 2012

Background.—Loosening of the glenoid component continues to be the foremost cause of medium and long-term failure of shoulder replacements. The purpose of this study was to evaluate the clinical and radiographic results of a minimally cemented all-polyethylene pegged glenoid component designed for biologic fixation.

Methods.—Forty-four shoulders in forty-one patients with a mean age of sixty-six years underwent total shoulder arthroplasty with a pegged bone-ingrowth glenoid component. Outcome data included the American Shoulder and Elbow Surgeons questionnaire, the Simple Shoulder Test, and visual analog scales. A detailed radiographic analysis was performed by two board-certified musculoskeletal radiologists who were blinded to clinical and patient-reported outcomes. The radiographs were evaluated with regard to the presence of radiolucent lines at the bone-cement interface, implant seating, and the radiodensity between the flanges of the central peg.

Results.—The mean duration of clinical follow-up was four years and the mean duration of radiographic follow-up was three years. Twenty shoulders had perfect seating and radiolucency grades, thirty had increased radiodensity between the flanges of the central peg, and three demonstrated osteolysis. Radiodensity about the uncemented central peg at the time of the latest follow-up was positively associated with perfect seating and radiolucency grades on the initial postoperative radiographs (p = 0.03, Fisher exact test). The Simple Shoulder Test score, the American Shoulder and Elbow Surgeons score, and all visual analog scale scores had improved significantly (p < 0.01) at the time of the latest follow-up.

Conclusions.—Total shoulder arthroplasty with a minimally cemented, all-polyethylene, pegged glenoid implant can yield stable and durable fixation at short to medium-term follow-up (mean, four years).

▶ The authors present the data from a well-organized study on the outcome of total shoulder arthroplasty with an all polyethylene pegged bone ingrowth glenoid component. This study provides useful information on the short-term to midterm clinical and radiographic survival of glenoid components. The study has particular merit because some surgeons continue to have concerns about glenoid component loosening. The data from this study reinforce the concept that the glenoid component survival is very good and provides durable pain relief.

J. W. Sperling, MD, MBA

A History of Reverse Total Shoulder Arthroplasty
Flatow EL, Harrison AK (Mount Sinai School of Medicine, NY)
Clin Orthop Relat Res 469:2432-2439, 2011

Background.—Management of the cuff-deficient arthritic shoulder has long been challenging. Early unconstrained shoulder arthroplasty systems were associated with high complication and implant failure rates. The evolution toward the modern reverse shoulder arthroplasty includes many variables of constrained shoulder arthroplasty designs.

Questions/Purposes.—This review explores the development of reverse shoulder arthroplasty, specifically describing (1) the evolution of reverse shoulder arthroplasty designs, (2) the biomechanical variations in the evolution of this arthroplasty, and (3) the current issues relevant to reverse shoulder arthroplasty today.

Methods.—Using a PubMed search, the literature was explored for articles addressing reverse shoulder arthroplasty, focusing on those papers with historical context.

Results.—Results of the early designs were apparently poor, although they were not subjected to rigorous clinical research and usually reported only in secondary literature. We identified a trend of glenoid component failure in the early reverse designs. This trend was recognized and reported by authors as the reverse shoulder evolved. Authors reported greater pain relief and better function in reverse shoulder arthroplasty with the fundamental change of Grammont's design (moving the center of rotation medially and distally). However, current reports suggest lingering concerns and challenges with today's designs.

Conclusions.—The history of reverse shoulder arthroplasty involves the designs of many forward-thinking surgeons. Many of these highly constrained systems failed, although more recent designs have demonstrated improved longevity and implant performance. Reverse shoulder arthroplasty requires ongoing study, with challenges and controversies remaining around present-day designs.

▶ This is an interesting article that presents the history of reverse total shoulder arthroplasty, discussing the various iterations beginning from the Mark I and evolving to the Delta III/Grammont design. This historical account aims to give insight as to why current designs have been clinically more successful than their predecessors. In addition, it provides a context through which we can understand current designs and future developments.

This article is of particular importance to specialists in shoulder and elbow as well as general orthopedists in that the historical evolution of the prosthesis provides a larger understanding of how technological developments occur in orthopedics.

N. Chen, MD

A Complication-based Learning Curve From 200 Reverse Shoulder Arthroplasties

Kempton LB, Ankerson E, Wiater JM (William Beaumont Hosp, Royal Oak, MI; William Beaumont Hosp Res Inst, Royal Oak, MI)
Clin Orthop Relat Res 469:2496-2504, 2011

Background.—Reported early complication rates in reverse total shoulder arthroplasty have widely varied from 0% to 75% in part due to a lack of standard inclusion criteria. In addition, it is unclear whether revision arthroplasty is associated with a higher rate of complications than primary arthroplasty.

Questions/Purpose.—We therefore (1) determined the types and rates of early complications in reverse total shoulder arthroplasty using defined criteria, (2) characterized an early complication-based learning curve for reverse total shoulder arthroplasty, and (3) determined whether revision arthroplasties result in a higher incidence of complications.

Patients and Methods.—From October 2004 to May 2008, an initial series of 200 reverse total shoulder arthroplasties was performed in 191 patients by a single surgeon. Forty of the 200 arthroplasties were revision arthroplasties. Of these, 192 shoulders were available for minimum 6-month followup (mean, 19.4 months; range, 6—49.2 months). We determined local and systemic complications and distinguished major from minor complications.

Results.—Nineteen shoulders involved local complications (9.9%), including seven major and 12 minor complications. Nine involved perioperative systemic complications (4.7%), including eight major complications and one minor complication. The local complication rate was higher in the first 40 shoulders (23.1%) versus the last 160 shoulders (6.5%). Seven of 40 (17.5%) revision arthroplasties involved local complications, including two major and five minor complications compared to 12 of 152 (7.9%) primary arthroplasties, including five major and seven minor complications. Nerve palsies occurred less frequently in primary arthroplasties (0.6%) compared to revisions (9.8%).

Conclusions.—The early complication-based learning curve for reverse total shoulder arthroplasty is approximately 40 cases. There was a trend toward more complications in revision versus primary reverse total shoulder arthroplasty and more neuropathies in revisions.

Level of Evidence.—Level IV, therapeutic study. See the guidelines online for a complete description of level of evidence.

▶ This article documents a large series of reverse total shoulder arthroplasties performed by a single surgeon, demonstrating a substantially higher complication rate in the first 40 arthroplasties and a subsequent decrease in complications following those initial surgeries. Complications were defined using alternative criteria in that an event was recorded if it resulted in an alteration of surgical or postoperative routine. Clinical outcomes data other than the incidence of complications were not reported.

This descriptive study provides insight into a single practice that has been successful in limiting the number of potential complications. In particular, the senior author demonstrated strict, well-defined indications for using reverse arthroplasty. Three different arthroplasty manufacturers were used throughout the series with similar results, suggesting that implant designs are relatively constant and design differences are relatively minor in affecting the incidence of complications.

N. Chen, MD

19 Shoulder: Arthroscopy

A New Method for Knotless Fixation of an Upper Subscapularis Tear
Denard PJ, Burkhart SS (Univ of Texas Health Science Ctr at San Antonio)
Arthroscopy 27:861-866, 2011

The advancement of shoulder arthroscopy has provided the opportunity to see the articular side of the rotator cuff and has led to increased recognition of subscapularis tears. One of the unique challenges to arthroscopic subscapularis repair is the small anterior space overlying the subscapularis. Whereas the subacromial space allows freedom of movement, the limited subcoracoid space makes visualization, instrument manipulation, and knot tying more difficult. We describe a technique for knotless restoration of the upper subscapularis footprint that eases some of the aforementioned difficulties. The technique is indicated for partial- or full-thickness tears of the upper 50% of the subscapularis tendon and therefore applies to the majority of tears involving the subscapularis tendon.

▶ The authors describe their knotless surgical technique of arthroscopic subscapularis repair. One of the challenges to arthroscopic subscapularis repair compared with superior rotator cuff repair is the small anterior space overlying the subscapularis. The limited space in the subcoracoid recess makes visualization, instrument manipulation, and knot tying more difficult. The authors offer technical pearls with a knotless anchor, which make this technique more expedient and attractive. All work is viewed from a standard posterior portal. The rotator interval is opened. The coracoid is identified, and keeping this landmark in view ensures safety of approach because all important neurovascular structures are more than 2.5 cm from the tip of the coracoid. The authors recommend decompression of a tight subcoracoid space with a high-speed burr, if necessary. This would make suture passage through the subscapularis easier. Sutures are passed from an anterosuperolateral working portal and retrieved through an anterior portal, which is just lateral to the tip of the coracoid. It is useful to switch to a 70-degree scope for final anchor placement. The knotless anchors are then placed through the anterior portal. The authors have found this technique to be such a reliable and efficient restoration of the subscapularis tendon footprint that it has become their procedure of choice for tears of the upper subscapularis tendon.

E. Cheung, MD

Agreement in the Classification and Treatment of the Superior Labrum

Wolf BR, for the MOON Shoulder Group (Univ of Iowa Hosps and Clinics; et al)

Am J Sports Med 39:2588-2594, 2011

Background.—The Snyder classification scheme is the most commonly used system for classifying superior labral injuries. Although this scheme is intended to be used for arthroscopic visual classification only, it is thought that other nonarthroscopic historical variables also influence the classification.

Purpose.—This study was conducted to evaluate the intrasurgeon and intersurgeon agreement in classifying variable presentations of the superior labrum and to evaluate the influence of clinical variables on the classification and treatment choices of surgeons.

Study Design.—Cohort study (diagnosis); Level of evidence, 3.

Methods.—A group of arthroscopic shoulder surgeons were asked to rank in order of importance clinical variables considered in diagnosing and treating the superior labrum. The surgeons then watched 50 arthroscopic videos of the superior labrum, ranging from normal to pathologic, on 3 different occasions. The first and third viewings were accompanied by no clinical information. The second viewing was accompanied by a detailed clinical vignette for each video. The surgeons selected a classification and treatment for each video.

Results.—A patient's job/sport, age, and physical examination findings were considered the most important clinical variables surgeons consider during management of the superior labrum. Comparing the 2 viewings without clinical information, surgeons selected a different classification 28.5% of the time from the first to the second time. A different classification was chosen 71.5% of the time when the surgeon was supplied a clinical vignette at the subsequent viewing. Similarly, the treatment selected changed in 36% and 69.1% of cases when viewed again without vignettes and with vignettes, respectively. Intersurgeon agreement was moderate without clinical vignettes and fair with vignettes. Historical, physical examination, and surgical observations were found to influence the odds of change of classification.

Conclusion.—There is significant intrasurgeon and intersurgeon variability in classification and treatment of the superior labrum. Clinical historical, examination, and surgical findings influence classification and treatment choices.

▶ This article adds to the growing literature about the accuracy and reliability in diagnosis and treatment of superior labral anterior to posterior tears. Prior literature has illustrated the unreliable nature of the physical examination in isolation and in combination for making this diagnosis. The authors take this a step further by evaluating other factors that may influence the diagnostic process. From the isolated perspective of surgical visualization, the authors showed great variability in classifying and treating this problem, but more interestingly, this changes significantly if the surgeon factors in history and physical examination findings. This study points out the most influential factors for diagnosis: job or athletic activity, age, and physical examination findings. The latter, physical examination, is of most interest since other recent studies have shown it to be unreliable. The study demonstrates the lack of consensus not only in the diagnosis but also in the fallacy of classification and how other factors contribute. Another interesting facet of this article is that the study group included orthopedic surgeons who had been trained by others within the group. This factor may have introduced a consensus bias from the authors. Consequently, inclusion of international authors or others outside the study group may produce different conclusions.

C. J. Tuohy, MD

Arthroscopic Basic Task Performance in Shoulder Simulator Model Correlates with Similar Task Performance in Cadavers
Martin KD, Belmont PJ Jr, Schoenfeld AJ, et al (William Beaumont Army Med Ctr, El Paso, TX; et al)
J Bone Joint Surg Am 93:e127.1-e127.5, 2011

Background.—Attainment of the technical skill necessary to safely perform arthroscopic procedures requires the instruction of orthopaedic surgery residents in basic arthroscopic skills. Although previous studies involving shoulder arthroscopy simulators have demonstrated a correlation between task performance and the level of prior arthroscopic experience, data demonstrating the correlation of simulator performance with arthroscopic skill in a surgical setting are scarce. Our goal was to evaluate the correlation between timed task performance in an arthroscopic shoulder simulator and timed task performance in a cadaveric shoulder arthroscopy model.

Methods.—Subjects were recruited from among residents and attending surgeons in an orthopaedic surgery residency program. Each subject was tested on an arthroscopic shoulder simulator and objectively scored on the basis of the time taken to complete a standardized object selection program. After an interval of at least two weeks, each subject was then tested on a cadaveric shoulder arthroscopy model designed to replicate the shoulder arthroscopy simulator testing protocol, and the time to completion was again recorded. Both testing protocols involved the simple task of placing a probe on a series of assigned locations in the glenohumeral joint. Spearman rank correlation analysis was performed, and regression analysis was used to determine the predictive ability of the simulator score.

Results.—The performance time on the simulation program was strongly correlated with the performance time on the cadaveric model ($r = 0.736$, $p < 0.001$). The time required to complete the simulator task was a significant predictor of the time required to complete the cadaveric task ($t = 4.48$, $p < 0.001$).

Conclusions.—These results demonstrated a strong correlation between performance of basic arthroscopic tasks in a simulator model and performance of the same tasks in a cadaveric model.

▶ This study seeks to establish a relationship between surgeons' performance of arthroscopic tasks in a nonbiologic shoulder model and a cadaver shoulder. Each participant was timed while placing a probe first on a series of anatomic locations in a shoulder simulator and then on a cadaver shoulder. The authors found that there was a strong correlation between these 2 times. As a result, they conclude that a nonbiologic shoulder model can be a useful tool for training residents in basic arthroscopic skills.

This article touches on the larger question of how to train residents to perform surgical procedures while minimizing potential harm to patients. Training on arthroscopic simulators has previously been shown to be superior to no training for novice surgeons. Although such models allow practice in manipulating arthroscopic instruments in space and performing simple tasks, such as placing a probe in specific locations (as in this study) or knot tying, they do not allow for true replication of more complex procedures such as labral repair. The fact that even the novice users in this study completed the task in a mean time of just over 2 minutes suggests that the required task was simple and not necessarily representative of an arthroscopic procedure that would be performed in orthopedic practice. In addition, the preexisting portals in such models do not allow the resident to practice the critical skill of portal placement.

This study cannot answer how effective practice on the shoulder model is at teaching arthroscopic surgery skills. Novice surgeons took about 50% longer to perform the same task in a cadaver shoulder, suggesting that even under the most standardized conditions, the use of a true human shoulder introduces complexities not replicable in the arthroscopic simulator.

C. M. Ward, MD

A Magnetic Resonance Imaging Study of 100 Cases of Arthroscopic Acromioplasty
Koh KH, Laddha MS, Lim TK, et al (Sungkyunkwan Univ School of Medicine, Seoul, Korea)
Am J Sports Med 40:352-358, 2012

Background.—A hooked-type acromion has been suspected to correlate with higher rotator cuff tear or impingement syndrome. However, correlation of acromial shape after acromioplasty with the rotator cuff retears and clinical results has not been studied before.

Purpose.—To assess the shape of the acromion after arthroscopic acromioplasty and to see if there is any relation with the rotator cuff retears and clinical results.

Study Design.—Case series; Level of evidence, 4.

Methods.—One hundred consecutive patients who underwent acromioplasty using a posterior cutting block technique accompanied by rotator cuff repair were included in this study. The decision was made to perform acromioplasty intraoperatively after confirmation of external impingement. Postoperative acromial shape was evaluated according to whether the acromion was flat, curved, or hooked on coronal and sagittal planes on magnetic resonance imaging (MRI) at a mean 13.4 months after surgery. Retear rates and clinical scores were compared between the hooked acromion and the others on postoperative MRI.

Results.—Preoperatively, only 29 patients had a hooked acromion on either coronal or sagittal plane MRI. After acromioplasty of those 100 patients, 23 still showed a hooked acromion. Twenty-six of 29 preoperatively hooked acromions were changed to nonhooked acromions, and 20 of 23 postoperatively hooked acromions had been nonhooked acromions preoperatively. No difference was found in the retear rate with respect to the postoperative acromial shape. Clinically, the American Shoulder and Elbow Surgeons (ASES) score was not different between the hooked acromion and the other group (82 vs 85, $P = .099$). However, the Constant score of the hooked acromion group was lower than that of the other group (74 vs 85, $P = .036$). Ninety-four of 100 patients were contacted again for the evaluation of the ASES score at a mean 36.5 months (range, 29-45 months) and showed no difference between the hooked acromion and the other group (87 vs 87, $P = .903$).

Conclusion.—Even with a standard posterior cutting block technique during acromioplasty, 23% of patients still showed a hooked acromion after arthroscopic acromioplasty. Using the signs of coracoacromial ligament impingement as an indication for acromioplasty might lead to hooked acromions postoperatively, which were nonhooked acromions preoperatively. However, the retear rate showed no difference according to the postoperative acromial shape.

▶ In this article, the authors report on their experience of 100 patients who underwent an arthroscopic acromioplasty at the time of their arthroscopic rotator cuff repair. They examined the acromioplasties with postoperative MRI to evaluate the shape of the acromion following acromioplasty and collected American Shoulder and Elbow Scores (ASES) and Constant scores. Interestingly, despite a diligent technique, they found 23% of the patients had a hooked acromion postoperatively. No differences in retear rate or final ASES were seen between the hooked and nonhooked acromion groups. The overall retear rate in this article was low, and patients showed significant improvement from preoperative outcome scores. This article highlights the need for a diligent technique of performing a subacromial decompression and the importance of making a clinical diagnosis of impingement. It also highlights that an increase in retear rate or decreased outcome measures are not observed in patients with postoperative hooking of the acromion.

J. Macalena, MD

Clinical outcomes of suprascapular nerve decompression

Shah AA, Butler RB, Sung S-Y, et al (Massachusetts General Hosp, Boston; Brigham and Women's Hosp, Boston, MA)
J Shoulder Elbow Surg 20:975-982, 2011

Background.—While the incidence and prevalence of suprascapular neuropathy (SSN) remains largely unknown, the evaluation and treatment of SSN appears to be increasing. Despite multiple technique articles demonstrating nerve decompression, there has been no clinical evidence to support the efficacy of SSN decompression in the absence of rotator cuff disease.

Methods.—Between October 2006 and February 2010, 27 patients underwent arthroscopic suprascapular nerve decompression at the suprascapular and/or spinoglenoid notch. Eighty-nine percent (24/27) of patients had preoperative positive electromyography and nerve conduction EMG/NCV studies documenting suprascapular nerve pathology. All patients had either a computed tomography (CT) arthrogram or magnetic resonance imaging (MRI) documenting rotator cuff integrity. All patients were evaluated with pre and postoperative subjective shoulder values (SSV) and American Shoulder and Elbow Society (ASES) self-assessment scores. Additionally, patients were questioned whether they would have the procedure again and approximately at what week they experienced noticeable pain relief.

Results.—The 27 patients were followed for an average of 22.5 months (range, 3-44). Three patients were lost to follow-up. Seventy-one percent (17/24) of patients reported pain relief (VAS [Visual Analogue Scales] pain scale) that was statistically significant ($P = .0001$) at an average of 9.4 weeks from surgery. Seventy-five percent (18/24) and 71% (17/24) had statistically significant improvement in ASES ($P = .0001$) and SSV scores ($P = .0014$), respectively. Seventy-one percent (17/24) would have the surgery again.

Conclusion.—The present study demonstrates a large series of patients treated for SSN without rotator cuff pathology. Our results show statistically significant improvement in VAS, ASES, and SSV.

▶ The diagnosis and treatment of suprascapular neuropathy have gained attention over the past decade, and this study represents the largest report of subjective patient-reported clinical outcomes to date. This retrospective case series involved 24 patients without rotator cuff pathology who underwent arthroscopic suprascapular nerve decompression for the primary treatment of neuropathic shoulder pain. Average follow-up was just under 2 years.

Approximately 75% of the patients had statistically significant pain relief, improvements in subjective shoulder values, and increased American Shoulder and Elbow Society self-assessment scores, and they reported they were pleased with their decision to have the surgery. Regression analysis determined that patients who had symptoms for less than 1 year trended toward improved pain relief and clinical outcomes. Male gender, spontaneous symptom onset, and non-worker's compensation cases also predicted better outcomes. No major complications were reported. The only other comparable case study by Lafosse et al[1] described the arthroscopic technique, reported excellent pain relief in 9 of 10 patients, and distinctly showed normalization of suprascapular motor latency by follow-up electrodiagnostic study.

The authors conclude that the short-term results of this procedure are promising in well-selected patients; however, the overall utility of this study is overtly limited by the simultaneously treated pathology (subacromial impingement, acromioclavicular osteoarthritis, proximal biceps tendinopathy, etc), which obfuscates the direct results of suprascapular nerve decompression and should therefore be interpreted with caution. Any study of this condition will likely be subject to this limitation, a known problem in studying the outcomes of treatment for rare conditions. Nonetheless, this study does at least bring added attention to a condition once considered a diagnosis of exclusion.

L. Brunton, MD

Reference

1. Lafosse L, Tomasi A, Corbett S, Baier G, Willems K, Gobezie R. Arthroscopic release of suprascapular nerve entrapment at the suprascapular notch: technique and preliminary results. *Arthroscopy.* 2007;23:34-42.

20 Shoulder: Rotator Cuff

Rotator Cuff Repair Healing Influenced by Platelet-Rich Plasma Construct Augmentation
Barber FA, Hrnack SA, Snyder SJ, et al (Plano Orthopedic Sports Medicine and Spine Ctr, Plano, TX; Southern California Orthopedic Inst, Van Nuys; et al)
Arthroscopy 27:1029-1035, 2011

Purpose.—To assess the effect of platelet-rich plasma fibrin matrix (PRPFM) construct augmentation on postoperative tendon healing as determined by magnetic resonance imaging (MRI) and clinical outcome of arthroscopic rotator cuff repair.

Methods.—A comparative series of patients undergoing arthroscopic rotator cuff repair was studied. Two matched groups of patients (20 each) were included: rotator cuff repairs without PRPFM augmentation (group 1) and rotator cuff repairs augmented with 2 sutured platelet-rich plasma (PRP) constructs (group 2). A single-row cuff repair to the normal footprint without tension or marrow vents was performed by a single surgeon. Postoperative rehabilitation was held constant. Postoperative MRI scans were used to evaluate rotator cuff healing. Outcome measures included American Shoulder and Elbow Surgeons, Rowe, Single Assessment Numeric Evaluation, Simple Shoulder Test, and Constant scores.

Results.—We followed up 40 patients (2 matched groups with 20 patients each) with a mean age of 57 years (range, 44 to 69 years) for a mean of 31 months (range, 24 to 44 months). Postoperative MRI studies showed persistent full-thickness tendon defects in 60% of controls (12 of 20) and 30% of PRPFM-augmented repairs (6 of 20) ($P = .03$). Of the control group tears measuring less than 3 cm in anteroposterior length, 50% (7 of 14) healed fully, whereas 86% of the PRPFM group tears measuring less than 3 cm in anteroposterior length (12 of 14) healed fully ($P < .05$). There was no significant difference between groups 1 and 2 in terms of American Shoulder and Elbow Surgeons (94.7 and 95.7, respectively; $P = .35$), Single Assessment Numeric Evaluation (93.7 and 94.5, respectively; $P = .37$), Simple Shoulder Test (11.4 and 11.3, respectively; $P = .41$), and Constant (84.7 and 88.1, respectively; $P = .19$) scores. The Rowe scores (84.8 and 94.9, respectively; $P = .03$) were statistically different.

Conclusions.—The addition of 2 PRPFM constructs sutured into a primary rotator cuff tendon repair resulted in lower retear rates identified

195

on MRI than repairs without the constructs. Other than the Rowe scores, there was no postoperative clinical difference by use of standard outcome measures.

Level of Evidence.—Level III, case-control study.

▶ The authors compared 2 matched series of prospectively followed patients to evaluate the effectiveness of adding a platelet-rich plasma construct to the suture site during arthroscopic repair of full thickness rotator cuff tears. Patients were selected after applying restrictive inclusion and exclusion criteria, including nonsmokers, nondiabetic patients under age 70 with no history of blood disease or any other past problem in their operated shoulders, and having a full thickness 10 mm to 50 mm in width rotator cuff tear independent of the existence of retraction and having up to stage 2 fatty infiltration based on MRI studies. Although patient characteristics are well described, information regarding selection of treatment type in each patient, such as how many patients could have been included on the study and were not, and the reasons for possible exclusions in this setting, is not available. Patient-matching protocol seemed to include tear size, defined as greater or less than 3 cm in width, but the mean tear size in each group is not provided, and statistical analysis did not include paired tests, so it is not clear if tear size was equivalent in each group. Clinical follow-up is also heterogeneous and not provided for each group, with a wide range including patients with almost double follow-up time compared to others.

The primary endpoint was the presence or absence of a retear as detected by an MRI performed at 4 months' follow-up, read by a radiologist blinded as to which study group the patient belonged. The secondary endpoint was the clinical assessment of the patient's outcome. Repairs consisted of a standard technique of single-row sutures using 1 or 2 bioabsorbable anchors, adding margin converging stitches when necessary. Study group patients received 2 platelet-rich plasma construct augments. Postoperative rehabilitation protocol was identical in all patients.

The authors found a lesser proportion of retears among patients treated with the platelet-rich constructs; however, no clinical differences were found on clinical outcomes. Despite this decreased retear rate, concerns regarding patient selection and methodology warrant cautious interpretation of the results of the present study.

A. M. Foruria, MD, PhD

Inter-Rater Agreement of the Goutallier, Patte, and Warner Classification Scores Using Preoperative Magnetic Resonance Imaging in Patients With Rotator Cuff Tears
Lippe J, Spang JT, Leger RR, et al (Univ of Connecticut Health Ctr, Farmington; Univ of North Carolina, Chapel Hill)
Arthroscopy 28:154-159, 2012

Purpose.—The purpose of this study was to determine the interobserver reliability of 3 commonly used classification systems in describing preoperative magnetic resonance imaging (MRI) studies of patients undergoing surgery for full-thickness rotator cuff tears.

Methods.—Thirty-one patients who underwent arthroscopic rotator cuff repair and had preoperative MRI studies available were selected over a 2-year period. Three board-certified shoulder surgeons independently reviewed these images. Each was instructed in the published method for determining the Patte score on the T2 coronal images, supraspinatus and infraspinatus atrophy on the T1 sagittal images as described by Warner et al., and the Goutallier score of fatty infiltration of the supraspinatus on the T1 coronal/sagittal images. Statistical analysis was then performed to determine the interobserver agreement using the κ statistic, with the level of significance set a priori at $P < .01$.

Results.—None of the classification systems studied yielded excellent or high interobserver reliability. The strongest agreement was found with the Patte classification assessing tendon retraction in the frontal plane ($\kappa = 0.58$). The Goutallier classification, which grades fatty infiltration of the supraspinatus, showed moderate interobserver agreement ($\kappa = 0.53$) when dichotomized into none to mild (grades 0, 1, and 2) and moderate to severe (grades 3 and 4). Muscle atrophy of both the supraspinatus and infraspinatus yielded the worst interobserver reliability, with only 28% agreement.

Conclusions.—The Goutallier, Patte, and Warner MRI classification systems for describing rotator cuff tears did not have high interobserver reliability among 3 experienced orthopaedic surgeons. Fatty infiltration of the supraspinatus and tendon retraction in the frontal planes showed only moderate reliability and moderate to high reliability, respectively. These findings have potential implications in the evaluation of the literature regarding the preoperative classification of rotator cuff tears and subsequent treatment algorithms.

Level of Evidence.—Level III, diagnostic agreement study with nonconsecutive patients.

▶ The authors evaluated the interobserver reliability of 3 rotator cuff tear classification systems. The systems evaluate the tear characteristics of tendon retraction (Patte), fatty infiltration of the muscle (Goutallier), and muscle atrophy (Warner). Previous studies have evaluated the observer agreement on the classification by Patte and Goutallier, but no studies have been performed for the Warner system. It is important to recognize that age, tear retraction, fatty infiltration, diabetes mellitus, and smoking have been confirmed factors that affect repair healing and clinical outcome. The authors found that none of these systems has better than moderate interobserver agreement. Interestingly, they grouped Goutallier's system into 2 groups, but this did not further improve the reliability past moderate. One of the strengths of this study was the inclusion of orthopedic shoulder specialists as evaluators. However, only selected images were shown to these evaluators in PowerPoint presentations. Furthermore, these images were chosen by an independent author whose qualifications were not specified. This individual may or may not have had the necessary experience to select the appropriate images. Lastly, the study did not include a power analysis and thus may have not included enough patients (n = 31). Despite these limitations, these findings raise concerns about the present classification systems and their applicability to guide treatment for rotator cuff tears.

C. J. Tuohy, MD

Comparable Biomechanical Results for a Modified Single-Row Rotator Cuff Reconstruction Using Triple-Loaded Suture Anchors Versus a Suture-Bridging Double-Row Repair

Lorbach O, Kieb M, Raber F, et al (Saarland Univ, Homburg/Saar, Germany; et al)
Arthroscopy 28:178-187, 2012

Purpose.—To compare the biomechanical properties and footprint coverage of a single-row (SR) repair using a modified suture configuration versus a double-row (DR) suture-bridge repair in small to medium and medium to large rotator cuff tears.

Methods.—We created 25- and 35-mm artificial defects in the rotator cuff of 24 human cadaveric shoulders. The reconstructions were performed as either an SR repair with triple-loaded suture anchors (2 to 3 anchors) and a modified suture configuration or a modified suture-bridge DR repair (4 to 6 anchors). Reconstructions were cyclically loaded from 10 to 60 N. The load was increased stepwise up to 100, 180, and 250 N. Cyclic displacement and load to failure were determined. Furthermore, footprint widths were quantified.

Results.—In the 25-mm rupture, ultimate load to failure was 533 ± 107 N for the SR repair and 681 ± 250 N for the DR technique ($P \geq .21$). In the 35-mm tear, ultimate load to failure was 792 ± 122 N for the SR reconstruction and 891 ± 174 N for the DR reconstruction ($P \geq .28$). There were no statistically significant differences for both tested rupture sizes. Cyclic displacement showed no significant differences between the tested configurations at 60 N ($P = .563$), 100 N ($P = .171$), 180 N ($P = .211$), and 250 N ($P = .478$) for the 25-mm tear. For the 35-mm tear, cyclic displacement showed significantly lower gap formation for the SR reconstruction at 180 N ($P = .037$) and 250 N ($P = .020$). No significant differences were found at 60 N ($P = .296$) and 100 N ($P = .077$). A significantly greater footprint width ($P = .028$) was seen for the DR repair (16.2 mm) compared with the SR repair (13.8 mm). However, both reconstructions were able to achieve complete footprint coverage compared with the initial footprint.

Conclusions.—The tested SR repair using a modified suture configuration was similar in load to failure and cyclic displacement to the DR suture-bridge technique independent of the tested initial sizes of the rupture. The tested DR repair consistently restored a larger footprint than the SR method. However, both constructs achieved complete footprint coverage.

Clinical Relevance.—SR repairs with modified suture configurations might combine the biomechanical advantages and increased footprint coverage that are described for DR repairs without increasing the overall costs of the reconstruction.

▶ The authors of this article present a novel repair technique for rotator cuff tears. In this biomechanical study, they have compared their repair design with an appropriate standard-of-care repair technique, the double-row suture bridge. Outcomes evaluated include repair strength, gap formation, and footprint restoration. Their article demonstrated comparable ultimate strength and footprint restoration in the repair designs. Interestingly and importantly, their technique decreased gap formation. The evaluation of gap formation is an essential and often overlooked outcome factor in rotator cuff repair techniques. The importance of gap formation has been illustrated in flexor tendon repairs. It should be recognized by the reader that the maximum gap formation that compromises healing is not known. Furthermore, neither technique reduced gap formation under 3 mm, which in flexor tendon repair has been shown to compromise healing. The other limitations include no clinical correlation to healing and the repairs being performed almost immediately after injury, which provides the most tension-free repair. Both of these issues raise questions of clinical applicability of the conclusions. The authors positively demonstrated comparable repair strength and footprint area with a less costly implant technique. Despite the limitations of the study, the authors have provided a reasonable and thought-provoking method for rotator cuff repair that should be considered with the escalating costs in health care.

C. J. Tuohy, MD

Comparison of a Novel Bone-Tendon Allograft With a Human Dermis— Derived Patch for Repair of Chronic Large Rotator Cuff Tears Using a Canine Model

Smith MJ, Cook JL, Kuroki K, et al (Univ of Missouri, Columbia)
Arthroscopy 28:169-177, 2012

Purpose.—This study tested a bone-tendon allograft versus human dermis patch for reconstructing chronic rotator cuff repair by use of a canine model.

Methods.—Mature research dogs (N = 15) were used. Radiopaque wire was placed in the infraspinatus tendon (IST) before its transection. Three weeks later, radiographs showed IST retraction. Each dog then underwent 1 IST treatment: debridement (D), direct repair of IST to bone with a suture bridge and human dermis patch augmentation (GJ), or bone-tendon allograft (BT) reconstruction. Outcome measures included lameness grading, radiographs, and ultrasonographic assessment. Dogs were killed 6 months after surgery and both shoulders assessed biomechanically and histologically.

Results.—BT dogs were significantly ($P = .01$) less lame than the other groups. BT dogs had superior bone-tendon, tendon, and tendon-muscle integrity compared with D and GJ dogs. Biomechanical testing showed that the D group had significantly $(P = .05)$ more elongation than the other groups whereas BT had stiffness and elongation characteristics that most closely matched normal controls. Radiographically, D and GJ dogs showed significantly more retraction than BT dogs $(P = .003$ and $P = .045$, respectively) Histologically, GJ dogs had lymphoplasmacytic infiltrates, tendon degeneration and hypocellularity, and poor tendon-bone integration. BT dogs showed complete incorporation of allograft bone into host bone, normal bone-tendon junctions, and well-integrated allograft tendon.

Conclusions.—The bone-tendon allograft technique re-establishes a functional IST bone-tendon-muscle unit and maintains integrity of repair in this model.

Clinical Relevance.—Clinical trials using this bone-tendon allograft technique are warranted.

▶ The authors present interesting and important findings with a novel repair technique in canines. They used an animal model in a delayed repair manner (3 weeks postinjury) that may correlate to the clinical situation, since human rotator cuff repairs are usually treated after a delay. Their technique using a bone tendon allograft showed better healing integrity but, more importantly, improved biomechanical properties (elongation and stiffness) than the dermal patch. Although not evaluated in the article, the improvement in relation to elongation and stiffness may result in a repair that provides better in vivo muscle function due to the better maintenance of sarcomere length. The limitations in the study include the inherent aspects of using a canine model compared to humans in both the manner of healing but also their manner of ambulation. This article provides further evidence that the present delayed repair techniques may not provide a method that restores in vivo characteristics of the rotator cuff.

C. J. Tuohy, MD

Does Platelet-Rich Plasma Accelerate Recovery After Rotator Cuff Repair? A Prospective Cohort Study

Jo CH, Kim JE, Yoon KS, et al (Seoul Natl Univ College of Medicine, Korea)
Am J Sports Med 39:2082-2090, 2011

Background.—Platelet-rich plasma (PRP) has been recently used to enhance and accelerate the healing of musculoskeletal injuries and diseases, but evidence is still lacking, especially on its effects after rotator cuff repair.

Hypothesis.—Platelet-rich plasma accelerates recovery after arthroscopic rotator cuff repair in pain relief, functional outcome, overall satisfaction, and enhanced structural integrity of repaired tendon.

Study Design.—Cohort study; Level of evidence, 2.

Methods.—Forty-two patients with full-thickness rotator cuff tears were included. Patients were informed about the use of PRP before surgery and decided themselves whether to have PRP placed at the time of surgery.

Nineteen patients underwent arthroscopic rotator cuff repair with PRP and 23 without. Platelet-rich plasma was prepared via plateletpheresis and applied in the form of a gel threaded to a suture and placed at the interface between tendon and bone. Outcomes were assessed preoperatively and at 3, 6, 12, and finally at a minimum of 16 months after surgery (at an average of 19.7 ± 1.9 months) with respect to pain, range of motion, strength, and overall satisfaction, and with respect to functional scores as determined using the following scoring systems: the American Shoulder and Elbow Surgeon (ASES) system, the Constant system, the University of California at Los Angeles (UCLA) system, the Disabilities of the Arm, Shoulder and Hand (DASH) system, the Simple Shoulder Test (SST) system, and the Shoulder Pain and Disability Index (SPADI) system. At a minimum of 9 months after surgery, repaired tendon structural integrities were assessed by magnetic resonance imaging.

Results.—Platelet-rich plasma gel application to arthroscopic rotator cuff repairs did not accelerate recovery with respect to pain, range of motion, strength, functional scores, or overall satisfaction as compared with conventional repair at any time point. Whereas magnetic resonance imaging demonstrated a retear rate of 26.7% in the PRP group and 41.2% in the conventional group, there was no statistical significance between the groups ($P = .388$).

Conclusion.—The results suggest that PRP application during arthroscopic rotator cuff repair did not clearly demonstrate accelerated recovery clinically or anatomically except for an improvement in internal rotation. Nevertheless, as the study may have been underpowered to detect clinically important differences in the structural integrity, additional investigations, including the optimization of PRP preparation and a larger randomized study powered for healing rate, are necessary to further determine the effect of PRP.

▶ To date, the enthusiasm for using platelet-rich plasma (PRP) to treat everything from Achilles tendonitis to lateral epicondylitis has outstripped any research we have to identify appropriate indications for this rather expensive treatment. This article examines if the addition of PRP to a standard arthroscopic rotator cuff repair provides any benefit.

In this study design, the patients were not blinded to the use of PRP in their treatment. In fact, patients were allowed to choose whether to have PRP incorporated in their surgical cuff repair. The two groups were very similar with regard to baseline demographics. Although those patients who selected PRP tended to have a longer duration of symptoms (40.9 vs 25.9 months) and larger tears (35 × 21 vs 26 × 15 mm), neither of these differences reached statistical significance.

Interestingly, there was no significant difference in outcomes between the two groups with regard to reported pain or function using multiple shoulder outcome tools, such as the American Shoulder and Elbow Surgeon system, the Constant system, the University of California at Los Angeles system, the Disabilities of the Arm, Shoulder and Hand system, the Simple Shoulder Test system, or the Shoulder Pain and Disability Index. Even with patients aware of the use of PRP in the shoulder, there did not appear to be a significant placebo effect. There was a higher retear rate (as determined by MRI) in the non-PRP group (41% vs 27%), but this did not reach statistical significance.

Although the patients were not blinded or randomized in this study, this report strongly suggests that PRP does not have a significant effect on the outcome of rotator cuff repair.

C. Ward, MD

National Trends in Rotator Cuff Repair
Colvin AC, Egorova N, Harrison AK, et al (Mount Sinai School of Medicine, NY)
J Bone Joint Surg Am 94:227-233, 2012

Background.—Recent publications suggest that arthroscopic and open rotator cuff repairs have had comparable clinical results, although each technique has distinct advantages and disadvantages. National hospital and ambulatory surgery databases were reviewed to identify practice patterns for rotator cuff repair.

Methods.—The rates of medical visits for rotator cuff pathology, and the rates of open and arthroscopic rotator cuff repair, were examined for the years 1996 and 2006 in the United States. The national incidence of rotator cuff repairs and related data were obtained from inpatient (National Hospital Discharge Survey, NHDS) and ambulatory surgery (National Survey of Ambulatory Surgery, NSAS) databases. These databases were queried with use of International Classification of Diseases, Ninth Revision (ICD-9) procedure codes for arthroscopic (ICD-9 codes 83.63 and 80.21) and open (code 83.63 without code 80.21) rotator cuff repair. We also examined where the surgery was performed (inpatient versus ambulatory surgery center) and characteristics of the patients, including age, sex, and comorbidities.

Results.—The unadjusted volume of all rotator cuff repairs increased 141% in the decade from 1996 to 2006. The unadjusted number of arthroscopic procedures increased by 600% while open repairs increased by only 34% during this time interval. There was a significant shift from inpatient to outpatient surgery (p < 0.001).

Conclusions.—The increase in national rates of rotator cuff repair over the last decade has been dramatic, particularly for arthroscopic assisted repair.

▶ The authors present a thorough review of the frequency of 2 common techniques used in the management of rotator cuff tears: arthroscopic and open surgical repair. They compared the relative frequency of these procedures at 2 historical time points: 1996 and 2006. Publicly available databases were queried and the results were presented. The authors found a large increase in the number of visits for rotator cuff tear and an increased frequency of surgeries performed per nonoperative visit (26 nonoperative visits per 1 surgery in 1996 and 16 nonoperative visits per 1 surgery in 2006). A large increase in the rate of open (43%) and arthroscopic (600%) rotator cuff repair compared to open rotator cuff repairs was also noted over the same interval. The authors also demonstrated increased operative times for arthroscopic rotator cuff repairs and a movement toward regional anesthesia and outpatient surgery. This article nicely highlights the growing trends in the surgical management of arthroscopic rotator cuff repairs and defines some of the societal implications of those trends.

J. Macalena, MD

Predictors of Pain and Function in Patients With Symptomatic, Atraumatic Full-Thickness Rotator Cuff Tears: A Time-Zero Analysis of a Prospective Patient Cohort Enrolled in a Structured Physical Therapy Program

Harris JD, The MOON (Multicenter Orthopedic Outcomes Network) Shoulder Group (Ohio State Univ Med Ctr, Columbus)
Am J Sports Med 40:359-366, 2012

Background.—Although the prevalence of full-thickness rotator cuff tears increases with age, many patients are asymptomatic and may not require surgical repair. The factors associated with pain and loss of function in patients with rotator cuff tears are not well defined.

Purpose.—To determine which factors correlate with pain and loss of function in patients with symptomatic, atraumatic full-thickness rotator cuff tears who are enrolled in a structured physical therapy program.

Study Design.—Cross-sectional study; Level of evidence, 3.

Methods.—A multicenter group enrolled patients with symptomatic, atraumatic rotator cuff tears in a prospective, nonrandomized cohort study evaluating the effects of a structured physical therapy program. Time-zero patient data were reviewed to test which factors correlated with Western Ontario Rotator Cuff (WORC) index and American Shoulder and Elbow Surgeons (ASES) scores.

Results.—A total of 389 patients were enrolled. Mean ASES score was 53.9; mean WORC score was 46.9. The following variables were associated with higher WORC and ASES scores: female sex ($P = .001$), education level (higher education, higher score; $P < .001$), active abduction (degrees; $P = .021$), and strength in forward elevation ($P = .002$) and abduction ($P = .007$). The following variables were associated with lower WORC and ASES scores: male sex ($P = .001$), atrophy of the supraspinatus ($P = .04$) and infraspinatus ($P = .003$), and presence of scapulothoracic dyskinesia ($P < .001$). Tear size was not a significant predictor (WORC) unless comparing isolated supraspinatus tears to supraspinatus, infraspinatus, and subscapularis tears ($P = .004$). Age, tear retraction, duration of symptoms, and humeral head migration were not statistically significant.

Conclusion.—Nonsurgically modifiable factors, such as scapulothoracic dyskinesia, active abduction, and strength in forward elevation and abduction, were identified that could be addressed nonoperatively with therapy. Therefore, physical therapy for patients with symptomatic rotator cuff tears should target these modifiable factors associated with pain and loss of function.

▶ In this well-performed review of a cohort of patients with full thickness rotator cuff tears, the authors demonstrate the modifiable factors that are associated with a worse outcome as judged by American Shoulder and Elbow and Western Ontario Rotator Cuff scores. The factors that predicted a worse outcome include the presence of scapulothoracic dyskinesis, loss of range of motion in active abduction and forward elevation, and loss of strength in abduction and forward elevation. These factors are all potentially modifiable factors that suggest a target for nonsurgical management for patients with symptomatic pathology. The factors found to *not* affect outcome include patient age, duration of symptoms, race, tear size, degree of tear retraction, presence of superior humeral head migration, smoking status, supraspinatus strength, and strength in external rotation. It should be noted that the limitations of this study include a "time-zero" selection point without follow-up as well as a low rate of enrollment of available patients (19%), which lead to potential selection bias.

J. Macalena, MD

Repair Integrity and Functional Outcome After Arthroscopic Rotator Cuff Repair: Double-Row Versus Suture-Bridge Technique

Kim KC, Shin HD, Lee WY, et al (Chungnam Natl Univ, Daejeon, Korea)
Am J Sports Med 40:294-299, 2012

Background.—Only a few studies have examined repair integrity and functional outcome after arthroscopic suture-bridge rotator cuff repair procedure. In addition, no reported study has compared outcomes between the suture-bridge and double-row techniques.

Purpose.—This study compared the functional outcome and repair integrity of arthroscopic double-row and conventional suture-bridge repair in full-thickness rotator cuff tears.

Study Design.—Cohort study; Level of evidence, 2.

Methods.—Fifty-two consecutive full-thickness rotator cuff tears with 1 to 4 cm of anterior to posterior dimension that underwent arthroscopic rotator cuff repair were included. A double-row technique was used in the first 26 consecutive shoulders, and a conventional suture-bridge technique was used in the next 26 consecutive shoulders. Fifty shoulders (92.5%) underwent magnetic resonance imaging or ultrasonography postoperatively. Clinical outcomes were evaluated a minimum 2 years (mean, 37.2 months; range, 24-54) postoperatively using the University of California at Los Angeles (UCLA), American Shoulder and Elbow Surgeons (ASES), and Constant scores. The postoperative cuff integrity was evaluated a mean of 33.0 (range, 10-54) months postoperatively.

Results.—At the final follow-up, the average UCLA, ASES, and Constant scores improved significantly, to 32.3, 90.5, and 80.7, respectively, in the double-row group and to 30.6, 88.5, and 74.0, respectively, in the suture-bridge group. The UCLA, ASES, and Constant scores improved in both groups postoperatively (all $P < .001$); however, there was no significant difference between the 2 groups at final follow-up ($P = .185$, .585, and .053, respectively). The retear rate was 24% in the shoulders that underwent double-row repair and 20% in the shoulders that underwent suture-bridge repair; this difference was not statistically significant ($P = .733$).

Conclusion.—The arthroscopic conventional suture-bridge technique resulted in comparable patient satisfaction, functional outcome, and rates of retear compared with the arthroscopic double-row technique in full-thickness rotator cuff tears (Figs 1 and 2).

▶ This prospective study of 52 patients who underwent arthroscopic rotator cuff repair shows no difference between 2 techniques of rotator cuff fixation. The 2 techniques evaluated were a double row construct and a suture bridge.

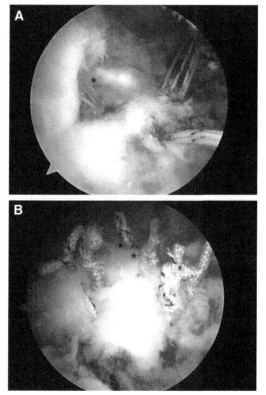

FIGURE 1.—(A) Arthroscopic view shows a rotator cuff tear involving the supraspinatus. One suture anchor was placed in the medial row and 2 suture anchors were placed in the lateral row. The sutures were passed through the reduced tendon. (B) The arthroscopic view from the lateral portal shows the completed repair of a rotator cuff tear (* indicates medial row). (Reprinted from Kim KC, Shin HD, Lee WY, et al. Repair integrity and functional outcome after arthroscopic rotator cuff repair: double-row versus suture-bridge technique. *Am J Sports Med.* 2012;40:294-299, with permission The Author.)

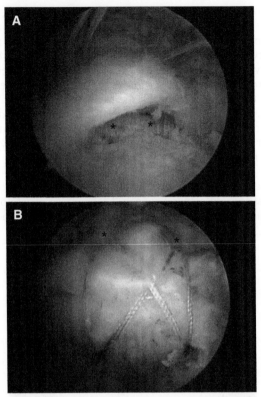

FIGURE 2.—(A) Arthroscopic view shows a rotator cuff tear involving the supraspinatus. Two suture anchors were placed in the medial row. Sutures were passed through the reduced tendon in a mattress configuration. (B) The arthroscopic view from the lateral portal shows the completed repair of a rotator cuff tear with 2 PushLock anchors (* indicates medial row). (Reprinted from Kim KC, Shin HD, Lee WY, et al. Repair integrity and functional outcome after arthroscopic rotator cuff repair: double-row versus suture-bridge technique. *Am J Sports Med.* 2012;40:294-299, with permission The Author.)

Advocates of a suture bridge technique highlight certain advantages, including compression of the rotator cuff by the medial row, a reduction in the surgical steps and reduced knot impingement. Figs 1 and 2 highlight the arthroscopic appearance of the double row technique (Fig 1) versus suture bridge (Fig 2). There were no differences in outcome measures at final follow-up or in the rate of retear between the 2 groups. The authors did not provide data on the length of surgery, complications of surgery (besides retear) or on the relative cost between these 2 groups. Those variables will also be important for future studies to address. As we await more data on these evolving techniques, it appears that both a suture bridge technique and a double row technique provide similar outcomes.

J. Macalena, MD

A Prospective, Randomized Evaluation of Acellular Human Dermal Matrix Augmentation for Arthroscopic Rotator Cuff Repair

Barber FA, Burns JP, Deutsch A, et al (Plano Orthopedic Sports Medicine and Spine Ctr, Plano, TX; Southern California Orthopedic Inst, Van Nuys; Kelsey-Seybold Clinic of Orthopaedics, Houston, TX; et al)
Arthroscopy 28:8-15, 2012

Purpose.—To prospectively evaluate the safety and effectiveness of arthroscopic acellular human dermal matrix augmentation of large rotator cuff tear repairs.

Methods.—A prospective, institutional review board—approved, multi-center series of patients undergoing arthroscopic repair of 2-tendon rotator cuff tears measuring greater than 3 cm were randomized by sealed envelopes opened at the time of surgery to arthroscopic single-row rotator cuff repair with GraftJacket acellular human dermal matrix (Wright Medical Technology, Arlington, TN) augmentation (group 1) or without augmentation (group 2). Preoperative and postoperative functional outcome assessments were obtained by use of the American Shoulder and Elbow Surgeons (ASES), Constant, and University of California, Los Angeles scales. Gadolinium-enhanced magnetic resonance imaging (MRI) evaluation of these repairs was obtained at a mean of 14.5 months (range, 12 to 24 months). Adverse events were recorded.

Results.—There were 22 patients in group 1 and 20 in group 2 with a mean age of 56 years. The mean follow-up was 24 months (range, 12 to 38 months). The ASES score improved from 48.5 to 98.9 in group 1 and from 46.0 to 94.8 in group 2. The scores in group 1 were statistically better than those in group 2 ($P = .035$). The Constant score improved from 41.0 to 91.9 in group 1 and from 45.8 to 85.3 in group 2. The scores in group 1 were statistically better than those in group 2 ($P = .008$). The University of California, Los Angeles score improved from 13.3 to 28.2 in group 1 and from 15.9 to 28.3 in group 2 ($P = .43$). Gadolinium-enhanced MRI scans showed intact cuffs in 85% of repairs in group 1 and 40% in group 2 ($P < .01$). No adverse events were attributed to the presence of the matrix grafts.

Conclusions.—Acellular human dermal matrix augmentation of large (>3 cm) cuff tears involving 2 tendons showed better ASES and Constant scores and more frequent intact cuffs as determined by gadolinium-enhanced MRI. Intact repairs were found in 85% of the augmented group and 40% of the nonaugmented group ($P < .01$). No adverse events related to the acellular human dermal matrix were observed.

Level of Evidence.—Level II, lesser-quality randomized controlled trial.

▶ I find that there are 2 interesting observations that arise from this study: (1) as has been demonstrated in past studies, complete repair or partial repair without augmentation has impressive short-term clinical results as seen by the substantial improvement of American Shoulder and Elbow Surgeons scores and (2) postoperative MRI at 1 year demonstrates that there is a decreased incidence of recurrent defect.

It is important to note that the absence of recurrent defect does not necessarily mean that the initial defect has healed or the material at the location of the old defect is functional; however, the findings are encouraging. Certainly long-term follow-up will be helpful in understanding whether the clinical results are durable in the no augmentation group. Recent studies demonstrate reasonable clinical outcomes for partial repair even at midterm follow-up; however, if there is a significant clinical difference between the groups without additional complications at 7- to 10-year follow-up, this would provide a strong rationale for augmentation in large rotator cuff tears.

N. Chen, MD

A Radiographic Classification of Massive Rotator Cuff Tear Arthritis
Hamada K, Yamanaka K, Uchiyama Y, et al (Hakone Natl Hospl, Kanagawa, Japan; Yamanaka Orthopaedic Clinic, Shikichi, Shizuoka, Japan; Tokai Univ School of Medicine, Isehara, Kanagawa, Japan; et al)
Clin Orthop Relat Res 469:2452-2460, 2011

Background.—In 1990, Hamada et al. radiographically classified massive rotator cuff tears into five grades. Walch et al. subsequently subdivided Grade 4 to reflect the presence/ absence of subacromial arthritis and emphasize glenohumeral arthritis as a characteristic of Grade 4.

Questions/Purposes.—We therefore determined (1) whether patient characteristics and MRI findings differed between the grades at initial examination and final followup; (2) which factors affected progression to a higher grade; (3) whether the retear rate of repaired tendons differed among the grades; and (4) whether the radiographic grades at final followup differed from those at initial examination among patients treated operatively.

Patients and Methods.—We retrospectively reviewed 75 patients with massive rotator cuff tears. Thirty-four patients were treated nonoperatively and 41 operatively.

Results.—Patients with Grade 3, 4, or 5 tears had a higher incidence of fatty muscle degeneration of the subscapularis muscle than patients with Grade 1 or 2 tears. In 26 patients with Grade 1 or 2 tears at initial examination, duration of followup was longer in patients who remained at Grade 1 or 2 than in those who progressed to Grade 3, 4, or 5 at final followup. The retear rate of repaired supraspinatus tendon was more frequent in Grade 2 than Grade 1 tears. In operated cases, radiographic grades at final followup did not develop to Grades 3 to 5.

Conclusions.—We believe cuff repair should be performed before acromiohumeral interval narrowing. Our observations are consistent with the temporal concepts of massive cuff tear pathomechanics proposed by Burkhart and Hansen et al.

Level of Evidence.—Level III, Therapeutic study. See Guidelines for Authors for a complete description of levels of evidence.

▶ This is an interesting revisit of the Hamada classification for rotator cuff arthropathy. Although retrospective in nature, these data suggest that the Hamada classification reflects some temporal characteristics in that the higher the grade, the longer the patient had been afflicted with the arthropathy. The authors admit that there is some substantial attrition in their series, but the observations are still noteworthy. Patients with a higher radiographic grade did not regress to a lower grading, patients who were Grades 3 to 5 had a higher mean age, and some patients with Grade 1 or 2 changes progressed to higher grades.

Thirty-four of 75 patients were treated nonoperatively. Forty-one were treated with rotator cuff repair, partial repair, or tendon transfer. Of those patients treated operatively, the authors found there was no progression above Grade 2 changes. These retrospective data suggest that rotator cuff repair in the setting of early cuff arthropathy may retard disease progression, but these data are not conclusive.

N. Chen, MD

Anabolic Steroids Reduce Muscle Damage Caused by Rotator Cuff Tendon Release in an Experimental Study in Rabbits
Gerber C, Meyer DC, Nuss KM, et al (Univ of Zürich, Switzerland)
J Bone Joint Surg Am 93:2189-2195, 2011

Background.—Muscles of the rotator cuff undergo retraction, atrophy, and fatty infiltration after a chronic tear, and a rabbit model has been used to investigate these changes. The purpose of this study was to test the hypothesis that the administration of anabolic steroids can diminish these muscular changes following experimental supraspinatus tendon release in the rabbit.

Methods.—The supraspinatus tendon was released in twenty New Zealand White rabbits. Musculotendinous retraction was monitored over a period of six weeks. The seven animals in group I had no additional intervention, the six animals in group II had local and systemic administration of nandrolone decanoate, and the seven animals in group III had systemic administration of nandrolone decanoate during the six weeks. Two animals (group III) developed a postoperative infection and were excluded from the analysis. At the time that the animals were killed, in vivo muscle performance as well as imaging and histological muscle changes were investigated.

Results.—The mean supraspinatus retraction was higher in group I (1.8 cm; 95% confidence interval: 1.64, 2.02 cm) than in group II (1.5 cm; 95% confidence interval: 1.29, 1.81 cm) or III (1.2 cm; 95% confidence interval: 0.86, 1.54 cm). Histologically, no fatty infiltration was measured in either treated group II (mean, 2.2%; range, 0% to 8%) or III (mean, 1%; range, 0% to 3.4%), but it was measured in the untreated group I (mean, 5.9%; range, 0% to 14.1%; p = 0.031). The radiographic cross-sectional area indicating atrophy and the work of the respective muscle during one standardized contraction with supramaximal stimulation decreased in all groups, but the work of the muscle was ultimately highest in group III.

Conclusions.—To our knowledge, this is the first documentation of partial prevention of important muscle alterations after retraction of the supraspinatus musculotendinous unit caused by tendon disruption. Nandrolone decanoate administration in the phase after tendon release prevented fatty infiltration of the supraspinatus muscle and reduced functional muscle impairment caused by myotendinous retraction in this rabbit rotator cuff model, but two of seven rabbits that received the drug developed infections.

▶ This elegant animal study is the first of its kind to evaluate the efficacy of anabolic steroids on muscular changes associated with chronic retraction following sectioning of New Zealand White rabbits. The authors devised a clever study that monitored 3 groups of rabbits following sectioning of the supraspinatus tendon. As noted in the abstract, 1 group received no additional intervention, while the remaining 2 groups received either local and systemic administration of nandrolone decanoate or system nandrolone decanoate alone. Once the animals were sacrificed, outcome measures included in vivo muscle performance as well as imaging and histologic muscle change investigation. Interestingly, in the treated groups (groups 2 and 3), there was no histologic evidence of fatty infiltration. There was also greater retraction of the supraspinatus muscle in the untreated group. This study represents a potential breakthrough in the possible pharmacologic treatment of rotator cuff injury. However, as the authors correctly indicate, this model may be representative but not indicative of similar results in the human model. Furthermore, 2 of the rabbits in the treatment group experienced postoperative infection, a finding that may certainly be extrapolated in the human model. At the very least, this creative study should serve as the impetus for investigation of other pharmacologic agents, including growth hormones, β_2 agonists, and others that may influence the development, growth, and reparative capabilities of muscle. Finally, it should be noted that the authors examined the effect of a steroid on muscle tissue and not tendon substance. Nonetheless, this type of study will serve as a template for translational medicine investigations in the future.

S. M. Jacoby, MD

21 Shoulder: Trauma

Hemiarthroplasty versus nonoperative treatment of displaced 4-part proximal humeral fractures in elderly patients: a randomized controlled trial
Olerud P, Ahrengart L, Ponzer S, et al (Stockholm Söder Hosp, Sweden)
J Shoulder Elbow Surg 20:1025-1033, 2011

Background.—The aim of the study was to report the 2-year outcome after a displaced 4-part fracture of the proximal humerus in elderly patients randomized to treatment with a hemiarthroplasty (HA) or nonoperative treatment.

Patients and Methods.—We included 55 patients, mean age 77 (range, 58-92) years, 86% being women. Follow-up examinations were done at 4, 12, and 24 months. The main outcome measures were health-related quality of life (HRQoL) according to the EQ-5D and the DASH and Constant scores.

Results.—At the final 2-year follow-up the HRQoL was significantly better in the HA group compared to the nonoperative group, EQ-5D$_{index}$ score 0.81 compared to 0.65 ($P=.02$). The results for DASH and pain assessment were both in favor of the HA group, DASH score 30 versus 37 ($P=.25$) and pain according to VAS 15 versus 25 ($P=.17$). There were no significant differences regarding the Constant score or range of motion (ROM). Both groups achieved a mean flexion of approximately 90-95° and a mean abduction of 85-90°. The need for additional surgery was low: 3 patients in the HA group and 1 patient in the nonoperative group.

Conclusion.—The results of the study demonstrated a significant advantage in quality of life in favor of HA, as compared to nonoperative treatment in elderly patients with a displaced 4-part fracture of the proximal humerus. The main advantage of HA appeared to be less pain while there were no differences in ROM.

▶ The authors present the best prospective, randomized trial of operative versus nonoperative management of 4-part proximal humerus fractures in elderly patients to date. At 2-year follow-up, there was a significantly better health-related quality of life (as measured by EQ-5D index scores) in patients treated with hemiarthroplasty. Although there were trends toward less pain and lower Disabilities of the Arm, Shoulder and Hand scores in the hemiarthroplasty group, constant scores and final range of motion were not different between groups. The main advantages of this study were the use of a modern prosthesis in the surgical group and the use of validated outcome measurement tools for both groups. Furthermore, the surgeries were performed by 2 surgeons, neither of whom performed the final follow-up evaluation.

Persistent pain and dysfunction remain pervasive in the treatment of these challenging fractures. Despite the overall trend toward better outcome in the hemiarthroplasty group (especially after 4 months), the authors admitted that their results are still largely unsatisfactory at 2-year follow-up. On the other hand, the patients treated nonoperatively actually deteriorated over time. The authors conclude that pain relief after hemiarthroplasty is more predictable and largely responsible for the differences elicited in their study. I would agree that the gain in pain relief and quality of life after hemiarthroplasty by an experienced shoulder surgeon is probably justified in patients who are fit for surgery, but conservative management is adequate for those with multiple comorbidities and low functional demands.

Although there has been great interest in the use of reverse shoulder prostheses as an alternative to hemiarthroplasty for proximal humerus fractures in this particular patient population, the authors discuss the limited case series data available (which show largely similar short-term outcomes compared with other forms of treatment) and the current lack of prospective, randomized data comparing the reverse prosthesis with either nonoperative treatment or surgical treatment with hemiarthroplasty.

J. Isaacs, MD

Nonoperative Treatment of Proximal Humerus Fractures: A Systematic Review

Iyengar JJ, Devcic Z, Sproul RC, et al (Univ of California, San Francisco)
J Orthop Trauma 25:612-617, 2011

Background.—Proximal humerus fractures are common in the setting of osteopenia and osteoporosis and can often be treated nonoperatively. There are few studies that evaluate the long-term outcomes of nonoperative treatment of these fractures. We performed a systematic review of the literature to examine the results of nonoperative treatment of proximal humerus fractures.

Methods.—The PubMed search engine and EMBASE database were used. Inclusion criteria were: 1) proximal humerus fractures resulting from trauma; 2) age older than 18 years; 3) more than 15 patients in the study; 4) greater than 1 year follow-up; 5) at least one relevant functional outcome score; and 6) a quality outcome score of at least a 5 of 10 according to previously published scoring system.

Results.—We identified 12 studies that included 650 patients with a mean age of 65.0 years (range, 51–75 years) and a mean follow-up of 45.7 months (range, 12–120 months). There were 317 one-part fractures, 165 two-part fractures, 137 three-part fractures, and 31 four-part fractures. The rate of radiographic union was 98% and the complication rate 13%. The average range of motion reported in five studies was 139° forward flexion, 48° external rotation, and 52° internal rotation.

The average Constant score reported in six studies was 74 (range, 55—81). Varus malunion was the most common complication reported, whereas avascular necrosis was uncommon (13 cases).

Conclusions.—We conclude that our systematic review of the literature on the nonoperative treatment of proximal humerus fractures demonstrates high rates of radiographic healing, good functional outcomes, and a modest complication rate.

▶ The authors perform a systematic review of nonoperative management of proximal humerus fractures. They compiled data from 12 studies that met their inclusion criteria with 650 patients. Union rates were extremely high at 98%, even when only 3-part and 4-part fractures were included. Varus malunion was the most common complication (23%). It was surprising that the avascular necrosis rate in this nonoperative group was high (14%). The overall Constant score was very good for these more complex fractures (67). The authors suggest, based on this review, that nonoperative management may be an acceptable treatment option even in 3-part and 4-part fractures with complication rates similar to those of internal fixation. Clearly this study is not designed to answer the question of whether open reduction and internal fixation is superior or inferior to nonoperative management, so the conclusion in the discussion should be interpreted with caution. Nevertheless, it appears from this review that nonoperative management of proximal humerus fractures, even for 3-part and 4-part fractures, is a viable option with acceptable results for pain and function, but it has a high rate of malunion.

T. Wright, MD

22 Soft Tissue

Comparison of glenohumeral and subacromial steroid injection in primary frozen shoulder: a prospective, randomized short-term comparison study
Oh JH, Oh CH, Choi J-A, et al (Seoul Natl Univ Bundang Hosp, Seongnam-si, Gyeonggi-do, South Korea; S-Seoul Hosp, Suwon-si, Gyeonggi-do, South Korea; et al)
J Shoulder Elbow Surg 20:1034-1040, 2011

Background.—Glenohumeral (GH) joint steroid injection is one of the most well-known treatments for frozen shoulder. However, the low accuracy of GH joint injections and the improvement of symptoms after subacromial (SA) steroid injections led us to design a study that compares the efficacy of a steroid injection for primary frozen shoulder according to the injection site.

Materials and Methods.—Patients with primary frozen shoulder were randomly divided into 2 groups according to the location of the injection: a GH group of 37 for the glenohumeral joint and an SA group of 34 for the subacromial space. Injections were completed using ultrasonographic guidance. Evaluations using a visual analog scale (VAS) for pain, the Constant score, and passive range of motion (ROM) were completed at 3, 6, and 12 weeks after the injection.

Results.—The GH group showed lower pain VAS at 3 weeks, but no statistical difference was found between the 2 groups at 6 and 12 weeks. Improvement in pain was evident at every follow-up visit compared with the preinjection evaluation. There was no significant difference between the 2 groups with respect to the Constant score or ROM at serial follow-up.

Conclusions.—The GH steroid injection was not superior to a SA injection for patients with primary frozen shoulder even though injection at the GH joint led to earlier pain relief compared with the SA injection. SA steroid injection along with a GH injection is an alternative modality, and the treatment should be individualized and tailored appropriately.

▶ Although the beneficial effect of corticosteroid injection to reduce pain in patients with adhesive capsulitis has been well described, it is unclear which tissue the steroid is working on to achieve this effect. Given the low accuracy of unguided glenohumeral injections, the higher accuracy and familiarity of subacromial injections, and the observation of improvement in patients with adhesive capsulitis treated with subacromial injection, the conclusions of this article have an impact on our day-to-day practice.

The authors randomized patients to receive either glenohumeral or subacromial injection of 40 mg triamcinolone. All injections were done under ultrasound guidance, and all patients were prescribed antiinflammatories and instructed in an at-home exercise program. No difference was seen between the groups in regard to pain, range of motion, or Constant score at 6-week and 12-week follow-ups. The main pitfall of the study was the lack of a control group receiving a placebo injection, so it is unknown whether the benefits seen would have occurred regardless of the cortisone injection as a result of time, home exercises, and medication.

Despite the article's limitations, the authors provide level 1 evidence that there is no added benefit of intraarticular glenohumeral corticosteroid injection, compared to subacromial injection, in patients with adhesive capsulitis. Given the difficulty in confirming intraarticular glenohumeral placement of injections without radiographic guidance, this article makes a compelling case to inject subacromially when treating patients with adhesive capsulitis with injectable steroids.

F. T. D. Kaplan, MD

Assessing the Impact of Antibiotic Prophylaxis in Outpatient Elective Hand Surgery: A Single-Center, Retrospective Review of 8,850 Cases

Bykowski MR, Sivak WN, Cray J, et al (Dept of Plastic and Reconstructive Surgery, Pittsburgh, PA; Hand and Upper Extremity Ctr, Wexford, PA; Johns Hopkins Univ School of Medicine, Baltimore, MD)
J Hand Surg 36A:1741-1747, 2011

Purpose.—Prophylactic antibiotics have been shown to prevent surgical site infection (SSI) after some gastrointestinal, orthopedic, and plastic surgical procedures, but their efficacy in clean, elective hand surgery is unclear. Our aims were to assess the efficacy of preoperative antibiotics in preventing SSI after clean, elective hand surgery, and to identify potential risk factors for SSI.

Methods.—We queried the database from an outpatient surgical center by Current Procedural Terminology code to identify patients who underwent elective hand surgery. For each medical record, we collected patient demographics and characteristics along with preoperative, intraoperative, and postoperative management details. The primary outcome of this study was SSI, and secondary outcomes were wound dehiscence and suture granuloma.

Results.—From October 2000 through October 2008, 8,850 patient records met our inclusion criteria. The overall SSI rate was 0.35%, with an average patient follow-up duration of 79 days. The SSI rates did not significantly differ between patients receiving antibiotics (0.54%; 2,755 patients) and those who did not (0.26%; 6,095 patients). Surgical site infection was associated with smoking status, diabetes mellitus, and longer procedure length irrespective of antibiotic use. Subgroup analysis revealed that prophylactic antibiotics did not prevent SSI in male patients, smokers, or diabetics, or for procedure length less than 30 minutes, 30 to 60 minutes, and greater than 60 minutes.

Conclusions.—Prophylactic antibiotic administration does not reduce the incidence of SSI after clean, elective hand surgery in an outpatient population. Moreover, subgroup analysis revealed that prophylactic antibiotics did not reduce the frequency of SSI among patients who were found to be at higher risk in this study. We identified 3 factors associated with the development of SSI in our study: diabetes mellitus status, procedure length, and smoking status. Given the potential harmful complications associated with antibiotic use and the lack of evidence that prophylactic antibiotics prevent SSIs, we conclude that antibiotics should not be routinely administered to patients who undergo clean, elective hand surgery.

Type of Study/Level of Evidence.—Therapeutic III.

▶ This is a retrospective review of almost 9000 outpatient elective hand surgeries to assess the impact of prophylactic antibiotics on preventing surgical site infection (SSI). Just more than 30% of this population received antibiotics with a rate of SSI of 0.54%, while the majority of patients received no prophylaxis and had an SSI rate of 0.26%. The authors did find SSI rates correlated with smoking, the presence of diabetes mellitus, and length of procedure.

The article has the obvious shortcoming that it is not a prospective or randomized trial. Clearly, a prospective, randomized trial would address the science of this issue more definitively. This article should have a sizable impact on hand surgery practice but I suspect will have a lesser impact in practice than it might. First, we are commonly more easily influenced by anecdotal evidence than by scientific reports. While there are potentially serious side effects of prophylactic antibiotics, the practicing surgeon rarely sees these; I cannot remember the last serious "M and M" related to prophylactic antibiotics in our group, which performs a similar number of orthopedic surgeries on an annual basis. And SSIs are seen by every surgeon. Second, prophylactic antibiotics have become a part of the expected routine by surgeons, operating room staff, and patients as well as a part of preoperative protocols in hospitals and surgery centers. In one site where I operate, if a surgeon chooses to not give a patient preoperative antibiotics, an order to not give the antibiotics must be written. Because clean elective hand surgery is likely only a small percentage of the surgical cases done at most operating rooms, modifying these practices is unlikely to be easy. Lastly, there is a perception of a medicolegal issue. I suspect many of us are uncomfortable with having to respond to an attorney (or a patient or family member) asking the question, "Might a dose of preoperative antibiotics have prevented Mrs. Smith's devastating infection?," irrespective of the strong evidence in this article.

P. Blazar, MD

23 Arthritis

Incidence and Risk Factors for the Development of Radiographic Arthrosis After Traumatic Elbow Injuries
Guitton TG, Zurakowski D, van Dijk NC, et al (Massachusetts General Hosp, Boston; Children's Hosp Boston, MA; and Academic Med Ctr Amsterdam, The Netherlands)
J Hand Surg 35A:1976-1980, 2010

Purpose.—Radiographic arthrosis is a common sequela of elbow trauma. Few studies have addressed risk factors for radiographic arthrosis after elbow injury, especially in the long term. Data from multiple long-term follow-up studies of patients with surgically treated elbow fractures provided us with an opportunity to assess risk factors for long-term radiographic arthrosis after elbow injury.

Methods.—During a 5-year period, we obtained radiographs during a research-specific evaluation of 139 patients (81 men and 58 women) 10 or more years (median, 19.5 y; range, 10–34 y) after surgical treatment of an elbow fracture as part of multiple retrospective studies. Radiographic arthrosis was graded according to the system of Broberg and Morrey. Bivariate and multivariable analyses evaluated risk factors for radiographic arthrosis.

Results.—Of 139 patients, 75 had radiographic evidence of arthrosis at final evaluation and 32 had moderate or severe radiographic arthrosis. Mechanism of injury, age, gender, follow-up time, occupation, and limb dominance were not associated with radiographic arthrosis. Multiple logistic regression analysis identified the type of injury as the only independent predictor of moderate to severe radiographic arthrosis. Patients with a bicolumnar fracture of the distal humerus, a capitellum/trochlear fracture, or an elbow fracture–dislocation were 8.0, 7.3, and 5.2 times more likely (odds ratio), respectively, to develop radiographic evidence of moderate or severe radiographic arthrosis than the average patient in this cohort.

Conclusions.—Distal humerus fractures (both columnar and capitellum/trochlea) and elbow fracture–dislocations are more likely than fractures of the olecranon and radial head to develop moderate or severe radiographic arthrosis in the long term.

Type of Study/Level of Evidence.—Prognostic IV.

▶ The purpose of this study was only to document arthrosis; there was no attempt to measure or report symptoms or dysfunction.

Utilizing data from 7 other studies, the authors assessed radiographic arthrosis after elbow trauma. At a mean of 19 years (range, 10-34) after surgical treatment, there were 139 patients, of which, 32 had moderate or severe arthrosis and 107 had mild to no arthrosis.

Not surprisingly, the higher-energy injuries demonstrated more arthrosis, with the radial head fractures and proximal ulna/olecranon fractures having the least. Patients with distal humeral fractures, capitellar and trochlear fractures, and fracture dislocations demonstrated a significantly higher rate of arthrosis than the average patient in the study. This correlation (fracture type to arthrosis) was the only significant one found after rigorous statistical analysis.

There were no correlations between arthrosis and follow-up, mechanism of injury, dominance, gender, age, or occupation. These last 2 categories present an important clinical finding. While we may not be able to alter the appearance or progression of arthrosis, this study suggests that clinicians need not counsel young patients to avoid rigorous avocations or occupations after these injuries.

R. F. Papandrea, MD

Biomechanical Effect of Increasing or Decreasing Degrees of Freedom for Surgery of Trapeziometacarpal Joint Arthritis: A Simulation Study

Domalain MF, Seitz WH, Evans PJ, et al (Cleveland Clinic, OH)
J Orthop Res 29:1675-1681, 2011

Osteoarthritis of the trapeziometacarpal (TMC) joint can be treated by arthrodesis and arthroplasty, which potentially decreases or increases the degrees of freedom (DoF) of the joint, respectively. The aim of our study was to bring novel biomechanical insights into these joint surgery procedures by investigating the influence of DoF at the TMC joint on muscle and joint forces in the thumb. A musculoskeletal model of the thumb was developed to equilibrate a 1 N external force in various directions while the thumb assumed key and pulp pinch postures. Muscle and joint forces were computed with an optimization method. In comparison to that of the 2-DoF (intact joint) condition, muscle forces slightly decreased in the 0-DoF (arthrodesis) condition, but drastically increased in the 3-DoF (arthroplasty) condition. TMC joint forces in the 3-DoF condition were 12 times larger than the 2-DoF joint. This study contributes to a further understanding of the biomechanics of the intact and surgically repaired TMC joint and addresses the biomechanical consequences of changing a joint's DoF by surgery.

▶ This study demonstrated strong forces loaded to the trapeziometacarpal (TMC) joint after removal of the trapezium followed by suspension arthroplasty. Narrowing of the joint space after suspension arthroplasty or destruction of artificial TMC joint prostheses is understandable because of the huge compression force applied to the TMC joint after removal of the trapezium. Narrowing of the space of the TMC joint sometimes results in a severe rigid deformity of the thumb. It is important to retain the height of the joint space during suspension arthroplasty surgery to prevent the deformity of the thumb. My opinion is that suspension arthroplasty alone is best indicated for older people. For young people having stage 4 arthritis of the TMC joint (which involves both the scaphotrapezial and TMC joints), I usually perform an interposition arthroplasty procedure combined with suspension arthroplasty. My preferential procedure for young patients is tendon interposition of the flexor carpi radialis (FCR) and abductor pollicis longus (APL) bound by using a half strip of the FCR[1] and suspension arthroplasty using a part of the APL.[2]

R. Kakinoki, MD, PhD

References

1. Kleinman WB, Eckenrode JF. Tendon suspension and sling arthroplasty for thumb trapeziometacarpal arthritis. *J Hand Surg Am.* 1991;16:983-991.
2. Thompson JS. Surgical treatment of trapeziometacarpal arthrosis. *Adv Orthop Surg.* 1986;10:105.

24 Neural Integration, Pain and Anesthesia

Is it true that injecting palmar finger skin hurts more than dorsal skin? New level 1 evidence
Wheelock ME, Leblanc M, Chung B, et al (Dalhousie Univ, Halifax, Canada)
Hand 6:47-49, 2011

Background.—Since the first texts on local anesthesia were written in the early 1900s, it has been widely quoted and believed that dorsal finger skin is less sensitive to needlestick pain than volar finger skin. The result is that the most commonly used finger block for local anesthesia is the dorsal two injection technique.

Methods.—In this study, the needlestick discomfort associated with dorsal and volar finger skin was compared in a group of 78 volunteers who had the long finger of both hands poked with a 25 G needle; one in the midline of the volar side and the other in the lateral web space of the dorsal side. Volunteers then completed a pain scale for each needlestick and ranked which technique they would prefer for future injections.

Results.—We found that there was no significant difference in needle-stick pain or preference of future needle location between the dorsal and volar aspects of the finger.

Conclusions.—We provide level 1 evidence that the needlestick of the SIMPLE block which has one needlestick on the volar side of the finger is not more painful than the needlestick of the dorsal finger block.

▶ The authors have once again exposed a surgical truism as being false. In this article, the authors question the common perception that a dorsal injection causes less pain than a volar injection. Although other studies have examined pain with injection into different parts of the hand, this article only looks at the needle sticks. Like most of the other articles, this study shows no advantage in dorsal injections. I am not sure the study adds to those already done (after all, the real question is related to the whole injection experience—needle stick plus infiltration), but it does continue to bring attention to the many misconceptions regarding digital blocks. Unfortunately, there does not seem to be any way to make digital blocks or injections in general pain free.

J. Frankenhoff, MD

Complex Regional Pain Syndrome of the Upper Extremity
Patterson RW, Li Z, Smith BP, et al (Wake Forest Univ School of Medicine, Winston-Salem, NC)
J Hand Surg 36A:1553-1562, 2011

The diagnosis and management of complex regional pain syndrome is often challenging. Early diagnosis and intervention improve outcomes in most patients; however, some patients will progress regardless of intervention. Multidisciplinary management facilitates care in complex cases. The onset of signs and symptoms may be obvious or insidious; temporal delay is a frequent occurrence. Difficulty sleeping, pain unresponsive to narcotics, swelling, stiffness, and hypersensitivity are harbingers of onset. Multimodal treatment with hand therapy, sympatholytic drugs, and stress loading may be augmented with anesthesia blocks. If the dystrophic symptoms are controllable by medications and a nociceptive focus or nerve derangement is correctable, surgery is an appropriate alternative. Chronic sequelae of contracture may also be addressed surgically in patients with controllable sympathetically maintained pain.

▶ This article makes a worthwhile attempt to define the subjective and objective manifestations of complex regional pain syndrome, to outline diagnostic criteria, to discuss nonoperative and operative treatment options, to elucidate common myths and misconceptions, and to delineate standard of care issues. The breadth of this subject makes it understandably difficult to summarize in one short review article.

A lot of the nuances of the various components outlined above are lost as a result, making the reading actually more difficult than the slightly longer chapter in Green's sixth edition,[1] which was written by substantially the same group of authors. However, there are a few must-read sections, such as their cogent descriptions of subgroups of patients based on physiology. Likewise, the section outlining the guidelines for initial treatment based on physiologic staging is concise and clear.

The main problem with the article is that the references to the psychological aspects of the syndrome and to the role of psychologically-directed treatment options are quite limited. Hopefully, future studies will explore this mind–body aspect and will shed more light on this important connection. As Ring et al[2] state in their review, "An improved conception and communication of the cognitive and behavioral aspects of illness should help to overcome the false dichotomy of mind versus body and facilitate such collaboration. In addition to placebo-controlled clinical trials to determine treatment efficacy (eg, sham vs active nerve simulation), the comparative effectiveness of various paradigms and their resulting treatments should be compared (eg, nerve stimulation therapies vs cognitive behavioral therapy)."

J. Frankenhoff, MD

References

1. Koman LA, Poehling GG, Smith BP, Smith TL, Chloros G. Green's Operative Hand Surgery, 6th edition. 2011;59:1959-1988.
2. Ring D, Barth R, Barsky A. Evidence-based medicine: disproportionate pain and disability. *J Hand Surg Am.* 2010;35:1345-1347.

25 Peripheral Nerve Injury and Repair

Cubital Tunnel Syndrome Caused by Amyloid Elbow Arthropathy in Long-term Hemodialysis Patients: Report of 4 Cases
Shinohara T, Tatebe M, Okui N, et al (Nagoya Univ, Japan)
J Hand Surg 36A:1640-1643, 2011

Carpal tunnel syndrome occurs frequently in long-term hemodialysis patients. However, the literature contains few detailed reports of other nerve entrapment syndromes of the upper extremity in these patients. We encountered 4 cases in which cubital tunnel syndrome occurred in long-term hemodialysis patients. In all cases, a hypertrophic synovial mass projecting from the humeroulnar joint compressed the ulnar nerve, and Congo red staining revealed that the mass contained amyloid deposition. Synovial proliferation resulting from amyloid arthropathy of the elbow joint appears to be the primary cause of this disease.

▶ In presenting a series of cubital tunnel syndrome secondary to extrinsic compression from amyloid deposition in hemodialysis patients, the authors bring attention to other less common etiologies of ulnar nerve compression. Four patients, with an average time on hemodialysis of 24.5 years and average duration of symptoms of 4 months, were reviewed. All patients had operative findings of proliferative synovitis with amyloid deposition expanding from the medial ulnohumeral joint directly compressing the ulnar nerve. Preoperative findings included sensory loss and intrinsic atrophy in all patients, and although the authors note improvement in numbness, no muscle recovery was seen at up to 7 years. Unfortunately, the authors do not provide baseline or follow-up sensory measurements for comparison, only indicating that "improvement" occurred. Similarly, we are left to wonder what the duration of follow-up was for each patient. Despite these deficiencies, the authors highlight the importance of close observation for compressive neuropathy in patients on chronic hemodialysis because of the potential for poor functional recovery.

F. T. D. Kaplan, MD

Biomedical and Psychosocial Factors Associated with Disability After Peripheral Nerve Injury
Novak CB, Anastakis DJ, Beaton DE, et al (Univ of Toronto, Ontario, Canada; Washington Univ School of Medicine, St Louis, MO)
J Bone Joint Surg Am 93:929-936, 2011

Background.—The purpose of this study was to evaluate the biomedical and psychosocial factors associated with disability at a minimum of six months following upper-extremity nerve injury.

Methods.—This cross-sectional study included patients who were assessed between six months and fifteen years following an upper-extremity nerve injury. Assessment measures included patient self-report questionnaires (the Disabilities of the Arm, Shoulder and Hand Questionnaire [DASH]; pain questionnaires; and general health and mental health questionnaires). DASH scores were compared by using unpaired t tests (sex, Workers' Compensation/litigation, affected limb, marital status, education, and geographic location), analysis of variance (nerve injured, work status, and income), or correlations (age and time since injury). Multivariable linear regression analysis was used to evaluate the predictors of the DASH scores.

Results.—The sample included 158 patients with a mean age (and standard deviation) of 41 ± 16 years. The median time from injury was fourteen months (range, six to 167 months). The DASH scores were significantly higher for patients receiving Workers' Compensation or involved in litigation ($p = 0.02$), had a brachial plexus injury ($p = 0.001$), or were unemployed ($p < 0.001$). There was a significant positive correlation between the DASH scores and pain intensity ($r = 0.51$, $p < 0.001$). In the multivariable regression analysis of the predictors of the DASH scores, the following predictors explained 52.7% of the variance in the final model: pain intensity (Beta $= 0.230$, $p = 0.006$), brachial plexus injury (Beta $= -0.220$, $p = 0.000$), time since injury (Beta $= -0.198$, $p = 0.002$), pain catastrophizing score (Beta $= 0.192$, $p = 0.025$), age (Beta $= 0.187$, $p = 0.002$), work status (Beta $= 0.179$, $p = 0.008$), cold sensitivity (Beta $= 0.171$, $p = 0.015$), depression score (Beta $= 0.133$, $p = 0.066$), Workers' Compensation/litigation (Beta $= 0.116$, $p = 0.049$), and female sex (Beta $= -0.104$, $p = 0.090$).

Conclusions.—Patients with a peripheral nerve injury report substantial disability, pain, and cold sensitivity. Disability as measured with the DASH was predicted by brachial plexus injury, older age, pain intensity, work status, time since injury, cold sensitivity, and pain catastrophizing.

▶ This is an interesting cross-sectional study of patients with peripheral nerve injuries who attended clinics in 2 different centers within the study period. The authors' findings suggest that such injuries can cause substantial disability, pain, and cold sensitivity. In analysis, the authors also found multiple factors associated with disability. Their findings corroborate that of other researchers who showed similar morbidity in their group of patients using a different study design.[1]

The cross-sectional design of this study introduces some limitations. The patient population mix may be unique. There is a tendency of the study to be overrepresented by patients with persistent disability who continue to seek treatment in the clinic. Patients who have recovered or improved substantially following such injuries may have been more likely to be lost to follow-up. In addition, because patients with injuries that had occurred 6 months or more prior to the study were included, some patients may not have completed their recovery at the study's end.

A. Chong, MD

Reference

1. Ciaramitaro P, Mondelli M, Logullo F, et al. Italian Network for Traumatic Neuropathies. Traumatic peripheral nerve injuries: epidemiological findings, neuropathic pain and quality of life in 158 patients. *J Peripher Nerv Syst.* 2010; 15:120-127.

Comparisons of Outcomes from Repair of Median Nerve and Ulnar Nerve Defect with Nerve Graft and Tubulization: A Meta-Analysis

Yang M, Rawson JL, Zhang EW, et al (Univ of Mississippi Med Ctr, Jackson; et al)
J Reconstr Microsurg 27:451-460, 2011

In this study, an updated meta-analysis of all published human studies was presented to evaluate the recovery of the median and the ulnar nerves in the forearm after defect repair by nerve conduit and autologous nerve graft. Up to June of 2010, search for English language articles was conducted to collect publications on the outcome of median or ulnar nerve defect repair. A total of 33 studies and 1531 cases were included in this study. Patient information was extracted from these publications and the postoperative outcome was analyzed using meta-analysis. There was no significant difference in the postoperative recovery between the median and the ulnar nerves (odds ratio = 0.98). Sensory nerves were found to achieve a more satisfactory recovery after nerve defect repair than motor nerves ($p < 0.05$). Median nerve can also achieve more satisfactory recovery in both sensory and motor function than ulnar nerve ($p < 0.05$). There was no statistical difference between tubulization and autologous nerve graft in repairing defects less than 5 cm. Based on the results of this study, a median nerve with sensory impairment was associated with improved postoperative prognosis, while an ulnar nerve with motor nerve damage was prone to a worse prognosis. Tubulization can be a good alternative in the reconstruction of small defects.

▶ This article pooled the data on repair of injured nerves with gaps in the forearm and assessed functional outcomes. The analysis compared recovery for (1) ulnar versus median nerve injuries, (2) sensory versus motor, and (3) conduit versus autograft repairs. They found that overall recovery of ulnar and median nerves was similar, sensory nerve recovery was better than motor, and conduits were similar to autografts for gaps less than 5 cm.

The article adds to the literature and updates previous studies that pooled nerve repair data. The study also highlights the major difficulty in pooling nerve repair data: heterogeneity. Heterogeneity of nerve injuries (eg, location of injury, age of patient) within the comparison groups presents a large barrier and limits the strength of the findings. Pooling of data is attractive to try and smooth out these differences, but, as this study showed, only the broadest analysis (comparing overall outcomes of ulnar and median nerve repairs) were homogeneous enough to perform meta-analysis comparisons.

Bridging nerve gaps is a challenge that continues to vex surgeons. Autograft remains the "gold standard," but the added operating time and donor site morbidity make this option less than perfect. Nerve conduits are attractive for short gaps, and this article suggests that the results may be comparable to those of autograft. However, these results should be interpreted with caution. In this study, the nerve conduits had smaller nerve gaps than the autografts (many gaps in the conduit group were less than 1 cm, whereas the majority of the autografts were greater than 2 cm and none less than 1 cm.) There is a substantial difference in the nerve regenerative capacities across a smaller than 1-cm versus greater than 2-cm nerve gap. For longer gaps, the nerve increasingly relies on internal scaffolding and Schwann cells to regenerate, neither of these are present in conduits. This has led to recommendations that conduits generally be used only for small short sensory nerve gaps.[1]

C. Curtin, MD

Reference

1. Boyd KU, Nimigan AS, Mackinnon SE. Nerve reconstruction in the hand and upper extremity. *Clin Plast Surg.* 2011;38:643-660.

Outcome After Delayed Oberlin Transfer in Brachial Plexus Injury
Sedain G, Sharma MS, Sharma BS, et al (All India Inst of Med Sciences, New Delhi)
Neurosurgery 69:822-828, 2011

Background.—Nerve transfers following traumatic brachial plexus injuries are infrequently operated on after 6 months of injury because myoneural degeneration may set in before nerve regeneration can occur. An exception may lie in transferring healthy donor nerve fascicles directly onto an injured recipient nerve close to the motor point. This is especially true of the Oberlin transfer in which ulnar nerve fascicle(s) are transferred onto the damaged nerve to the biceps.

Objective.—This retrospective observational study evaluated the outcome of the Oberlin transfer on bicipital power in patients with upper trunk/C5,6,7 root level injuries operated on after 6 months of injury.

Methods.—Using a standard infraclavicular exposure, the musculocutaneous nerve was followed to its branch to the biceps. Distal to this, the ulnar nerve was skeletonized and a constituent motor fascicle was transferred onto the nerve to biceps. Medical Research Council (MRC) motor power grading was assessed every 3 months following surgery. Patients with a follow-up less than 12 months were excluded.

Results.—Nine patients operated on after an average of 12.2 months (range, 7-24 months) following injury qualified for the study. At an average follow-up of 26.7 months (range, 12-41 months), all patients had ≥2/5 biceps power. Seven patients (77.8%) had useful biceps function ≥3/5 MRC score. A single patient operated on 24 months after injury gained 4/5 MRC biceps power.

Conclusion.—The Oberlin transfer is a useful salvage procedure in patients presenting after 6 months of a brachial plexus injury.

▶ This article would have been better as an interesting case report. Although the authors report on "delayed" nerve transfers, only 3 of 9 patients had denervation greater than 12 months. The others had overall good results (5 of 6 patients M4 or better), but this is nothing new. Out of the truly delayed transfers, only 1 of 3 patients had worthwhile recovery. What is interesting is that this 1 patient was 24 months postinjury. Of note, he had a pan-plexus injury with significant distal recovery, which suggests that some nerve fibers may have reached the biceps (perhaps preserving the muscle). Regardless, transferring that far out is typically viewed as hopeless, and transferring a "regenerated" nerve is typically not considered a good idea. The take-home message may be that "hopeless" is not always "hopeless," although clearly reinnervation greater than 12 months post-injury had a lower chance of being successful.

J. Isaacs, MD

Repair of nerve defect with acellular nerve graft supplemented by bone marrow stromal cells in mice
Zhao Z, Wang Y, Peng J, et al (General Hosp of Chinese PLA, Beijing, People's Republic of China)
Microsurgery 31:388-394, 2011

The acellular nerve graft that can provide internal structure and extracellular matrix components of the nerve is an alternative for repair of peripheral nerve defects. However, results of the acellular nerve grafting for nerve repair still remain inconsistent. This study aimed to investigate if supplementing bone marrow mesenchymal stromal cells (MSCs) could improve the results of nerve repair with the acellular nerve graft in a 10-mm sciatic nerve defect model in mice. Eighteen mice were divided into three groups ($n = 6$ for each group) for nerve repairs with the nerve autograft, the acellular nerve graft, and the acellular nerve graft by supplemented with MSCs (5×10^5) fibrin glue around the graft. The mouse static sciatic index was evaluated by walking-track testing every 2 weeks. The weight preservation of the triceps surae muscles and histomorphometric assessment of triceps surae muscles and repaired nerves were examined at week 8. The results showed that the nerve repair by the nerve autografting obtained the best functional recovery of limb. The nerve repair with the acellular nerve graft supplemented with MSCs achieved better functional recovery and higher axon number than that with the acellular nerve graft alone at week 8 postoperatively. The results indicated that supplementing MSCs might help to improve nerve regeneration and functional recovery in repair of the nerve defect with the acellular nerve graft.

▶ Acellular nerve allograft offers the advantage of scaffolding for Schwann cell and axonal migration over hollow tube conduits. Autograft is still superior in supporting nerve regeneration partly because the Schwann cells are already present and do not need to migrate in. The idea in this article is to supplement allograft with marrow-derived mesenchymal stem cells, which have the potential to support axonal regeneration in a manner similar to Schwann cells. This strategy has been shown to have promise in other studies, including in a primate.[1] One of the differences in this study is that the stem cells are supplied via a fibrin glue substrate basically squirted along the allograft. This study does suggest a slight benefit from the stem cells, as evidenced primarily by increased axon counts (although not necessarily improved myelination, which is unfortunate because this may be one of the key potential benefits lost by the lack of Schwann cells). The authors fail to demonstrate migration of the stem cells into the graft, which I think might be a key step in really solving the problem of allograft versus autograft. This idea, while interesting, is still completely confined to the lab, with no or at least minimal impending clinical applications.

J. Isaacs, MD

Reference

1. Wang J, Ding F, Gu Y, Liu J, Gu X. Bone marrow mesenchymal stem cells promote cell proliferation and neurotrophic function of Schwann cells in vitro and in vivo. *Brain Res.* 2009;1262:7-15.

Radial nerve palsy associated with humeral shaft fracture. Is the energy of trauma a prognostic factor?
Venouziou AI, Dailiana ZH, Varitimidis SE, et al (Univ of Thessalia, Biopolis, Larissa, Greece)
Injury 42:1289-1293, 2011

Background.—Radial nerve palsy associated with humeral shaft fractures is the most common nerve lesion complicating fractures of long bones. The purpose of the study was to review the outcome of surgical management in patients with low energy and high energy radial nerve palsy after humeral shaft fractures.

Methods.—Eighteen patients were treated operatively for a humeral shaft fracture with radial nerve palsy. The mean age was 32.2 years and the mean follow up time was 66.1 months (range: 30–104). The surgical management included fracture fixation with early nerve exploration and repair if needed. The patients were divided in two groups based on the energy of trauma (low vs. high trauma energy). The prevalence of injured and unrecovered nerves and time to nerve recovery were analysed.

Results.—Five patients sustained low and 13 high energy trauma. All patients with low energy trauma had an intact (4) or entrapped (1) radial nerve and recovered completely. Full nerve recovery was also achieved in five of 13 patients with high energy trauma where the nerve was found intact or entrapped. Signs of initial recovery were present in a mean of 3.2 weeks (range: 1−8) for the low energy group and 12 weeks (range: 3−23) for the high energy group ($p = 0.036$). In these patients, the average time to full recovery was 14 and 26 weeks for the low and high energy trauma group respectively. Eight patients with high energy trauma had severely damaged nerves and failed to recover, although microsurgical nerve reconstruction was performed in 4 cases. Patients with high energy trauma had a prolonged fracture healing time (18.7 weeks on average) compared to those with low energy fractures (10.4 weeks), ($p = 0.003$).

Conclusions.—The outcome of the radial nerve palsy following humeral fractures is associated to the initial trauma. Palsies that are part of a low energy fracture uniformly recover and therefore primary surgical exploration seems unnecessary. In high energy fractures, neurotmesis or severe contusion must be expected. In this case nerve recovery is unfavourable and the patients should be informed of the poor prognosis and the need of tendon transfers.

▶ This article is one of many regarding the treatment of radial nerve palsy after humerus fracture. It continues to be a vexing problem in the world of trauma and nerve surgery. As other investigators have found, low-energy fractures with radial nerve palsy do not necessarily require surgical exploration since the incidence of spontaneous recovery is quite high. The authors, however, found that one of the low-energy fractures had the radial nerve entrapped within the fracture site. It is unclear whether this would have spontaneously recovered if it had been left alone. Unfortunately, all of theses cases were ones that had open reduction internal fixation of the humerus; what would have been interesting would have been including the series of patients with low-energy closed injuries with radial nerve palsy who did not have surgery. Did they all spontaneously recover? The series also included 9 of 18 patients with open fractures—5 were grade IIIC and 2 were IIB. There was a high number of severe open fractures, causing concern of selection bias. In the high-energy cases, 4 had lacerated nerves and 4 had "irreparable" nerves. For the lacerated nerves, 3 had end-to-end repair and 1 had nerve grafting. For the lacerated nerves, it seems questionable that end-to-end repair could be performed without tension. A nerve that is lacerated by high-energy trauma will usually have a traction or crush component to it, requiring nerve grafting in all cases, in my experience. It is no surprise that their results were poor. For the "irreparable" nerves, this is an arbitrary distinction. With enough segmental resection to good fascicular pattern on either end, the injuries could all have been grafted. Others have demonstrated and I have seen in my own series of long nerve grafts for brachial plexus injuries that grafts of 13 to 15 cm can work. They take a long time to recover, but they can recover. In my practice, I would explore high-energy injuries, resect injured segments, and perform nerve graft. Tendon transfers can always be performed in the future; I would wait at least 1.5 years before abandoning the nerve grafts to perform secondary tendon transfer.

J. Yao, MD

An in vivo engineered nerve conduit—fabrication and experimental study in rats
Penna V, Munder B, Stark G-B, et al (Albert-Ludwigs Univ, Freiburg, Germany; Sana Clinic Gerresheim, Germany; et al)
Microsurgery 31:395-400, 2011

Background.—Several types of nerve conduits have been used for peripheral nerve gap bridging. This study investigated the in vivo engineering of a biological nerve conduit and its suitability for nerve gap bridging.

Material and Methods.—A 19-mm long polyvinyl chloride (PVC) tube was implanted parallely to the sciatic nerve. After implantation, a connective tissue cover developed around the PVC-tube, the so-called biogenic conduit. Histological cross-sections were performed after 1, 2, 3, and 4 weeks. Wall thicknesses were measured and all vessels per cross-section were counted. The biogenic conduit filled with fibrin was used to bridge a 15-mm long nerve gap in the sciatic lesion model of the rat ($n = 8$). The results of nerve repair with the conduit were compared to the autologous nerve graft ($n = 8$). Sciatic functional index (SFI), nerve area, axon count, myelination index, and ratio of total myelinated fiber area/nerve area (N-ratio) were analyzed after 4 weeks.

Results.—The wall thickness of biogenic conduits increased over the 4 weeks implantation time. Biogenic conduits revealed highest number of vessels per cross-section after 4 weeks. The results of SFI analysis did not show significant difference between the repairs with biogenic conduit and autologous nerve graft. Nerve area and axon count in the biogenic conduit group were significantly lower than in the autologous nerve group ($P < 0.001$). The biogenic conduit group showed significant higher myelination values, but lower N-ratio when compared to the nerve graft group ($P < 0.001$).

Conclusions.—The in vivo engineered conduits allow nerve gap bridging of 15 mm. However, quality of regeneration after 4 weeks observation time is not comparable to autologous nerve grafts. Whether biogenic conduits might be a suitable alternative to artificial and biological conduits for gap bridging will have to be evaluated in further studies (Fig 1).

▶ This is an interesting study, primarily to readers with basic science interest toward nerve regeneration and conduit development. Citing improved vascularity as a primary advantage of this technique, the authors introduce a strategy

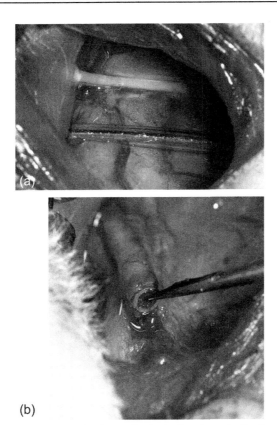

(b)

FIGURE 1.—(a) Implanted PVC tube; (b) 4 weeks after implantation, tube-like fibrous tissue (biogenic conduit). [Color figure can be viewed in the online issue, which is available at wileyonlinelibrary.com.] (Reprinted from Penna V, Munder B, Stark G-B, et al. An in vivo engineered nerve conduit—fabrication and experimental study in rats. *Microsurgery.* 2011;31:395-400, with permission from Wiley-Liss, Inc.)

of in vivo bioengineering a vascularized conduit—a polyvinyl chloride tube is implanted next to the rodent sciatic nerve. After 4 weeks, the hindlimb was reopened, the polyvinyl chloride (PVC) tube removed, and the biogenic remaining tube (tube-shaped fibrous tissue that had formed around the PVC) was filled with commercially available fibrin glue (to prevent the biogenic tube from collapsing; Fig 1). The sciatic nerve was transected and repaired to either end of the tube (15 mm long regeneration length). This was compared with a 15-mm autologous tube model. Recovery was assessed at only 4 weeks after repair, which seems a little early for assessment. This is an interesting idea but didn't really work (low axon counts) and, from a clinical standpoint, would be completely impractical (2-stage surgery, implanting next to the area that requires repair).

V. Penna, MD

FIGURE 23-... (figure caption illegible)

V. Penna, MD

26 Rehabilitation, Outcomes and Assessment

Conflicts of Interest With the Hand Surgeon's Relationship With Industry
Delsignore JL, Goodman MJ (Univ of Rochester School of Medicine, NY; Salem Orthopaedic Surgeons, MA)
J Hand Surg 37A:179-183, 2012

Many advances in hand surgery have been supported and enabled by the integral relationship that exists between the profession of hand surgery and industry. This relationship takes many forms, including medical education, development of new technology and methodology, research, and opportunities for patient education. As with all of these endeavors, the primary focus of both the physician and industry must be the care of the patient. When a collaborative relationship exists between physicians and industry, a conflict of interest is present and must be recognized as such and managed to avoid any detriment to patient care. Although the hand surgeon, the patient, and industry share the common interest of advancement of patient care, there does exist real and potential conflicts of interest, which are unavoidable, but not necessarily undesirable. Multiple guidelines exist to govern relationships between industry and physicians. The cooperative relationship between the physician and industry is not only helpful, but it can be critical to the advancement of and innovations in patient care. When properly managed, collaboration between the physician and industry can effectively achieve the common goal of serving the best interest of the patient.

▶ The front door of a nearby restaurant reads, on 1 side, "This restaurant is good for your diet." On the other side: "This restaurant is bad for your diet." All sorts of healthy, and indulgent, options are available—the choice is yours. So might read a similar signpost for our discipline: "Industry is good for hand surgery." Alternatively, "Industry is bad for hand surgery." Of course, the answer lies somewhere between. The choice is ours, and authors DelSignore and Goodman remind us that the patient and the patient's needs must always come first. (The word "patient" appears 37 times in the article, so the message is clear.) This article serves as an excellent primer for the laws and history of ethics in the medical profession, especially related to the Department of Justice rulings in 2007. It reviews the American Society for Surgery of the Hand and the American Academy of Orthopaedic Surgeons code of ethics and rationale and guidelines on how to proceed in relating with industry in an ethical manner. The authors cite Stanford University as one of the first institutions to enforce strict conflict of interest policies. As an employee of Stanford and having lived with these guidelines for more than a decade, it is possible to maintain relationships with industry for educational and professional support befitting the university policies. These relationships are pursued carefully; the mantra in mind, as these authors will remind you, is always, "The Patient Comes First."

A. Ladd, MD

Factors Associated With Patient Satisfaction
Vranceanu AM, Ring D (Massachusetts General Hosp, Boston)
J Hand Surg 36A:1504-1508, 2011

Purpose.—This investigation tested the null hypothesis that psychological factors have no effect on patient satisfaction in a hand and upper limb practice.

Methods.—The Center for Epidemiologic Studies Depression Scale, the Pain Catastrophizing Scale, and the Disabilities of the Arm, Shoulder, and Hand questionnaire were administered to 248 new patients presenting to a hand and upper limb practice. After the appointment, the treating physician was asked to rate the patient's uneasiness with his or her symptoms. The Consumer Assessment of Health Care Providers and Systems questionnaire was mailed to patients 2 weeks after their visit. A total of 178 patients returned this questionnaire.

Results.—There were small but significant correlations between (1) depression and perception of how well the doctor (a) listens carefully, (b) gives easy-to-understand instructions, and (c) spends enough time; (2) pain catastrophizing and the degree to which doctor gives enough information about a procedure; and (3) the doctor's perception of inordinate patient concern and (a) the impression that the doctor gives easy-to-understand explanations, (b) the impression that the doctor listens carefully, (c) the impression that the doctor gives enough information about surgical procedures, and (d) the patient's overall rating of the doctor. In multivariable models, the doctor's perception of disproportionate uneasiness was the only significant predictor of "doctor gave enough information" and "doctor listened carefully."

Conclusions.—In this study, the provider's sense that the patient was disproportionately uneasy with his or her symptoms was the only significant predictor of patient satisfaction, and this accounted for a small percentage of the variance in responses to these items. Patient satisfaction is complex, and the divide between medical advice and a patient's expectations are not easily reduced to one or more disease-specific or patient-specific factors.

TABLE 1.—Multivariable Model for Patients' Rating of "Frequency That Doctors Give Enough Information About Surgery Procedures"

Independent Variable	R^2	F	β	P Value
Entire model	.14	6.49		.003
Pain catastrophizing			.15	.24
Overall health			.06	.63
Uneasiness			−.59	.003

TABLE 2.—Multivariable Model for Patients' Response to "Frequency With Which Doctors Give Easy to Understand Instructions"

Independent Variable	R^2	F	β	P Value
Entire model	.04	3.53		.05
Depression			.86	.26
Uneasiness			−.30	.05

Type of Study/Level of Evidence.—Prognostic II (Tables 1-3).

▶ This particular study is one of very few that attempts to analyze some of the more qualitative (as opposed to quantitative) aspects of the care that is provided by hand surgeons. It attempts to determine what factors might be associated with patient satisfaction (or dissatisfaction as it were) in the outpatient clinic setting. The study was understandably somewhat narrow in scope in that it did not analyze factors associated with surgical treatment for hand problems.

Nearly 200 patients enrolled and completed study procedures. On the day of enrollment (which was also the time of initial consultation), patients completed questionnaires on pain catastrophizing, depression, and disability (DASH survey). Two weeks after the initial visit, patients were mailed the Consumer Assessment of Health Care Providers and Systems (CAHPS) questionnaire. These surveys were then correlated for each patient.

The results of the study give credence to some of the patient—physician dynamic factors that many of us have surely noted anecdotally. Specifically, the authors found that depressive symptoms and pain catastrophizing negatively correlated with patient satisfaction. Similarly, the physicians' perception that a patient is inordinately concerned about the problem was correlated with lower patient satisfaction. In this particular group of patients (for whom doctors rated them as overly concerned), many felt that the doctors were not sufficiently concerned about their problem(s). One can see how this factor alone could lead to a rapidly deteriorating patient—physician relationship. The authors also used multivariable analysis on 3 models (doctor gives information about surgery, doctor listens carefully, and doctor gives easy-to-understand instructions) to find factors associated with each. "Uneasiness" correlated with all 3 models, and depression correlated with the first 2 (Tables 1-3).

TABLE 3.—Multivariable Model for Patients' Responses to "Frequency With Which Doctors Listen Carefully"

Independent Variable	R^2	F	β	P Value
Entire model	.02	3.61		.04
Depression			.15	.10
Uneasiness			−.49	.04

Interestingly, the results of the study also showed there were no significant differences in individual provider satisfaction scores and that satisfaction more strongly correlated with the psychological factors mentioned. This was somewhat unexpected, and it suggests that individual patients' coping skills and overall psychological milieu are more important in determining how a patient perceives the physician–patient interaction. Ultimately, the authors suggest that patient satisfaction as a quality-of-care indicator should perhaps be prorated or adjusted based on individual psychosocial characteristics. However, while plausible, this weighting of patient satisfaction scores will likely not be feasible in most institutions simply because of limited resources. Perhaps a more proactive approach in which physicians briefly analyze psychosocial characteristics prior to the patient interaction will allow them to tailor the physician–patient interaction individually, thereby leading to higher patient satisfaction scores.

J. Freidrich, MD

Static Versus Dynamic Splinting for Proximal Interphalangeal Joint Pyrocarbon Implant Arthroplasty: A Comparison of Current and Historical Cohorts

Riggs JM, Lyden AK, Chung KC, et al (Univ of Michigan Health System, Ann Arbor; Univ of Michigan, Ann Arbor; Univ of Michigan Med School, Ann Arbor)

J Hand Ther 24:231-239, 2011

Study Design.—Nonrandomized mixed current and historical cohort follow-up study. The purpose of the study was to test the effectiveness of static splinting after arthroplasty in patients with osteoarthritis. Dynamic splinting is recommended after proximal interphalangeal joint pyrocarbon implant arthroplasty; however, static splinting may be more feasible to deliver. Nine consecutive patients received static splinting in this study. These patients were compared with those of a historical control group ($n = 10$) who received dynamic splinting. Function and performance variables were measured preoperatively and 3 months after surgery. All patients underwent surgery by the same hand surgeon, and most of the patients were treated by the same certified hand therapist. Both static and dynamic groups showed improvement on several function and performance measures. Compared with the dynamic group, the static group showed greater improvements in the Michigan. Hand Outcomes Questionnaire subset of work performance (21.00 ± 14.75 vs 3.13 ± 14.13, p < 0.05) and Jebsen-Taylor Test (−11.58 ± 5.44 vs −2.81 ± 3.23, p < 0.03). Patients who received static splinting had similar outcomes to those who received the dynamic splinting. Static splinting requires less therapist training and offers greater patient convenience and is a promising protocol that should be evaluated in a larger study (Fig 1, Table 2).

▶ This excellent study compares 2 splinting/orthotic approaches for the post-operative management of pyrocarbon proximal interphalangeal (PIP) joint implants. The standard protocol currently used by certified hand therapists consists of combined daytime dynamic splinting with nighttime static splinting. This is often a difficult routine for the patients, as it involves donning and doffing 2 different splints numerous times during the day as well as having to adjust the dynamic splint tension correctly. It is also a more technically demanding protocol for the therapist. The authors used exceptional clinical reasoning to determine that static orthoses alone combined with protected range-of-motion exercises may be clinically similar to the combined dynamic and static orthotic device approach. All participants used in this study underwent PIP joint arthroplasty from the same surgeon. The static orthotic group was evaluated prospectively, and the dynamic orthotic group, which was part of a previous study, was

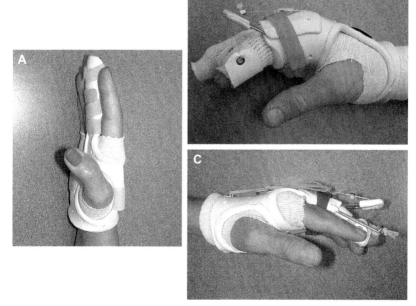

FIGURE 1.—(A) Static extension splint; (B) dynamic PIP joint extension splint; (C) dynamic PIP joint extension splint with PIP extension block. PIP = proximal interphalangeal. (Reprinted from Riggs JM, Lyden AK, Chung KC, et al. Static versus dynamic splinting for proximal interphalangeal joint pyrocarbon implant arthroplasty: a comparison of current and historical cohorts. *J Hand Ther*. 2011;24:231-239, with permission from Hanley & Belfus, an imprint of Elsevier Inc.)

TABLE 2.—Static and Dynamic Splinting Approaches

Postoperative Period	Static Splinting Approach	Dynamic Splinting Approach
4–7 d	Fabricate hand-based volar static extension gutter splint with PIP in slight flexion, worn between exercises during the day and at night.	Fabricate hand-based clamshell dynamic PIP extension splint allowing 30° arc with precaution not to hyperextend implant, worn during the day and gradually adjusting to allow for 45° by 3 wk postoperation.
	Gradually adjust goniometer or cardboard template to allow for a 30° arc initially and progress to 45° by 3 wk postoperation.	
	If hyperextension exists, fit in a dorsal blocking splint with PIP at 30° worn during the day.	If hyperextension exists, add PIP extension block at 30°.
	Initiate active flexion and passive extension hourly using goniometer to MCP/PIP/DIP.	Fabricate hand-based (originally forearm-based) volar static extension gutter splint with PIP in slight flexion, worn at night.
		Initiate AROM hourly within splint to PIP and DIP.
10–14 d	Scar management initiated after suture removal	Scar management initiated after suture removal
3 wk	Goal: 45° of PIP flexion	Goal: 45° of PIP flexion
	Active extension initiated	Active–assisted extension initiated in dynamic splint
4 wk	Goal: 60° of PIP flexion	Goal: 60° of PIP flexion
	May reduce static splinting during the day and replace with buddy strap to radial border digit or hinged PIP splint for index.	May discontinue dynamic splint and replace with buddy strap to radial border digit or hinged PIP splint for index
	A blocking splint may be fabricated to enhance PIP flexion and reverse blocking.	
6 wk	Goal: 15/75° at PIP.	Goal: 0/75° at PIP
	Replace with buddy straps to a radial border digit if not already done.	
	Gentle passive range of motion initiated.	Gentle passive range of motion initiated
	Encourage light use of digit using joint protection principles and avoiding lateral pressure to digit.	Encourage light use of digit using joint protection principles and avoiding lateral pressure to digit
8 wk	Gentle strengthening initiated	Gentle strengthening initiated
	Encourage continued use of night splint for 3+ mo.	Encourage continued use of night splint for 3+ mo.

MCP = metacarpal phalangeal; PIP = proximal interphalangeal; DIP = distal interphalangeal.

evaluated retrospectively. The results of this study indicated similarity in outcomes among the 2 treatment groups.

Due to the small number of cases studied, a larger trial including a multicenter study is in order. Until more evidence is available, I recommend that the treating therapist make a case-by-case decision as to which protocol to use. If the patient will have difficulty donning a dynamic splint, will be treated by a therapist close to home that does not have dynamic splinting experience, or needs additional lateral support for the surgical digit, then the static orthotic model is the appropriate choice.

S. J. Clark, OTR/L, CHT

27 Diagnostic Imaging

---

de Quervain Disease: US Identification of Anatomic Variations in the First Extensor Compartment with an Emphasis on Subcompartmentalization
Choi S-J, Ahn JH, Lee Y-J, et al (Univ of Ulsan College of Medicine, Gangwon-do, Korea; Hanyang Univ Hosp, Seoul, Korea)
Radiology 260:480-486, 2011

Purpose.—To demonstrate the usefulness of ultrasonography (US) in the detection of anatomic variations in the first extensor compartment of the wrist in patients with de Quervain disease.

Materials and Methods.—The institutional review board approved this study protocol and waived the informed consent requirement. Fifteen wrists in 13 women (age range, 41–62 years) in whom de Quervain disease was clinically diagnosed and who underwent surgery for intractable pain were included. A musculoskeletal radiologist performed US before surgery. The absence or presence and extent of subcompartmentalization within the first extensor compartment and the number of abductor pollicis longus (APL) and extensor pollicis brevis (EPB) tendon slips were evaluated and recorded. Preoperative US findings were compared with surgical records and photographs.

Results.—Subcompartmentalization within the first extensor compartment was observed during surgery in 11 of the 15 wrists (73 %), including four (27%) that had subcompartmentalization only in the distal portion of this compartment. US was used to identify all 11 wrists showing subcompartmentalization within this compartment (sensitivity, 100%; 95% confidence interval [CI]: 74%, 100%), as well as three of the four wrists with distal incomplete subcompartmentalization. There was one wrist with false-positive distal incomplete subcompartmentalization. US had a positive predictive value in the detection of subcompartmentalization of 73% (95% CI: 47%, 91%). The number of tendon slips in this compartment detected with US was identical to that identified at surgery with one exception.

Conclusion.—US can be used to depict various types of anatomic variations in the first extensor compartment in patients with de Quervain disease.

▶ In this study, patients with the clinical diagnosis of de Quervain disease underwent sonographic examination of the first extensor compartment of the wrist. All patients received conservative therapy. Of the 40 wrists included in this investigation, 15 were operated on because of failure of conservative therapy. The operative findings in this subgroup were compared with the sonographic results with emphasis on subcompartmentalization of the first extensor compartment.

All patients with intracompartmental septation were identified preoperatively (sensitivity 100%). One patient was false-positively identified to have a partial septation. The number of tendon slips was also predicted quite accurately.

There have already been a couple of articles dealing with sonographic evaluation of the first dorsal compartment of the wrist. The authors remind us once again of the possibility of subcompartmentalization of this compartment and the multiple slips of the abductor pollicis longus (up to 4) and extensor pollicis brevis (EPB) (up to 2 in this study) tendons that may be contained in the compartment. They point out that subcompartmentalization may be the cause for failure of injection therapy and even surgical treatment, if the EPB, which lies deeper, remains untreated.[1,2]

The etiologic relationship between this kind of variation and the disease as suggested by Loomis and others still remains to be clarified.[3,4]

Sonography prior to any treatment appears to be helpful, as septated patients, which are potential nonresponders to the injection, can be screened before the initial therapy. These patients should be injected under sonographic guidance to inject both subcompartments or primarily operated on with the intent to completely release the compartment along with the intracompartmental septum.

M. Choi, MD

References

1. Kwon BC, Choi SJ, Koh SH, Shin DJ, Baek GH. Sonographic identification of the intracompartmental septum in de Quervain's disease. *Clin Orthop Relat Res.* 2010;468:2129-2134.
2. Witt J, Pess G, Gelberman RH. Treatment of de Quervain tenosynovitis. A prospective study of the results of injection of steroids and immobilization in a splint. *J Bone Joint Surg Am.* 1991;73:219-222.
3. Jackson WT, Viegas SF, Coon TM, Stimpson KD, Frogameni AD, Simpson JM. Anatomical variations of the first extensor compartment of the wrist. A clinical and anatomical study. *J Bone Joint Surg Am.* 1986;68:923-926.
4. Loomis LK. Variations of stenosing tenosynovitis at the radial styloid process. *J Bone Joint Surg Am.* 1951;33-A:340-346.

Defining Ulnar Variance in the Adolescent Wrist: Measurement Technique and Interobserver Reliability
Goldfarb CA, Strauss NL, Wall LB, et al (Washington Univ School of Medicine, St Louis, MO)
J Hand Surg 36A:272-277, 2011

Purpose.—The measurement technique for ulnar variance in the adolescent population has not been well established. The purpose of this study was to assess the reliability of a standard ulnar variance assessment in the adolescent population.

Methods.—Four orthopedic surgeons measured 138 adolescent wrist radiographs for ulnar variance using a standard technique. There were 62 male and 76 female radiographs obtained in a standardized fashion for subjects aged 12 to 18 years. Skeletal age was used for analysis. We determined mean variance and assessed for differences related to age and gender. We also determined the interrater reliability.

Results.—The mean variance was −0.7 mm for boys and −0.4 mm for girls; there was no significant difference between the 2 groups overall. When subdivided by age and gender, the younger group (≤15 y of age) was significantly less negative for girls (boys, −0.8 mm and girls, −0.3 mm, p<.05). There was no significant difference between boys and girls in the older group. The greatest difference between any 2 raters was 1 mm; exact agreement was obtained in 72 subjects. Correlations between raters were high (r_p 0.87—0.97 in boys and 0.82—0.96 for girls). Interrater reliability was excellent (Cronbach's alpha, 0.97—0.98).

Conclusions.—Standard assessment techniques for ulnar variance are reliable in the adolescent population. Open growth plates did not interfere with this assessment. Young adolescent boys demonstrated a greater degree of negative ulnar variance compared with young adolescent girls.

▶ The authors present a retrospective radiographic analysis of 138 adolescent wrists in which they used a similar technique for measuring ulnar variance to that commonly used for adults (the method of perpendiculars). Prior to this study, only 1 study had proposed a technique specific for adolescents, one that is not familiar to most hand surgeons, which produced values that are not comparable to those reported for adults.[1] The authors report on the outcome and excellent interobserver reliability among 4 orthopedic surgeons at varying levels of training and experience. There is a succinct review of previous reports on comparison of measurement techniques as well as reports on average ulnar variance in adults. They note that the mean adolescent ulnar variance in this study was consistent with values found in 2 studies in the normal adult population. The authors appropriately cite the limitation of a primarily white patient base (116 of 138 patients), so with no other published study defining racial or ethnic differences in ulnar variance, applying the values of mean variance to a nonwhite population should be done with caution. This is a well-conceived contribution confirming that by using a familiar measuring technique, ulnar variance in adolescents can be reliably and accurately determined. This will prove useful when treating adolescent patients with conditions such as growth arrest, Kienböck's disease, and Madelung's deformity.

R. C. Chadderdon, MD

Reference

1. Hafner R, Poznanski AK, Donovan JM. Ulnar variance in children—standard measurements for evaluation of ulnar shortening in juvenile rheumatoid arthritis, hereditary multiple exostosis and other bone or joint disorders in childhood. *Skeletal Radiol.* 1989;18:513-516.

28 Miscellaneous

Cost-Effectiveness of Open Partial Fasciectomy, Needle Aponeurotomy, and Collagenase Injection for Dupuytren Contracture

Chen NC, Shauver MJ, Chung KC (Univ of Michigan Med School, Ann Arbor)
J Hand Surg 36A:1826-1834, 2011

Purpose.—We undertook a cost-utility analysis to compare traditional fasciectomy for Dupuytren with 2 new treatments, needle aponeurotomy and collagenase injection.

Methods.—We constructed an expected-value decision analysis model with an arm representing each treatment. A survey was administered to a cohort of 50 consecutive subjects to determine utilities of different interventions. We conducted multiple sensitivity analyses to assess the impact of varying the rate of disease recurrence in each arm of the analysis as well as the cost of the collagenase injection. The threshold for a cost-effective treatment is based on the traditional willingness-to-pay of $50,000 per quality-adjusted life years (QALY) gained.

Results.—The cost of open partial fasciectomy was $820,114 per QALY gained over no treatment. The cost of needle aponeurotomy was $96,474 per QALY gained versus no treatment. When we performed a sensitivity analysis and set the success rate at 100%, the cost of needle aponeurotomy was $49,631. When needle aponeurotomy was performed without surgical center or anesthesia costs and with reduced hand therapy, the cost was $36,570. When a complete collagenase injection series was priced at $250, the cost was $31,856 per QALY gained. When the injection series was priced at $945, the cost was $49,995 per QALY gained. At the market price of $5,400 per injection, the cost was $166,268 per QALY gained.

Conclusions.—In the current model, open partial fasciectomy is not cost-effective. Needle aponeurotomy is cost-effective if the success rate is high. Collagenase injection is cost-effective when priced under $945.

Type of Study/Level of Evidence.—Economic and Decision Analysis II.

▶ This high-caliber, thoroughly executed, cost-effectiveness analysis study is designed to help physicians and patients navigate the choices regarding Dupuytren treatment by comparing fasciectomy to needle aponeurotomy and collagenase injection. The study draws on health economics research and metrics to construct a custom utility survey that is based on a sophisticated decision model for use in policy and clinical decision making. The authors should be applauded for introducing a novel and important methodology to the hand surgery literature. Initial findings of this particular model must be interpreted with care as it is limited by a single case scenario to generate output and is unable to distinguish between clinical conditions. It should be viewed as an initial attempt to present a framework for a more comprehensive attempt to further identify factors to be used in clinical decision making in this diagnostic group.

A. Wolff, OTR, CHT

Assessing Physical Function in Adult Acquired Major Upper-Limb Amputees by Combining the Disabilities of the Arm, Shoulder and Hand (DASH) Outcome Questionnaire and Clinical Examination
Østlie K, Franklin RJ, Skjeldal OH, et al (Innlandet Hosp Trust, Ottestad, Norway; Innlandet Hosp Trust, Brumunddal, Norway; et al)
Arch Phys Med Rehabil 92:1636-1645, 2011

Objectives.—To describe physical function in adult acquired major upper-limb amputees (ULAs) by combining self-assessed arm function and physical measures obtained by clinical examinations; to estimate associations between background factors and self-assessed arm function in ULAs; and to assess whether clinical examination findings may be used to detect reduced arm function in unilateral ULAs.

Design.—Survey: postal questionnaires and clinical examinations.

Setting.—Norwegian ULA population. Clinical examinations performed at 3 clinics.

Participants.—Questionnaires: population-based sample (n = 224; 57.4% response rate). Clinical examinations: combined referred sample and convenience sample of questionnaire responders (n = 70; 83.3% of those invited). Survey inclusion criteria: adult acquired major upper-limb amputation, resident in Norway, mastering of spoken and written Norwegian.

Interventions.—Not applicable.

Main Outcome Measures.—The Disabilities of the Arm, Shoulder and Hand (DASH) Outcome Questionnaire, and clinical examination of joint motion and muscle strength with and without prostheses.

Results.—Mean DASH score was 22.7 (95% confidence interval [CI], 20.3—25.0); in bilateral amputees, 35.7 (95% CI, 23.0—48.4); and in unilateral amputees, 22.1 (95% CI, 19.8—24.5). A lower unilateral DASH score (better function) was associated with paid employment (vs not in paid employment: adjusted regression coefficient [aB] = −5.40, $P = .033$; vs students: aB = −13.88, $P = .022$), increasing postamputation time (aB = −.27, $P = .001$), and Norwegian ethnicity (aB = −14.45, $P < .001$). At clinical examination, we found a high frequency of impaired neck mobility and varying frequencies of impaired joint motion and strength at the shoulder, elbow, and forearm level. Prosthesis wear was associated with impaired joint motion in all upper-limb joints ($P < .006$) and with reduced shoulder abduction strength ($P = .002$). Impaired without-prosthesis joint motion in shoulder flexion (ipsilateral: aB = 12.19, $P = .001$) and shoulder abduction (ipsilateral: aB = 12.01, $P = .005$; contralateral: aB = 28.82, $P = .004$) was associated with increased DASH scores.

Conclusions.—Upper-limb loss clearly affects physical function. DASH score limitation profiles may be useful in individual clinical assessments. Targeted clinical examination may indicate patients with extra rehabilitational needs. Such examinations may be of special importance in relation to prosthesis function.

▶ This study reports the Disabilities of the Arm, Shoulder and Hand (DASH) scores and clinical examination findings in patients with upper limb amputations. Patients with a history of amputation through or proximal to the wrist were asked to complete a mail questionnaire including the DASH survey. A portion of this group also underwent clinical examination of range of motion of the neck, shoulder, elbow, and forearm.

Surprisingly, unilateral arm amputees in this study reported DASH scores similar to those in patients with Dupuytren disease. This suggests that either hand amputation is less disabling than we would suspect or, more likely, the DASH is not the most useful instrument for assessing difficulties due to amputation. Most unilateral amputees adapt to performing most of the DASH activities (prepare a meal, carry an object) with their intact hand. Presumably, an instrument that asked questions about activities that required bimanual function would detect differences between a patient with an amputation and patients with other common hand problems.

Results in this study may be biased toward more functional patients, as higher-functioning patients may be more likely to complete and return the questionnaire. Indeed, the investigators found that patients who completed the DASH questionnaire were significantly younger, better educated, and more frequently in paid employment than those who did not complete the DASH.

Unilateral amputees demonstrated near-normal neck motion but did have diminished motion in the involved shoulder. Decreased shoulder flexion and abduction was associated with worse DASH scores.

C. M. Ward, MD

Upper Extremity-Specific Measures of Disability and Outcomes in Orthopaedic Surgery
Smith MV, Calfee RP, Baumgarten KM, et al (Washington Univ School of Medicine, Saint Louis, MO)
J Bone Joint Surg Am 94:277-285, 2012

➤ Outcome measures may consist of simple questions or they may be more complex instruments that evaluate multiple interrelated domains that influence patient function.

➤ Outcome measures should be relevant to patients, easy to use, reliable, valid, and responsive to clinical changes.

➤ The Disabilities of the Arm, Shoulder and Hand score can be used to measure disability for any region of the upper limb.

➤ Joint and disease-specific outcome measures have been developed for the shoulder, the elbow, and the wrist and hand. Many of these measures would benefit from further research into their validity, reliability, and optimal applicability.

▶ This article is a review of available outcome measures for evaluation of the patient with a hand or upper extremity complaint, including limitations and information regarding reliability, validity, and responsiveness. It is an excellent review that is helpful for both the interested research investigator, to better understand and appropriately use various outcome measures, and the interested reader who wishes to better understand and critically evaluate the medical literature. The authors note a wide variability in documentation of the validity, reliability, and applicability of commonly used outcome measures. The authors further suggest that when outcomes are reported, it may be helpful to consider including an evaluation of general health and the level of activity, as well as evaluation specific to the issue of concern. The desire to be thorough, however, needs to be balanced with the "responder burden" of responding to a long and detailed set of questions. This article may be considered required reading for trainees and those interested in outcomes' research.

J. Adams, MD

Arterial Grafts for Vascular Reconstruction in the Upper Extremity
Trocchia AM, Hammert WC (Univ of Rochester Med Ctr, NY)
J Hand Surg 36A:1534-1536, 2011

Background.—When direct arterial repair cannot be done to correct acute or chronic upper extremity ischemia, vascular grafts may be needed. Even if ischemia does not accompany isolated arterial injury, reconstruction can reduce symptoms such as cold intolerance. Grafts are ideally of the same diameter and vessel wall thickness as the original vessel, are readily available, are easy to harvest, and cause minimal donor site morbidity. Vein, artery, and synthetic grafts can be used, but generally the synthetic types are only used for larger vessels, such as the aorta, axillary, femoral, and popliteal vessels. A shift has occurred from vein grafts to arterial grafts. Each type of graft has advantages and disadvantages when used for vascular reconstruction in the upper extremity.

Vein Grafts.—Vein grafts offer the advantages of ease of harvest and ready accessibility. They can be harvested from the same extremity, with different vessels used based on size requirements. Challenges associated with their use include the need for separate incisions for the various vessels, which can increase the risk of graft compression and occlusion. Veins have valves so the surgeon must either reverse the graft or remove the valves to ensure patency. Graft reversal can produce size mismatches, requiring vein narrowing or end-to-side anastomosis, complicating the procedure. Vein walls are thinner than artery walls, which can complicate the anastomosis. Even experienced surgeons can be challenged by vein graft procedures. Vein grafts can twist on themselves; a longitudinal mark can help maintain the correct orientation.

Arterial Grafts.—Arterial grafts have higher patency rates than vein grafts and are appealing because they allow one to replace arteries with arteries, do not require reversal, and provide similar vessel wall thickness. An expendable artery must be available. The commonly used arterial grafts include the descending branch of the lateral femoral circumflex artery, the deep inferior epigastric artery, and the thoracodorsal artery. These provide the vascular supply to widely used free flaps and are familiar to surgeons who perform free tissue transfers. These arteries are reliable and are analyzed for patency only if the area has undergone previous surgery, trauma, or incisions. Arterial graft harvesting procedures are similar to those for vein graft harvesting, although arterial grafts are found in or deep to the muscles whereas vein grafts usually come from subcutaneous tissues and are more readily accessed. One or two venae comitantes usually accompany arteries, facilitating their identification. Hand-held Doppler probes can also be used. The artery is separated from the venae comitantes to the desired length, and side branches are ligated. Anticoagulation is not needed with arterial grafts.

Disadvantages associated with arterial grafts include remote donor site, more complex harvesting than for vein grafts, limited graft length, and fewer donor graft options. Specific to the distal upper extremity, most arterial reconstructions do not require substantial length, so donor sites are readily available. The preferred arterial graft is the descending branch of the lateral femoral circumflex artery, which is harvested in a supine position, is located away from major vessels, and is in an area well-known to orthopedic and plastic surgeons. Grafts can be harvested proximal or distal along the course of this artery. Side branches can also be used, especially for digital reconstruction.

Conclusions.—Hand surgery literature documents the usefulness of arterial grafts. Patient factors, surgeon's experience, and anatomic awareness are important contributing factors when planning arterial reconstructions. Currently arterial grafts are used for reconstructions for chronic conditions and some cases of acute ischemia. Prospective studies are needed to compare the results of various grafts in upper extremity procedures (Table 1).

▶ The authors provide a brief review of the use of arterial grafts for upper extremity vascular reconstruction. Vessel grafts can be necessary for acute or chronic vascular problems. The benefits of arterial grafts in upper extremity

TABLE 1.—Sizes of Commonly Used Arterial Grafts[4]

Graft	Flap Supplied	Length (cm)	Diameter (mm)
Descending branch of lateral femoral circumflex	Anterolateral thigh	15	2.0–2.5
Deep inferior epigastric artery	Rectus abdominis	10	2.0–2.7
Thoracodorsal artery	Latissimus dorsi	12	2.0–3.0

Editor's Note: Please refer to original journal article for full references.

reconstruction are, to some degree, extrapolated from the evolution of cardiac vascular reconstruction. While vein grafts were commonly used for cardiac bypass surgery, arterial grafts are currently more common. A chief reason for this shift is the higher patency rates seen with arterial grafts.

Vein grafts have disadvantages as pointed out by the authors. They often require a separate incision. If they are reversed for use in arterial reconstruction, there may be a vessel size mismatch at one or both ends. If the vein is not reversed, then the valves must be removed, which can be challenging.

The authors advocate using arterial grafts in the upper extremity to replace "like with like." They do acknowledge that arterial graft harvest may be more difficult, and there are less expendable arterial grafts available, in contrast to potential donor veins. The 3 common arterial grafts highlighted in this review are the descending branch of the lateral femoral circumflex artery, the deep inferior epigastric artery, and the thoracodorsal artery. It is not a coincidence that these vessels are the donor vessels for commonly used free flaps. A convenient table is provided giving average lengths and diameters of these donor arteries (Table 1). Ultimately, the authors state that their preferred arterial donor is the descending branch of the lateral femoral circumflex artery due to length, branching possibilities, and ability to harvest with the patient supine.

This is a thoughtful and succinct review of an interesting topic, and, as the authors state, it points out the need for definitive evidence about the safety and effectiveness of arterial grafts for upper extremity vascular reconstruction.

J. Freidrich, MD

Assessing the Impact of Antibiotic Prophylaxis in Outpatient Elective Hand Surgery: A Single-Center, Retrospective Review of 8,850 Cases

Bykowski MR, Sivak WN, Cray J, et al (Dept of Plastic and Reconstructive Surgery, Pittsburgh, PA; Hand and Upper Extremity Ctr, Wexford, PA; Johns Hopkins Univ School of Medicine, Baltimore, MD)
J Hand Surg 36A:1741-1747, 2011

Purpose.—Prophylactic antibiotics have been shown to prevent surgical site infection (SSI) after some gastrointestinal, orthopedic, and plastic surgical procedures, but their efficacy in clean, elective hand surgery is unclear. Our aims were to assess the efficacy of preoperative antibiotics in preventing SSI after clean, elective hand surgery, and to identify potential risk factors for SSI.

Methods.—We queried the database from an outpatient surgical center by Current Procedural Terminology code to identify patients who underwent elective hand surgery. For each medical record, we collected patient demographics and characteristics along with preoperative, intraoperative, and postoperative management details. The primary outcome of this study was SSI, and secondary outcomes were wound dehiscence and suture granuloma.

Results.—From October 2000 through October 2008, 8,850 patient records met our inclusion criteria. The overall SSI rate was 0.35%, with an average patient follow-up duration of 79 days. The SSI rates did not significantly differ between patients receiving antibiotics (0.54%; 2,755 patients) and those who did not (0.26%; 6,095 patients). Surgical site infection was associated with smoking status, diabetes mellitus, and longer procedure length irrespective of antibiotic use. Subgroup analysis revealed that prophylactic antibiotics did not prevent SSI in male patients, smokers, or diabetics, or for procedure length less than 30 minutes, 30 to 60 minutes, and greater than 60 minutes.

Conclusions.—Prophylactic antibiotic administration does not reduce the incidence of SSI after clean, elective hand surgery in an outpatient population. Moreover, subgroup analysis revealed that prophylactic antibiotics did not reduce the frequency of SSI among patients who were found to be at higher risk in this study. We identified 3 factors associated with the development of SSI in our study: diabetes mellitus status, procedure length, and smoking status. Given the potential harmful complications associated with antibiotic use and the lack of evidence that prophylactic antibiotics prevent SSIs, we conclude that antibiotics should not be routinely administered to patients who undergo clean, elective hand surgery.

Type of Study/Level of Evidence.—Therapeutic III (Table 1).

▶ The authors of this study completed an impressive analysis of the use of prophylactic perioperative antibiotics during elective hand surgery. While we tend to think of use of antibiotics as a low-risk practice, the authors rightly point out that, although rare, complications from the use of antibiotics can be severe. The types of procedures analyzed are a good representation of the most common elective hand surgical procedures (Table 1). Factors analyzed included patient demographics, type of surgery, selected comorbidities, and presence and characteristics of any postoperative infection. Their stratification of the surgeries based on time to completion makes the data more robust, as other studies have shown a correlation of operating time and infection incidence. To the degree that they can be, surgical site infections were objectively diagnosed based on Centers for Disease Control criteria.

The sheer numbers in the study are impressive: 8850 patient records met inclusion criteria. Of these, 2755 patients received prophylactic antibiotics

TABLE 1.—Audit of Type of Surgery in 8,850 Elective Cases

CPT Code	CPT Code Description	Total Cases (%)	Infection Rate
64721	Carpal tunnel release	43	0.24%
64719	Ulnar nerve neuroplasty at wrist	4	0.26%
64718	Ulnar nerve transposition at elbow	4	0.56%
26116	Excision tumor/malformation hand, subfascial	5	0.95%
26115	Excision tumor hand, subcutaneous	2	2.00%
26055	Tendon sheath incision (trigger finger)	23	0.50%
25111	Wrist ganglion excision	7	0.00%
25075	Excision forearm/wrist tumor, subcutaneous	0	0.00%
25000	de Quervain release	12	0.29%

CPT, Current Procedural Terminology.

and 6095 did not. It is worth noting that the administration of antibiotics was not standardized, rather it was the choice of the operating surgeon. This fact introduces potential bias and could be considered a weakness of the study. The surgical site infection rate for both groups was extremely small and overall was 0.35%. There were no significant differences in infection rate between antibiotic and no-antibiotic groups, and not surprisingly, the most common organism isolated was *staphylococcus aureus*. The authors found that multiple factors, including smoking status, diabetes, and length of procedure correlated with rate of infection, but, most importantly, antibiotic administration was not one of those factors. It is worth noting that although the authors found that longer procedure time correlated with infection, it did not appear that antibiotic administration had any effect on the infection risk in these longer procedures.

When analyzing this study, one can easily conclude that perioperative antibiotic administration is not necessary in clean, elective hand surgery cases. However, in the current climate of proliferating quality care indicators, perioperative antibiotic administration is one of the very few intraoperative indicators that are analyzed by quality improvement bodies.[1] Therefore, a nonstandardized approach to perioperative antibiotic administration for hand surgery may be difficult to reconcile with ongoing quality improvement efforts.

J. Freidrich, MD

Reference

1. Ingraham AM, Cohen ME, Bilimoria KY, et al. Association of surgical care improvement project infection-related process measure compliance with risk-adjusted outcomes: implications for quality measurement. *J Am Coll Surg*. 2010;211:705-714.

Single-Lead Percutaneous Peripheral Nerve Stimulation for the Treatment of Hemiplegic Shoulder Pain: A Case Report
Wilson RD, Bennett ME, Lechman TE, et al (Case Western Reserve Univ, Cleveland, OH; SPR Therapeutics (subsidiary of NDI Med), Cleveland, OH; et al)
Arch Phys Med Rehabil 92:837-840, 2011

Previous studies demonstrated the efficacy of 6 weeks of a 4-lead percutaneous, peripheral nerve stimulation system in reducing hemiplegic shoulder pain. This case report describes the first stroke survivor treated for 3 weeks with a less complex, single-lead approach. The participant was a 59-year-old male who developed hemiplegic shoulder pain shortly after his stroke 7.5 years prior to study enrollment and was treated with multiple modalities without sustained pain relief. After study enrollment, a single intramuscular lead was placed percutaneously into the deltoid muscle. He was treated 6 hours per day for 3 weeks and the lead was removed. The primary outcome measure was the Brief Pain Inventory (Short-Form) Question 3 (BPI-3), which queries the worst pain in the last week on a 0 to 10 numeric rating scale. At baseline, BPI 3 was an 8. At the end of treatment and at 1 and 4 weeks after treatment was completed, BPI 3 scores were 3, 2, and 2, respectively. Substantial improvements in quality of life measures were also observed. The participant remained infection-free and the lead was removed fully intact. After completing the study protocol, the participant was followed clinically for 13 months posttreatment with complete resolution of hemiplegic shoulder pain. This case report demonstrates the feasibility of a single-lead peripheral nerve stimulation for the treatment of chronic hemiplegic shoulder pain. Additional studies are needed to further demonstrate safety and efficacy, determine optimal dose, define optimal prescriptive parameters, expand clinical indications, and demonstrate long-term effect.

▶ The causes and treatment of hemiplegic shoulder pain could be debated endlessly, but that is irrelevant to the most engaging aspect of this short clinical note. This is indicative of another interesting use for percutaneous peripheral nerve stimulation or, more importantly, as a convenient form of functional electrical stimulation (FES). Using electrodes that are tunneled under the skin, one can stimulate nerves or motor points in muscles that have intact peripheral nerves but are not otherwise functional. This may be particularly helpful in upper motor nerve disorders. The most dramatic uses of this technique are diaphragmatic pacing in upper cervical tetraplegia[1,2] and neuroprosthetics for plegic upper and lower limbs.[3-5] Diaphragmatic pacing has dramatically improved the quality of life in many patients with higher cervical cord lesions. Previously, these people were wedded to a fairly large and ungainly mechanical ventilator for the rest of their lives. Now, with the use of a quite small battery pack, somewhat similar to a pacemaker, these patients are relatively untethered from a pulmonary standpoint despite their considerable motor disabilities.[1,2] The use of neuroprosthetics is still in a stage of development. However, such devices are already being used to facilitate grasp and release in hemiplegics with upper limb dysfunction.[3] Similarly, lower-extremity FES can be used to eliminate the need for an ankle-foot orthosis in hemiplegics with foot drop.[4] Further on the horizon, multichannel stimulators are being devised to aid in standing, transfers, and even walking in paraplegic patients.[5] For hand surgeons, this presents an opportunity and a challenge to develop new ways to use this technology to enhance the function of those with upper limb motor disorders.

K. A. Bengtson, MD

References

1. DiMarco AF, Onders RP, Ignagni A, Kowalski KE, Mortimer JT. Phrenic nerve pacing via intramuscular diaphragm electrodes in tetraplegic subjects. *Chest.* 2005;127:671-678.
2. Onders RP, Elmo MJ, Ignagni AR. Diaphragm pacing stimulation system for tetraplegia in individuals injured during childhood or adolescence. *J Spinal Cord Med.* 2007;30:S25-S29.
3. Kilgore KL, Peckham PH, Keith MW, et al. An implanted upper-extremity neuroprosthesis. Follow-up of five patients. *J Bone Joint Surg Am.* 1997;79:533-541.
4. Hausdorff JM, Ring H. Effects of a new radio frequency-controlled neuroprosthesis on gait symmetry and rhythmicity in patients with chronic hemiparesis. *Am J Phys Med Rehabil.* 2008;87:4-13.
5. Davis JA Jr, Triolo RJ, Uhlir JP, et al. Surgical technique for installing an eight-channel neuroprosthesis for standing. *Clin Orthop Relat Res.* 2001;385:237-252.

Complex Regional Pain Syndrome of the Upper Extremity

Patterson RW, Li Z, Smith BP, et al (Wake Forest Univ School of Medicine, Winston-Salem, NC)
J Hand Surg 36A:1553-1562, 2011

The diagnosis and management of complex regional pain syndrome is often challenging. Early diagnosis and intervention improve outcomes in most patients; however, some patients will progress regardless of intervention. Multidisciplinary management facilitates care in complex cases. The onset of signs and symptoms may be obvious or insidious; temporal delay is a frequent occurrence. Difficulty sleeping, pain unresponsive to narcotics, swelling, stiffness, and hypersensitivity are harbingers of onset. Multimodal treatment with hand therapy, sympatholytic drugs, and stress loading may be augmented with anesthesia blocks. If the dystrophic symptoms are controllable by medications and a nociceptive focus or nerve derangement is correctable, surgery is an appropriate alternative. Chronic sequelae of contracture may also be addressed surgically in patients with controllable sympathetically maintained pain.

▶ Reading a review of complex regional pain syndrome (CRPS) written by hand surgeons is like reading a review of distal radius fractures written by family practitioners. In one sense, this is a perfect pairing where the authors are intimately aware of the needs and tastes of their audience, since they are all part of the same professional group. The authors speak directly to the interests of the audience. Their salient points accurately find their targets. Everyone gets what he or she wants. For example, the audience is clearly being addressed in the section "Why should you care?" The authors state: "Patients with poor outcomes and CRPS may be litigious. Furthermore, patients with CRPS who prevail in court have increased monetary rewards." Clearly, these pearls have not been gleaned from the mainstream pain journals.

In the opposite sense, however, there is a vague sense of dissatisfaction, realizing that the knowledge expounded is somehow secondhand. I am assuming, perhaps wrongly, that hand surgeons at a tertiary care institution are not fumbling around with stellate ganglion blocks, therapeutic modalities, and neuromodulatory medications. Therefore, the writing lacks authenticity and authority. Ideally, since the authors are many in this case, the committee for such a review article would include hand surgeons as well as pain clinicians. This is apparent in the number of times that the antiquated practice of intravenous phentolamine is recommended.

One could dissect the many bits of misinformation scattered throughout the article, but these are of little consequence. Overall, the efforts of this group are to be applauded. They have distilled a messy and complex subject filled with controversial areas into a readable and helpful review. The closing sections, titled "Myths and Disinformation" and "Clinical Pearls," are especially terse and helpful. In the end, one must take it for what it is—an article written by experts who are slightly out of their comfort zone.

K. Bengtson, MD

Reductions in finger blood flow in men and women induced by 125-Hz vibration: association with vibration perception thresholds

Ye Y, Griffin MJ (Univ of Southampton, UK)
J Appl Physiol 111:1606-1613, 2011

Vibration of one hand reduces blood flow in the exposed hand and in the contralateral hand not exposed to vibration, but the mechanisms involved are not understood. This study investigated whether vibration-induced reductions in finger blood flow are associated with vibrotactile perception thresholds mediated by the Pacinian channel and considered sex differences in both vibration thresholds and vibration-induced changes in digital circulation. With force and vibration applied to the thenar eminence of the right hand, finger blood flow and finger skin temperature were measured in the middle fingers of both hands at 30-s intervals during seven successive 4-min periods: *1)* pre-exposure with no force or vibration, *2)* pre-exposure with force, *3)* *vibration 1*, *4)* rest with force, *5)* *vibration 2*, *6)* postexposure with force, and *7)* recovery with no force or vibration. A 2-N force was applied during *periods 2–6* and 125-Hz vibration at 0.5 and 1.5 ms^{-2} root mean square (r.m.s.; unweighted) was applied during *periods 3* and *5*, respectively. Vibrotactile thresholds were measured at the thenar eminence of right hand using the same force, contact conditions, and vibration frequency. When the vibration magnitude was greater than individual vibration thresholds, changes in finger blood flow were correlated with thresholds (with both 0.5 and 1.5 ms^{-2} r.m.s. vibration): subjects with lower thresholds showed greater reductions in finger blood flow. Women had lower vibrotactile thresholds and showed greater vibration-induced reductions in finger blood flow. It is concluded that mechanoreceptors responsible for mediating vibration perception are involved in the vascular response to vibration.

▶ The authors present their basic science follow-up on the effect of vibration stimuli on digit perfusion in humans. The clinical application served as a backdrop and is the potential for vibrational tools to cause digit vasoconstriction and a corresponding reduction in blood flow (vibration-induced white finger or hand-arm vibration syndrome). There is evidence that the reduction in blood flow even occurs in the nonexposed hand, mediated by the sympathetic nervous system through mechanoreceptors in the exposed hand. In this study, the authors further investigated two aspects of these previous findings. They hypothesized that the changes in digit blood flow would correlate with vibrotactile perception thresholds, and that these responses would differ between men and women. Essentially, the study shows that women have a lower perception threshold and consequently greater reductions in digit perfusion. The scientific design and study execution seem outstanding, but it is unlikely that practicing surgeons will find additional value in reading the details of this article. A perusal of the reference list for this article yields no pertinent related studies published in high-impact journals readily available to orthopedic or hand surgeons. The association between occupational exposure to vibration and carpal tunnel syndrome and hand-arm vibration syndrome is well known; however, the scientific conclusions from this study add very little to the diagnosis and treatment of these conditions.

L. Brunton, MD

Results of 189 wrist replacements. A report from the Norwegian Arthroplasty Register
Krukhaug Y, Lie SA, Havelin LI, et al (Haukeland Univ Hosp, Bergen, Norway)
Acta Orthop 82:405-409, 2011

Background and Purpose.—There is very little literature on the long-term outcome of wrist replacements. The Norwegian Arthroplasty Register has registered wrist replacements since 1994. We report on the total wrist replacements and their revision rates over a 16-year period.

Material and Methods.—189 patients with 189 primary wrist replacements (90 Biax prostheses (80 of which were cementless), 23 cementless Elos prostheses, and 76 cementless Gibbon prostheses), operated during the period 1994—2009 were identified in the Norwegian Arthroplasty Register. Prosthesis survival was analyzed using Cox regression analyses. The 3 implant designs were compared and time trends were analyzed.

Results.—The 5-year survival was 78% (95% CI: 70—85) and the 10-year survival was 71% (CI: 59—80). Prosthesis survival was 85% (CI: 78—93) at 5 years for the Biax prosthesis, 77% (CI: 30—90) at 4 years for the Gibbon prosthesis, and 57% (CI: 33—81) at 5 years for the Elos prosthesis. There was no statistically significant influence of age, diagnosis, or year of operation on the risk of revision, but females had a higher revision rate than males (RR = 3, CI: 1—7). The number of wrist replacements performed due to osteoarthritis increased with time, but no such change was apparent for inflammatory arthritis.

Interpretation.—The survival of the total wrist arthroplasties studied was similar to that in other studies of wrist arthroplasties, but it was still not as good as that for most total knee and hip arthroplasties. However, a failed wrist arthroplasty still leaves the option of a well-functioning arthrodesis.

▶ The authors present the outcome statistics from the Norwegian Arthroplasty Register for 189 total wrist replacements that were performed over a 16-year period from 1994 through 2009. The significance of the article is that it is the largest group of patients with total wrist replacements to be reported in the literature.

Three different wrist replacements were used: the Biax prosthesis, the Elos prosthesis, and the Gibbon prosthesis, but only the last one, which is manufactured in Sweden, is currently being used. The authors acknowledge that they were unable to provide any meaningful information regarding the specific prostheses, because the Biax was used only in patients with inflammatory arthritis, and the Elos was used only in patients with noninflammatory arthritis. Only the Gibbon prosthesis was used for both inflammatory and noninflammatory wrist arthritis. The authors report that total wrist replacements are being used with increasing frequency in Norway for noninflammatory arthritis. The only significant statistics were that women were 3 times more likely to require surgical revisions than men and that the necessity for revision was unrelated to the type of arthritis.

I agree with the conclusion of the article that "current evidence does not support widespread implementation" of total wrist replacement. While it appears that total wrist implants are being inserted with the same frequency in Norway as they were years ago and possibly are being inserted with greater frequency, as more are being used in patients with noninflammatory arthritis, the same is not true at many centers in the United States. Most wrist implants inserted at my institution were in patients with inflammatory arthritis, and many of these implants, especially the distal components, became unstable. Although current wrist implants are third generation, additional research is necessary to improve their long-term stability.

M. A. Posner, MD

Upper Extremity-Specific Measures of Disability and Outcomes in Orthopaedic Surgery
Smith MV, Calfee RP, Baumgarten KM, et al (Washington Univ School of Medicine, Saint Louis, MO)
J Bone Joint Surg Am 94:277-285, 2012

➤ Outcome measures may consist of simple questions or they may be more complex instruments that evaluate multiple interrelated domains that influence patient function.

➤ Outcome measures should be relevant to patients, easy to use, reliable, valid, and responsive to clinical changes.

➤ The Disabilities of the Arm, Shoulder and Hand score can be used to measure disability for any region of the upper limb.

➤ Joint and disease-specific outcome measures have been developed for the shoulder, the elbow, and the wrist and hand. Many of these measures would benefit from further research into their validity, reliability, and optimal applicability.

▶ For the most part, validated disability and outcome measures have been underutilized in clinical studies involving the upper extremity. The authors of this review stress the importance of not only utilizing outcome measures when studying the treatment of upper extremity disorders but also emphasize the need to use the most appropriate outcome tool given the clinical scenario.

Overall, the authors reviewed a total of 23 validated outcome and disability measures in this review, with 10 involving the shoulder, 8 the elbow, and only 5 involving the hand. The Disabilities of the Arm, Shoulder and Hand (DASH) is the only validated measurement tool reviewed that surveys the shoulder, elbow, and hand. In this article, the authors profile each of the measurement tools, including why they were developed and what they were designed to assess.

Also compared among the various tools is the so-called "response burden" of each measure. For the hand instruments, the Michigan Hand Outcome Questionnaire has the greatest response burden with 71 questions.

This article is by no means exhaustive in its review of upper extremity outcome and disability measurement tools. It does, however, review the more commonly used tools. As the authors mention, it is critically important to exercise caution when interpreting any of these measurement tools, as bias may be injected from physician-based rating scales. Outcomes tools that are the most effective should incorporate the evaluation of overall functional activity and generalized health and well-being to the assessment of success or failure of treatment for conditions of the upper extremity.

P. Murray, MD

Upper Extremity Function in Stroke Subjects: Relationships between the International Classification of Functioning, Disability, and Health Domains
Faria-Fortini I, Michaelsen SM, Cassiano JG, et al (Fundação Mineira de Educação e Cultura (FUMEC), Belo Horizonte, Brazil; Universidade do Estado de Santa Catarina, Florianópolis, Brazil; Universidade Federal de Minas Gerais, Belo Horizonte, Brazil)
J Hand Ther 24:257-265, 2011

Upper limb (UL) impairments are the most common disabling deficits after stroke and have complex relationships with activity and participation domains. However, relatively few studies have applied the ICF model to identify the contributions of specific UL impairments, such as muscular weakness, pain, and sensory loss, as predictors of activity and participation. The purposes of this predictive study were to evaluate the relationships between UL variables related to body functions/structures, activity, and participation domains and to determine which would best explain activity and participation with 55 subjects with chronic stroke. Body functions/structures were assessed by measures of grip, pinch, and UL strength, finger tactile sensations, shoulder pain, and cognition (MMSE); activity domain by measures of observed performance (BBT, NHPT, and TEMPA); and participation by measures of quality of life (SSQOL). Upper-limb and grip strength were related to all activity measures $(0.52 < r < 0.82, p < .0001)$. Shoulder pain $(r = -.39, p < .001)$ was the variable which was mostly related to participation. Grip strength alone accounted for 62%, 54%, and 36% of the variance in the activity measures (respectively TEMPA, BBT and NHPT). Shoulder pain accounted for 30% of the participation measure. Strength deficits and shoulder pain of the paretic UL demonstrated to be important targets for clinical interventions to improve activity and participation with chronic stroke subjects.
Level of Evidence.—2c.

▶ Overall, the general purpose of the study was to evaluate the relationship between upper limb variables in relation to function, activity, and participation using the International Classification of Functioning, Disability, and Health (this study was based on chronic stroke classification [> 6 months]). It also discussed the relation between grip and functional activities of daily living participation. It acknowledged a lacking in social factors with a focus on finger and hand dexterity and pinch strength.

ABSTRACT: Accurate.

INTRODUCTION: Purpose of study stated with reference to previous literature and where the results may lead to effective intervention strategies.

METHODS: Study design appropriate to achieve study objective. Clearly stated study population, sample size, and exclusion criteria. Statistical analyses appropriate and used appropriately. Very thorough inclusion of procedure, outcome measures, and data analyses. Tables included in the statistical reporting and analysis accurate and used appropriately.

RESULTS: Text statistics adequate and results clearly presented in tables with explanation grid.

DISCUSSION: Restated the study to achieve objective. Previous pertinent literature stated along with relationship to current study. References to previous studies and reasoning to as why this study finding varied and reinforced the hypothesis regarding other influences, such as environmental and personal factors. Cited cautions in the results of this study with the relatively young sample with mild impairments may not fully reflect the domain of participants.

CONCLUSIONS: Good conclusion; clearly stated in a concise manner.

FORM, STYLE, AND SUBSTANCE: Novel contribution to the literature. Length is appropriate. Written fairly clear; however, needed to frequently refer back and forth on multiple test names, acronyms.

REFERENCES: Relevant and comprehensive; correct format and up-to-date.

S. Kranz, CHT

Article Index

Chapter 1: Hand Trauma

Chapter 2: Hand: Arthritis and Arthroplasty

Chapter 3: Hand: Bone and Ligament

Chapter 4: Hand: Carpal Tunnel Syndrome

Chapter 5: Hand: Congenital Differences

Chapter 6: Hand: Microsurgery and Flaps

Chapter 7: Hand: Peripheral Nerve

Chapter 8: Hand: Tendon

Chapter 9: Dupuytren's Contracture

Chapter 10: Carpus

Chapter 11: Distal Radius

Chapter 12: Flexor Tendon

Chapter 13: Elbow

Chapter 14: Elbow: Trauma

Chapter 15: Brachial Plexus

Chapter 16: Arm and Humerus

Chapter 17: Shoulder: Anatomy and Instability

Chapter 18: Shoulder: Arthroplasty

Chapter 19: Shoulder: Arthroscopy

Chapter 20: Shoulder: Rotator Cuff

Chapter 21: Shoulder: Trauma

Chapter 22: Soft Tissue

Chapter 23: Arthritis

Chapter 24: Neural Integration, Pain and Anesthesia

Chapter 25: Peripheral Nerve Injury and Repair

Chapter 26: Rehabilitation, Outcomes and Assessment

Chapter 27: Diagnostic Imaging

Chapter 28: Miscellaneous

Author Index

Printed and bound by CPI Group (UK) Ltd, Croydon, CR0 4YY

08/05/2025

01864678-0006